Diagnosis-Related Groups in Europe

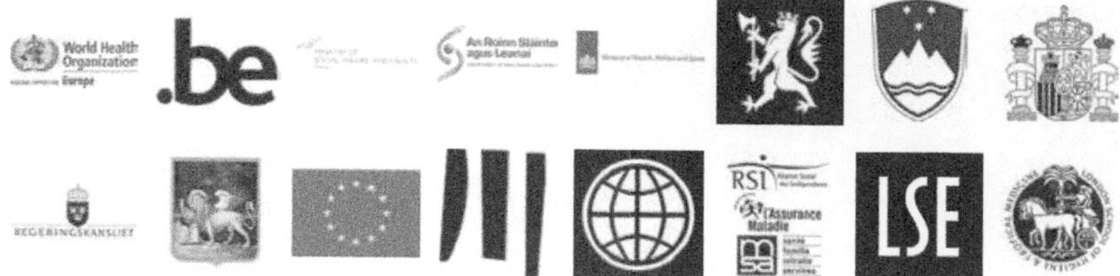

The European Observatory on Health Systems and Policies supports and promotes evidence-based health policy-making through comprehensive and rigorous analysis of health systems in Europe. It brings together a wide range of policy-makers, academics and practitioners to analyse trends in health reform, drawing on experience from across Europe to illuminate policy issues.

The European Observatory on Health Systems and Policies is a partnership between the World Health Organization Regional Office for Europe, the Governments of Belgium, Finland, Ireland, the Netherlands, Norway, Slovenia, Spain, Sweden and the Veneto Region of Italy, the European Commission, the European Investment Bank, the World Bank, UNCAM (French National Union of Health Insurance Funds), the London School of Economics and Political Science, and the London School of Hygiene & Tropical Medicine.

European Observatory on Health Systems and Policies

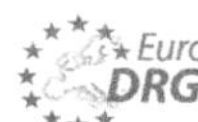

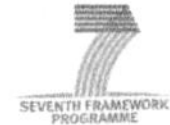

Diagnosis-Related Groups in Europe

Moving towards transparency, efficiency and quality in hospitals

Edited by

Reinhard Busse, Alexander Geissler, Wilm Quentin, Miriam Wiley

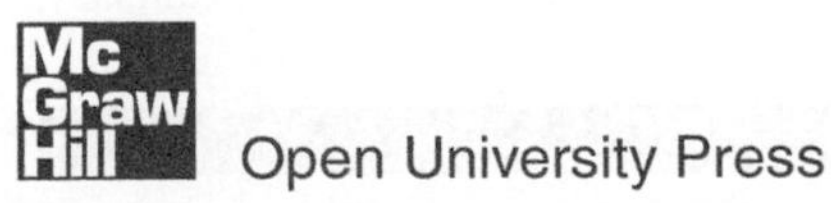

Open University Press
McGraw-Hill Education
McGraw-Hill House
Shoppenhangers Road
Maidenhead
Berkshire
England
SL6 2QL

email: enquiries@openup.co.uk
world wide web: www.openup.co.uk

and Two Penn Plaza, New York, NY 10121-2289, USA

First published 2011

A catalogue record of this book is available from the British Library

ISBN-13: 978-0-33-524557-4
ISBN-10: 0-33-524557-9
eISBN: 978-0-33-524558-1

Library of Congress Cataloging-in-Publication Data
CIP data applied for

Typeset by RefineCatch Limited, Bungay, Suffolk
Printed and bound by CPI Group (UK) Ltd, Croydon, CR0 4YY

The McGraw·Hill Companies

European Observatory on Health Systems and Policies Series

The European Observatory on Health Systems and Policies is a unique project that builds on the commitment of all its partners to improving health systems:

- World Health Organization Regional Office for Europe
- Government of Belgium
- Government of Finland
- Government of Ireland
- Government of the Netherlands
- Government of Norway
- Government of Slovenia
- Government of Spain
- Government of Sweden
- Government of Veneto Region of Italy
- European Commission
- European Investment Bank
- World Bank
- UNCAM (French National Union of Health Insurance Funds)
- London School of Economics and Political Science
- London School of Hygiene & Tropical Medicine

The series

The volumes in this series focus on key issues for health policy-making in Europe. Each study explores the conceptual background, outcomes and lessons learned about the development of more equitable, more efficient and more effective health systems in Europe. With this focus, the series seeks to contribute to the evolution of a more evidence-based approach to policy formulation in the health sector.

These studies will be important to all those involved in formulating or evaluating national health policies and, in particular, will be of use to health policy-makers and advisers, who are under increasing pressure to rationalize the structure and funding of their health system. Academics and students in the field of health policy will also find this series valuable in seeking to understand better the complex choices that confront the health systems of Europe.

The Observatory supports and promotes evidence-based health policy-making through comprehensive and rigorous analysis of the dynamics of health care systems in Europe.

Series Editors

Josep Figueras is Director of the European Observatory on Health Systems and Policies, and Head of the European Centre for Health Policy, World Health Organization Regional Office for Europe.

Martin McKee is Head of Research Policy and Head of the London Hub of the European Observatory on Health Systems and Policies. He is Professor of European Public Health at the London School of Hygiene & Tropical Medicine as well as a co-director of the School's European Centre on Health of Societies in Transition.

Elias Mossialos is the Co-director of the European Observatory on Health Systems and Policies. He is Brian Abel-Smith Professor in Health Policy, Department of Social Policy, London School of Economics and Political Science and Director of LSE Health.

Richard B. Saltman is Associate Head of Research Policy and Head of the Atlanta Hub of the European Observatory on Health Systems and Policies. He is Professor of Health Policy and Management at the Rollins School of Public Health, Emory University in Atlanta, Georgia.

Reinhard Busse is Associate Head of Research Policy and Head of the Berlin Hub of the European Observatory on Health Systems and Policies. He is Professor of Health Care Management at the Berlin University of Technology.

European Observatory on Health Systems and Policies Series
Series Editors: Josep Figueras, Martin McKee, Elias Mossialos, Richard B. Saltman and Reinhard Busse

Published titles

Regulating entrepreneurial behaviour in European health care systems
Richard B. Saltman, Reinhard Busse and Elias Mossialos (eds)

Hospitals in a changing Europe
Martin McKee and Judith Healy (eds)

Health care in central Asia
Martin McKee, Judith Healy and Jane Falkingham (eds)

Funding health care: options for Europe
Elias Mossialos, Anna Dixon, Josep Figueras and Joe Kutzin (eds)

Health policy and European Union enlargement
Martin McKee, Laura MacLehose and Ellen Nolte (eds)

Regulating pharmaceuticals in Europe: striving for efficiency, equity and quality
Elias Mossialos, Monique Mrazek and Tom Walley (eds)

Social health insurance systems in western Europe
Richard B. Saltman, Reinhard Busse and Josep Figueras (eds)

Purchasing to improve health systems performance
Josep Figueras, Ray Robinson and Elke Jakubowski (eds)

Human resources for health in Europe
Carl-Ardy Dubois, Martin McKee and Ellen Nolte (eds)

Primary care in the driver's seat
Richard B. Saltman, Ana Rico and Wienke Boerma (eds)

Mental health policy and practice across Europe: the future direction of mental health care
Martin Knapp, David McDaid, Elias Mossialos and Graham Thornicroft (eds)

Decentralization in health care
Richard B. Saltman, Vaida Bankauskaite and Karsten Vrangbæk (eds)

Health systems and the challenge of communicable diseases: experiences from Europe and Latin America
Richard Coker, Rifat Atun and Martin McKee (eds)

Caring for people with chronic conditions: a health system perspective
Ellen Nolte and Martin McKee (eds)

Nordic health care systems: recent reforms and current policy challenges
Jon Magnussen, Karsten Vrangbæk and Richard B. Saltman (eds)

Forthcoming titles

Migration and health in the European Union
Bernd Rechel, Philipa Mladovsky, Walter Devillé, Barbara Rijks, Roumyana Petrova-Benedict and Martin McKee (eds)

Contents

List of tables, figures and boxes

Tables

Figures

Boxes

Abbreviations

A&E	Accident & Emergency (department, services)
AC	Autonomous Community
ACCC	Australian Casemix Clinical Committee
ACHI	Australian Classification of Health Interventions
ACRA	Advisory Committee on Resource Allocation
ACSS	Central Administration of the Health System (Portugal)
ADRG	Adjacent DRG
AFS	Annual financial statement(s)
AFSSAPS	Agency for Safety of Medical Products (France)
(A)LOS	(Average) Length(s) of stay
AMI	Acute myocardial infarction
AN-DRG	Australian National DRG
AOTM	Health Technology Assessment Agency (Poland)
AP-DRG	All-Patient DRG
APG	Ambulatory Patient Group(s)
AR-DRG	Australian Refined DRG
ARH	Regional Hospital Agencies (France)
ARS	Regional Health Agencies (France)
ATIH	Technical Agency for Hospital Information (France)
ATU	Temporary access for treatment (France)
AWBZ	Exceptional Medical Expenses Act (Netherlands)
BQS	Federal Office for Quality Assurance (Germany)
CART	Classification and Regression Trees
CAT	Computerized axial tomography

CC	Complication and co-morbidity
CCAM	French classification of procedures (France)
CCSAE	Clinical Costing Standards Association of England
CED	Coverage with Evidence Development
CHS	Catalan Health Service
CM	Major category (France)
CMA	Severe/acute/complicated episode(s) (France)
CMBD	Joint standardized minimum basic dataset (Spain)
CMD	Major diagnostic categories (France)
CMI	Casemix index
CMS	Centers for Medicare and Medicaid Services
CMU	Casemix unit (Ireland)
COPD	Chronic obstructive pulmonary disease
CQUIN	Commissioning for Quality and Innovation (framework)
CT	Computerized tomography
CVZ	Healthcare Insurance Board (Netherlands)
DBC	Diagnosis–treatment combinations (Netherlands)
DBC-DIS	DBC information system (Netherlands)
DBC-O	DBC onderhoud (Netherlands DBC administrative organisation)
DEA	Data envelopment analysis
DG	Day grouper
DIM	Medical information units (France)
DIMDI	German Institute of Medical Documentation and Information
DoHC	Department of Health and Children (Ireland)
DPG	Day-patient grouper
DRG	Diagnosis-related group
ED	Emergency department
EHESP	*Ecole des hautes études en santé publique* (School of Public Health)
EHIF	Estonian Health Insurance Fund
ENC	National Cost Study (France)
ENCC	Hospital cost database (France)
ESRI	Economic and Social Research Institute (Ireland)
EU	European Union
EU15	European Union Member States prior to May 2004
FPG	Case Fees Act (Germany)
G-BA	Federal Joint Committee (Germany)
GHCA	General Health Care Act (Spain)
GHJ	Homogeneous groups of days (French patient classification tool)
GHM	Homogeneous groups of patients (French patient classification system)
GP	General practitioner
HAS	High Health Authority (France)
HCAT	HIPE Coding Audit Toolkit (Ireland)
HCFA	Health Care Financing Administration (United States)
HDG	Main diagnosis group (Austria)
HES	Hospital Episode Statistics
HIPE	Hospital In-Patient Enquiry (Ireland)
HNDP	Hospital Network Development Plan
HPID	Health Policy and Information Division (Ireland)

HRG	Healthcare Resource Group(s) (Ireland)
HRID	Health Research and Information Division (Ireland)
HSE	Health Service Executive
HTA	Health Technology Assessment
ICD	International Classification of Diseases (WHO)
ICD-9-CM	International Classification of Diseases, Ninth Revision, Clinical Modification
ICD-10	International Classification of Diseases, Tenth Revision
ICD-10-AM	International Classification of Diseases, Tenth Revision, Australia Modification
ICD-10-GM	International Classification of Diseases, Tenth Revision, German Modification
ICHI	International Classification of Health Interventions
ICPM	International Classification of Procedures in Medicine
ICS	Catalan Health Care Institute (Spain)
ICU	Intensive care unit
IGZ	Healthcare Inspectorate (Netherlands)
InEK	Institute for the Hospital Remuneration System (Germany)
IRDES	Institute for Research and Information in Health Economics (France)
IR-DRGs	International Refined DRGs
IRF-PPS	American Inpatient Rehabilitation Facility Prospective Payment System
IT	Information technology(ies)
JGP	Homogeneous groups of patients (Polish patient classification system)
KAKuG	Federal Hospitals Act (Austria)
KHEntgG	Hospital Remuneration Act (Germany)
KMÅ	Swedish national classification system for non-surgical procedures
KRUS	Agricultural Social Insurance Fund (Poland)
KVÅ	Swedish national classification system for surgery and non-surgical procedures
LDF	Procedure- and diagnosis-oriented case groups (Austria)
LKF	Performance-oriented hospital financing framework (Austria)
LTR	Swiss performance-oriented payment system for rehabilitation
MAS	Major ambulatory surgery
MBDS	Minimum basic dataset
MDC	Major diagnostic category
MEL	Single medical procedure (Austria)
MERRI	*Missions d'enseignement, de recherche, de reference et d'innovation* (teaching, research, recourse and innovation, France)
MFF	Market forces factor
MIGAC	Missions of general interest and assistance with contracting, including payments for education, research and public health programmes
MRI	Magnetic resonance imaging
MS-DRG	Medicare Severity DRG
NCECI	NOMESCO Classification of External Causes of Injury
NCSP	NOMESCO Classification of Surgical Procedures

NFZ	National Health Fund (Poland)
NHS	National Health Service
NOMESCO	Nordic Medico-Statistical Committee
NordDRG	Nordic patient classification system
NPR	National Patient Register
NUB	New Diagnostic and Treatment Methods Regulation (Germany)
NZA	Dutch Healthcare Authority
OECD	Organisation for Economic Co-operation and Development
OPCS	Office of Population Censuses and Surveys (British Classification of Surgical Operations and Procedures)
OPS	Procedure classification codes (Germany)
OR	Operating room
P4P	Pay for performance
PbR	Payment by Results
PCCL	Patient Clinical Complexity Level
PCS	Patient classification system
PCSI	Patient Classification Systems International
PCT	Primary Care Trust
PERFECT	PERFormance, Effectiveness and Cost of Treatment episodes
PLICS	Patient-Level Information and Costing Systems
PMSI	Hospital activity database (France)
PRIKRAF	Private Hospitals Financing Fund (Austria)
QMS	Quality management system(s) (Germany)
RBG	Rehabilitation Treatment Groups (Germany)
R&D	Research and development
RRI	Relative resource intensity
RSS	Patient discharge summary (France)
RUM	Departmental discharge summary (France)
RV	Relative value(s) (Ireland)
SALAR	Swedish Association of Local Authorities and Regions
SAM	State Agency of Medicines (Estonia)
SD	Skewed distribution
SGB V	German Social Law, Fifth book
SHF	State Health Fund (Austria)
SHI	Statutory health insurance
STAKES	National Research and Development Centre for Health and Welfare
TB	Tuberculosis
TUB	Berlin University of Technology
UBA	Basic Care Unit (Spain)
UMBDS	Uniform minimum basic datasets (Portugal)
VAT	Value-added tax
VHI	Voluntary health insurance
VWS	Ministry of Health, Welfare and Sport (Netherlands)
XHUP	Public Hospital Network (Spain)
ZBC	Independent Treatment Centre (Netherlands)
ZUS	Social Insurance Institution (Poland)
ZVW	Health Insurance Act (Netherlands)

Foreword 1

This book has global application; it will find an eager audience among policy leaders, technicians, hospitals, and physicians. In Organisation for Economic Co-operation and Development (OECD) countries, in which DRGs have been implemented since the 1980s, there is still little or no comparison three decades later across countries, in terms of key building blocks, and whether or how variations in design make a difference. How many categories are enough, and when are there too many? When do DRGs begin to look like a fee-for-service model? Which cost-accounting system works best? Almost all DRG experts are conversant in one or two, or perhaps a small number of systems, without any in-depth knowledge of the larger number of countries in the European Union (EU) which have implemented some form of DRGs.

As with other mechanisms and policies in the health sector, the book sheds light and presents evidence on the importance of history and context. As far as DRGs are concerned, the book suggests, there is no "one size fits all" situation. At least not yet. While a uniform approach across Europe may emerge at some point, it is clear that the experience of countries to date is defined by EU Member States taking different approaches in terms of clinical categories, patient classification systems, costing and allocation, quality, and their readiness to respond to the somewhat euphemistically termed "unintended consequences" that seem to emerge in every implementation process. The diagnostic across countries is both interesting and useful, and will be enlightening to students in any country looking for ways to improve the casemix system, either under design or already fully implemented. The variation in the short term takes the form of an opportunity to provide a menu of options for solving technical issues within each of the building blocks.

Still, it is remarkable that, from a broader vantage point, there is a path of convergence in payment models for hospitals across Europe, with some mix of DRGs and global budgets. Within the bigger picture, guidance is also given, not only on what to do about individual building blocks, but also in terms of the need to constantly "mind" or monitor and update the system in place. A former United States Medicare administrator in the late 1980s, Dr. William Roper, once argued that a system of DRGs would collapse under its own complicated and technocratic weight, to be replaced by a simpler and more powerful capitation model for the full benefits package. That day has not yet arrived, although the book competently offers a glimpse of the future, which shows a system that includes outpatient stays and the emergence of payment for entire episodes of care, as is the case in the Netherlands.

Yet, this book will be appreciated beyond the EU and other OECD countries. As a peripatetic World Bank health economist working in middle- and low-income countries since the 1990s, upon arriving in a country and visiting the leadership, a clear pattern of priorities emerges from the first meeting with a Minister of Health. The discussion typically starts with a series of questions about how to mobilize more funds for services in the health sector. This is often an ambiguous and meandering discussion, which highlights the need to assess fiscal space, and raises some questions (from me back to the Minister) regarding sectoral efficiency and performance. Resource allocation, not new money, quickly becomes front and centre. Like the Europeans and North Americans of the 1970s and 1980s, the Minister agrees that the system needs to restructure incentives to improve performance, while simultaneously facing a landscape of changing demographics, changing disease profiles, and increasing citizen dissatisfaction regarding responsiveness. Almost without exception, the Minister then pronounces that the sector needs DRGs for hospitals, and in quick succession wants to know in how many weeks might "we" (together) implement the system in the country. Such a scenario has often played out in the countries of the former USSR in the 1990s, in the Middle East in the first decade of this century, and in South and East Asia in the last few years. My colleagues report that examples of this type of discussion are increasing in number in Latin America and (most recently) Africa; for example, in Ghana, Kenya, and South Africa.

Starting with the hospital sector in non-OECD countries makes sense. That is where the money is. The share of expenditure for inpatient acute care is typically more than 50 per cent of all spending. In China, it is 58 per cent, in Brazil over 60 per cent and in the countries of the former USSR it was often above 70 per cent. Most countries face significant challenges with both technical and allocative efficiency. Some effort to move from line-item budgets and/or fee-for-service payment holds the promise of addressing multiple objectives related to improved sectoral performance.

At the same time, the move to some form of DRGs is not risk free. Non-OECD countries have often bought a software grouper from Australia, the United States or the Nordic countries. More recently, they have begun to download from the United States Medicare web site an open-source DRG grouper, with 350 categories and 3 levels of severity. "We can start right away" is often the remark heard from the Minister's staff. However, the European country experience is that this model takes time to implement well – typically 5–10 years, and it took even longer in the United States. This book is an insightful and helpful guide on the multiplicity of paths that need to be followed – at times in parallel, at times in concert – while at the same time providing options for finding the fastest and most direct path to implementation.

A few years ago, the World Bank published a manual to help countries design, build and implement new payment systems. The chapter on casemix was certainly the centerpiece of the book. The book was written because countries wanted to know not only "what" to do, but also "how" to do it. That book drew on a very small number of countries in Central Asia, but most OECD and non-OECD countries aspire to have a health sector similar to those found in Europe today. Countries such as Germany, the United Kingdom, the Netherlands, Denmark and Sweden have in place models that are often held up as examples, if not actually emulated. Estonia has become the prime example of what can be done well, from a rather dismal start point, and within a short space of time. This list and mix of advanced and yet relatively similar European countries identified in the book become an optimal platform from which to really assess the impact and potential of DRGs in terms of transparency, efficiency, quality, and so on. The book shows that, while there are predictable patterns of impact, such as reduced length of stay, changes in numbers of beds, admissions and occupancy, there are also significant variations across the EU. And while most of the world sees Europe as relatively homogeneous, the book also shows that organization, financing and delivery models continue to vary from country to country. Finally, the country case studies are quite rich in detailing the political, economic and technocratic approaches used in these individual countries, and (again) provide a strong message to learn from others, but perhaps also to develop unique and innovative solutions that reflect history and the special issues in any single country. The key message of good design is mingled well with certain "preconditions" of success relating to political support, the necessary legal framework, autonomy in the delivery system, good information systems, and proactive quality assurance systems.

Enjoy, learn, compare, and be careful at the design and implementation stages. The World Bank is a founding partner in the European Observatory on Health Systems and Policies, and Bank experts will greatly appreciate this work. With some Observatory books and publications, the experts contribute, but in every case we also learn. We learn along with our many client countries, most of which aspire to a system like those found in Europe today.

Jack Langenbrunner
The World Bank

Foreword 2

As a starting point, I think it is a good idea to use a private example to present a book dealing with issues common to, and important for, all European countries.

Since the 1990s, Bulgaria has moved from the socialist model of centrally planned health care to a single-payer health insurance system. The payment of hospitals, formerly based on annual line-item budgets, gradually began to be based on reported activities, known as "clinical pathways". Each of these pathways is defined for a set of similar diagnoses and has a fixed price. Prices were negotiated between the insurer and professional physicians' organizations. This was just the opposite of what had taken place for 40 years – after centrally planned budgets, prices and wages, the country set out optimistically, with the hope of a free market in hospital care! A few years later, however, it became clear that the agreed prices of clinical pathways were influenced by medical lobbyists and had no direct connection to the costs actually incurred in hospitals – neither in respect of the ratios between the different diagnoses and conditions, nor in terms of the varying degrees of severity within a diagnosis. This was due to the fact that the clinical pathways were based on the main diagnosis and procedure, but neglected the severity of the patient's condition and concomitant diseases. Thus, the more pathways a hospital reported, the more money it received, and the milder the cases that were treated, the more "cost-effective" (that is, profitable) the hospital was. As a result, within ten years hospitalizations in the country increased by 68 per cent and the statistics reported a "growth" in diagnoses, mainly for the well-paid clinical pathways. Part of this increase was also due to newly opened private hospitals specializing precisely in these well-paid areas. Paradoxically (or actually, not surprisingly), despite the increase in financial resources, citizens' dissatisfaction with the health care system also increased.

Given the rapidly increasing hospitalizations and associated costs, global budgets at hospital level were introduced, while the accounting continued to be carried out through clinical pathways. Immediately, questions emerged: how can we determine a fair global budget? How can we encourage those performing well and limit those that are inefficient? How can we ensure transparency? How can we ensure access and quality, without stimulating excessive consumption? The system of clinical pathways was not able to provide adequate answers to these questions, so Bulgaria began to look for alternatives, and intends to introduce a DRG-based payment system, following the example of many other countries in Europe. However, to reveal and compare the strengths, weaknesses, opportunities and threats of European DRG-systems, as well as their design – which is clearly different across countries due to their intended use – is a big challenge for countries such as Bulgaria that want to introduce DRG-based payments which are based on reliable data reflecting patient needs and actual costs, and which incentivize the provision of appropriate, high-quality and efficient care.

Therefore, this book – with Part One focusing on the main issues relating to DRGs, as well as Part Two presenting structured DRG system comparisons across twelve European countries – imparts extremely interesting information for countries which are about to introduce DRGs to finance hospitals. It will certainly be useful, not only for me, but for all others engaged with this issue. It is essential reading for people who ask questions, share problems, offer solutions and disseminate best practices.

Stefan Konstantinov
Minister of Health, Bulgaria

Acknowledgements

The editors would like to thank all EuroDRG project partners and related authors who contributed their knowledge and broad experiences to this book; their great patience with the editors ensured that countless reviews and revisions did not threaten its realization. We would like to give special thanks to Dana Forgione and Frank Hartmann, who reviewed some of the chapters in Part One, encouraging the authors to improve these chapters. Furthermore, we would like to thank Nicole Russell for the extensive editing work and Jonathan North for coordinating the production process.

As the EuroDRG workshops were fundamental for collaboration among project partners in order to develop this book, the editors would like to thank Alexandra Starke, Carola Haring, Esther Martinez Amor and Reelika Ermel, who organized the EuroDRG workshops in Potsdam (2009), Berlin (2009), Paris (2010), Barcelona (2010), Tallinn (2011) and Berlin (again, in 2011). We would also like to thank Pascal Garel, Bernhard Gibis, Luca Lorenzoni, Predrag Djukic and Predrag Stojicic, who participated in EuroDRG workshops and provided insight into related fields in different countries, which clearly contributed to the development of the project as a whole.

Earlier versions of various chapters were presented and discussed at numerous national and international conferences and workshops, such as the EHMA conference 'Hospital Financing: Diagnosis Related Groups – Leading the Debate' in Brussels (2009), the 4th Nordic Casemix Conference in Helsinki (2010), the EHMA Annual Conference in Lahti (2010), the 8th European Conference on Health Economics (ECHE) in Helsinki (2010), the 'Polish DRG System Directions of Future Developments' conference in Warsaw

(2010), the 'Funding Models to Support Quality and Sustainability – A Pan-Canadian Dialogue' conference in Edmonton/Canada (2010), the Patient Classification Systems International (PCSI) Winter School in Dublin (2011), the 3rd German Association of Health Economics Conference in Bayreuth (2011), the World Bank Workshop on 'Health Financing Reforms to Improve Efficiency and Quality of Care' in Moscow (2011), the 12th European Federation of National Associations of Orthopaedics and Traumatology (EFORT) congress in Copenhagen (2011), the European Observatory on Health Systems and Policies' policy dialogue 'Changing the Payment System for Hospital Care in Bulgaria to Improve Equity and Efficiency' in Sofia (2011) and the 8th World Congress on Health Economics in Toronto (2011). The editors would like to thank the auditorium of all these presentations for their inspiring thoughts, which have influenced the final versions presented in this volume.

European projects with multilateral relationships are subject to considerable financial administration efforts. The editors would therefore like to thank Anette Schade, Silke Hönert and Katrin Ludwig from the European liaison office at the Berlin University of Technology for their thoughts to clarify budget-related queries.

In addition, without funding from the European Commission (within the Seventh Framework Programme, research area HEALTH-2007-3.2-8, reference: 223300) the Diagnosis-Related Groups in Europe: towards efficiency and quality research project in this highly relevant area would never have begun.

Finally, the authors would like to thank the numerous supporters of the project, such as Philipp Seibert, Claudia Brendler, Claudia Reiche and Julia Röttger.

Reinhard Busse
Alexander Geissler
Wilm Quentin
Miriam Wiley

List of contributors

Ain Aaviksoo, PRAXIS Center for Policy Studies, Estonia
Tõnis Allik, North Estonian Medical Centre, Estonia
Martine Bellanger, National School of Public Health, France
Reinhard Busse, Berlin University of Technology, Germany
Montse Bustins, Catalan Health Service, Spain
Xavier Castells, Hospital del Mar Research Institute, Spain
Pietro Chiarello, Hospital del Mar Research Institute, Spain
Francesc Cots, Hospital del Mar Research Institute, Spain
Katarzyna Czach, National Health Fund, Poland
Alexander Geissler, Berlin University of Technology, Germany
Leona Hakkaart-van Roijen, Erasmus University Rotterdam, the Netherlands
Unto Häkkinen, National Institute for Health and Welfare, Finland
Mona Heurgren, National Board of Health and Welfare, Sweden
Kristiina Kahur, Estonian Health Insurance Fund, Estonia
Kirsi Kautiainen, National Institute for Health and Welfare, Finland
Katarzyna Klonowska, National Health Fund, Poland
Conrad Kobel, Innsbruck Medical University, Austria
Heli Laarmann, PRAXIS Center for Policy Studies, Estonia
Jorma Lauharanta, Hospital District of Helsinki and Uusimaa, Finland
Miika Linna, National Institute for Health and Welfare, Finland
Anne Mason, University of York, United Kingdom
Céu Mateus, Universidade Nova de Lisboa, Portugal
Brian McCarthy, Economic and Social Research Institute Dublin, Ireland
Zeynep Or, Institute of Research and Information on Health Economics, France

Jacqueline O'Reilly, Economic and Social Research Institute Dublin, Ireland
Gerli Paat, PRAXIS Center for Policy Studies, Estonia
Karl-Peter Pfeiffer, Innsbruck Medical University, Austria
Wilm Quentin, Berlin University of Technology, Germany
Ken Redekop, Erasmus University Rotterdam, the Netherlands
Xavier Salvador, Catalan Health Service, Spain
David Scheller-Kreinsen, Berlin University of Technology, Germany
Lisbeth Serdén, National Board of Health and Welfare, Sweden
Andrew Street, University of York, United Kingdom
Maria Świderek, National Health Fund, Poland
Siok Swan Tan, Erasmus University Rotterdam, the Netherlands
Josselin Thuilliez, National School of Public Health, France
Martin van Ineveld, Erasmus University Rotterdam, the Netherlands
Martti Virtanen, Nordic Casemix Centre, Finland
Padraic Ward, University of York, United Kingdom
Katarzyna Wiktorzak, National Health Fund, Poland
Miriam Wiley, Economic and Social Research Institute Dublin, Ireland

Part One

chapter one

From the origins of DRGs to their implementation in Europe

Miriam Wiley

1.1 The starting point

> Really the whole hospital problem rests on one question: What happens to the cases? [...] We must formulate some method of hospital report showing as nearly as possible what are the results of the treatment obtained at different institutions. This report must be made out and published by each hospital in a uniform manner, so that comparison will be possible. With such a report as a starting-point, those interested can begin to ask questions as to management and efficiency.
>
> (Dr Eugene Codman, Address to the Philadelphia County Medical Society, 1913)[1]

The 'hospital problem', as presented by Dr Codman – a surgeon at Massachusetts General Hospital – at the beginning of the 20th century continues to present a challenge today, almost 100 years later (Fetter, 1991). The work which was initiated by Codman was revisited and further developed by Professor Robert Fetter and his colleagues at Yale University in the late 1960s, when they were invited to assist with the development of a programme of utilization review and quality assurance for their local university hospital. The questions posed of Fetter and his team relating to their work on this issue began what he later described as a 20-year process of 'measuring hospital production as a means of evaluating what takes place in the hospital' (Fetter, 1991, p. 4). It is interesting that the original initiative was prompted by the requirements of registration for the Medicare Program, which had been established in 1965, and it was the Medicare Program in 1983 that first implemented the diagnosis-related group (DRG) system that emerged from this lengthy development process.

Because of the requirements to process very large sets of hospital data, developments in information technology (IT) were critical to the work that took place throughout the 1970s relating to 'finding a way to measure and cost the output of hospitals' (Fetter, 1993). The first version of what became the DRG system was developed in 1973 and comprised 54 major diagnostic categories (MDCs) and 333 final groups. The second version was developed for the Federal Social Security Administration and comprised 83 MDCs and 383 DRGs (Fetter et al., 1980), while the third version in 1978 was developed for the State of New Jersey, which was proceeding with putting in place a DRG-based hospital payment system. The final (original) version of the DRG system was developed by the Health Systems Management Group at Yale University within the framework of a contract with the Health Care Financing Administration (HCFA) for the purpose of developing 'an inpatient classification system that differentiated the amount of hospital resources required to provide care and was clinically coherent in the sense that the groups were expected to evoke a set of clinical responses which resulted in a similar pattern of resources' (Rodrigues, 1993). The so-called 'prospective payment system', which was introduced for the Medicare Program in 1983 mandated that payments for hospital services were determined on the basis of the first version of the HCFA-DRG system, which at that time comprised 470 groups across 23 MDCs.

The enactment of Medicare's prospective payment system was considered to be 'the single most influential post-war innovation in medical financing' by Mayes (2007, p. 21), who notes that 'Medicare's new prospective payment system with DRGs triggered a shift in the balance of political and economic power between the providers of medical care (hospitals and physicians) and those who paid for it – power that providers had successfully accumulated for more than half a century' (ibid, p. 21). The view put forward by Mayes that this change went virtually unnoticed by the general public is particularly interesting because what this book attempts to track is how this innovation worked its way around the world to the point where, almost 30 years later, the DRG system is the single most important patient classification system (PCS) in use internationally.

1.2 Crossing the Atlantic and the Pacific

Living, as we do, in an era of almost 'instant' communication, it would be easy to underestimate the significance of the international ripple-effect associated with the adoption of the DRG system by the United States Government in 1983. While we are now accustomed to being immediately informed about significant world events or important developments in our areas of interest, in the early 1980s we had to order journals by post, go to libraries to access literature and communicate with our international colleagues by fax or 'phone!

Despite such challenges, however, the international impact of the move to a prospective payment system by the United States Medicare Program was rapid, with developments in Europe and Australia proceeding quickly by the standards of the era (and even by current standards). In Europe, a meeting hosted by the Ministry of Health in France in 1984 included Professor Robert Fetter, the leader of the team which developed the DRG system, and involved five countries

(Belgium, France, Ireland, the Netherlands and Portugal). A further international meeting was held just two years later in Dublin, already involving 11 European countries. When 15 countries participated in a meeting in Lisbon in 1987, they agreed to set up a network for those interested in working on issues related to the classification of patients, and Patient Classification Systems International (PCSI)'s Patient Classification Systems Network continues to function today.[2]

In parallel with the European developments, a National Seminar on DRGs was held in Australia in 1984. Following this seminar, the funding of a number of research projects sowed the seeds which quickly flourished into a substantial research area, producing the evidence base on which subsequent developments in DRG systems and their applications in Australia were founded.

The momentum in international developments regarding the portability and suitability of DRGs for use in health systems outside of the United States was given some additional support from international meetings organized by the Yale development team in London in 1986, Washington in 1987, and Sydney in 1988. In addition to profiling the activities in an increasing number of countries, these conferences enabled the researchers and policy-makers to make personal contacts which facilitated more rapid exchange of information and sharing of experiences than would otherwise have been possible (in the era before the World Wide Web). These meetings, together with those organized by PCSI, helped to foster a spirit of cooperation amongst those in a position at the fore in this field, such that each new entrant could quickly benefit from those who had gone before.

The momentum for international collaboration on developments and applications for DRG-type systems also benefitted from initiatives supported by a number of international organizations. In 1985 the Council of Europe supported a review of the research being undertaken in Europe at that time on DRGs, while the Organisation for Economic Co-operation and Development (OECD) began to publish international comparisons of average lengths of stay by DRG (Rodrigues, 1989). The European Union (EU) programme of the late 1980s which was concerned with supporting medical and health research also supported a number of projects relating to costing and using DRGs, and supporting the development of PCSs appropriate for European hospitals (Casas & Wiley, 1993; Leidl et al., 1990). Over the same period, WHO supported a number of planning meetings regarding the use of DRGs for hospital budgeting and performance measurement (Wiley, 1990).

While the lead-in to the application of DRGs within the United States prospective payment system was not particularly lengthy when viewed in terms of the pace at which translating research into policy applications usually takes place, it is interesting to note that a much more truncated period predated the first national applications of DRG-based payment systems in Europe and Australia. In Europe, Portugal was the first country to begin operating a DRG-based hospital payment system for payments from occupational health insurance schemes in 1988 (see Chapter 21), which accounted for about 30 per cent of hospital activity at the time. Norway followed, with the introduction of a DRG-based payment system in selected hospitals in the period 1991–1993 (Magnussen & Solstad, 1994), and Ireland began the introduction of a

DRG-based budget allocation system for a limited number of acute care hospitals in 1993 (see Chapter 15). The first initiative in Australia dates back to 1988, when the then Australian Federal Health Department incorporated DRGs into the 1988–1993 Medicare Agreements between the Commonwealth and eight states and territories, and began funding the development of an Australian version of DRGs (Australian National (AN-)DRGs), introduced in 1992. Victoria was the first state to use DRGs (in 1993) to set budgets for its public hospitals (McNair & Duckett, 2002).

1.3 Where are we now? Aims of the book

It is evident that the development of the DRG casemix classification system – together with advancing a range of applications – could be described as an international phenomenon (Kimberly et al., 2008). It is rare in the world of health systems development to identify an initiative which has progressed so rapidly from the research phase to implementation and international dissemination. This book aims to bring readers up to date on developments in this field in European countries in more recent times. While it is clear that most countries have introduced DRG systems and DRG-based hospital payment systems with the aims of increasing transparency, improving efficiency and assuring quality in hospitals, it remains relatively unknown whether countries are really moving towards achieving these goals. This book therefore summarizes experiences and developments in European DRG systems.

The focus of the book on Europe relates to the fact that the EuroDRG project[3] that gave rise to this initiative has been funded by the Seventh Framework Programme (FP 7) of the EU. The 12 countries (Austria, England, Estonia, Finland, France, Germany, Ireland, the Netherlands, Poland, Portugal, Spain, Sweden) which take part in the EuroDRG project and which are included in this book were selected based on their geographical region (for example, Portugal versus Finland, and Poland versus France), health system typology (such as National Health Service (NHS) versus Statutory Health Insurance (SHI)) and their duration of affiliation to the EU (for example, Estonia versus the Netherlands), in order to ensure a comparison of countries with truly different characteristics. However, it is recognized that there would be scope for a companion volume tracking developments in Australia, Asia, Africa, and Central and South America.

The book is addressed to health policy-makers and researchers from Europe and beyond and is intended to contribute to the emergence of a 'common language' that will facilitate communication between those researchers and policy-makers, from different countries. Both the overview of the key issues (Part One) and the experience from the 12 countries analysed herein (Part Two) should be particularly useful for countries and regions that want to introduce, extend, or optimize their DRG systems. However, in the context of the increasing importance of cross-border movement of patients and payments, this book also aims to draw attention to the potential for coordinating and eventually harmonizing DRG systems and DRG-based hospital payment in Europe. Clearly, the book demonstrates that progress has been made since the work undertaken by Codman a century ago, and that countries are continuously striving to optimize their DRG systems in order to better understand what Robert Fetter termed 'the rather strange cost behaviour of hospitals' (Fetter, 1993, p. v).

1.4 Notes

1 See Codman, 1913–1917.
2 More information on the network can be found at the PCSI web site (www.pcsinternational.org, accessed 26 July 2011).
3 More information is available at the EuroDRG project web site (www.eurodrg.eu, accessed 26 July 2011).

1.5 References

Casas, M., Wiley, M., eds. (1993). *Diagnosis-Related Groups in Europe, Uses and Perspectives.* Berlin: Springer-Verlag.

Codman, E.A. (1913–1917). The product of a hospital (Philadelphia address) (Box 4, Folder 77), in E.A. Codman. *Ernest Amory Codman Papers, 1849–1981: Finding Aid.* Boston, MA: Boston Medical Library and Francis A. Countway Library of Medicine (B MS c60).

Fetter, R.B., ed. (1991). *DRGs: Their Design and Development.* Ann Arbor, MI: Health Administration Press.

Fetter, R.B. (1993). Foreword, in M. Casas, M. Wiley, eds. *Diagnosis-Related Groups in Europe, Uses and Perspectives.* Berlin: Springer-Verlag.

Fetter, R.B., Shin, Y., Freeman, J.L., Averill, R.F., Thompson, J.D. (1980). Casemix definition by diagnosis-related groups. *Medical Care,* 18(2):1–53.

Kimberly, J.R., de Pouvourville, G., D'Aunno, T., eds. (2008). *The Globalization of Managerial Innovation in Health Care.* Cambridge: Cambridge University Press.

Leidl, R., Potthoff, P., Schwefel, D., eds. (1990). *European Approaches to Patient Classification Systems.* Berlin: Springer-Verlag.

Magnussen, J., Solstad, K. (1994). Case-based hospital financing: the case of Norway, *Health Policy,* 28:23–36.

Mayes, R. (2007). The origins, development and passage of Medicare's revolutionary prospective payment system. *Journal of the History of Medicine and Allied Sciences,* 62(1):21–55.

McNair, P., Duckett, S. (2002). Funding Victoria's public hospitals: the casemix policy of 2000–2001. *Australian Health Review,* 25(1):72–99.

Rodrigues, J.M. (1989). L'Europe des DRG. *Sozial- und Präventivmedizin,* 34:152–5.

Rodrigues, J.M. (1993). DRGs: origin and dissemination throughout Europe, in M. Casas, M. Wiley, eds. *Diagnosis-Related Groups in Europe, Uses and Perspectives.* Berlin: Springer-Verlag.

Wiley, M. (1990). Patient classification systems: overview of experiments and applications in Europe, in R. Leidl, P. Potthoff, D. Schwefel, eds. *European Approaches to Patient Classification Systems.* Berlin: Springer-Verlag.

chapter two

Introduction to DRGs in Europe: Common objectives across different hospital systems

Alexander Geissler, Wilm Quentin, David Scheller-Kreinsen and Reinhard Busse

2.1 Introduction

Since 1983, when Medicare adopted diagnosis-related groups (DRGs) as the basis for paying hospitals in the United States, DRG-based hospital payment systems have become the basis for paying hospitals and measuring their activity in most high-income countries, albeit to different extents (Paris et al., 2010). However, the term DRG is widely used with different meanings across and within countries. Some countries use DRGs mostly as a measure for assessing hospital casemix (for example, Sweden and Finland), whereas in other countries DRGs are used as a synonym for payment rates (such as in France and Germany). This is partly due to different DRG implementation processes that took place in different decades, and partly due to the fact that DRG systems were adopted and designed primarily based on the needs of the health system concerned (Busse et al., 2006; Schreyögg et al., 2006).

The second section (2.2) of this chapter summarizes the purposes of the introduction of DRGs in European countries and the expectations associated with their implementation, as well as illustrating the complexity of this process by highlighting the extended periods of time that sometimes evolved from the initial application of DRGs in hospitals to their use for hospital payment. In many countries, this process was highly controversial because of the potential unintended consequences of DRG-based hospital payment systems (see Chapter 6), and it is difficult to understand the international success of these systems without being aware of the alternatives. Therefore, section 2.3 presents the basic incentives of fee-for-service systems and global budgets that were traditionally used in most countries. Section 2.4 then turns to the large structural differences in the hospital sector – both those that existed between countries at the time when DRGs were introduced for hospital payment and those that continue to persist today, despite the fact that DRGs are used for hospital payment in all countries. This serves to illustrate the original aim of this book; namely, to identify similarities and differences in the use of DRG systems across Europe. The chapter closes with a brief overview of the structure of this book.

2.2 Expectations and purposes of DRG introduction

Independent of the type of hospital system in place (see section 2.4), DRG systems were internationally introduced for similar reasons, which can be grouped into two broad categories: first, they should increase the transparency of services which are effectively provided in hospitals (that is, through patient classification, measuring hospital output, etc); and second, DRG-based payment systems should give incentives for the efficient use of resources within hospitals by paying hospitals on the basis of the number and type of cases treated. In addition, the combination of increased transparency and efficient use of resources was assumed to contribute to improving – or at least assuring – the level of quality of care.

Table 2.1 shows how the purpose of DRG introduction varied according to when the country in question introduced the DRG-based system. Interestingly,

Table 2.1 Years of introduction and purposes of DRG systems over time

Country	*Year of DRG introduction*	*Original purpose(s)*	*Principal purpose(s) in 2010*
Austria	1997	Budgetary allocation	Budgetary allocation, planning
England	1992	Patient classification	Payment
Estonia	2003	Payment	Payment
Finland	1995	Description of hospital activity, benchmarking	Planning and management, benchmarking, hospital billing
France	1991	Description of hospital activity	Payment
Germany	2003	Payment	Payment
Ireland	1992	Budgetary allocation	Budgetary allocation
Netherlands	2005	Payment	Payment
Poland	2008	Payment	Payment
Portugal	1984	Hospital output measurement	Budgetary allocation
Spain (Catalonia)	1996	Payment	Payment, benchmarking
Sweden	1995	Payment	Benchmarking, performance measurement

Source: Authors' own compilation based on information presented in the country-specific chapters of Part Two of this volume.

Note: Even if the stated original purpose was to pay hospitals on the basis of DRGs, most countries began this process only after a conversion period (see Figure 2.1).

countries that were early adopters of DRGs primarily did so with the aim of increasing transparency (such as Portugal and France). Countries that introduced DRGs later (such as the Netherlands and Poland) generally did so with the intention of paying hospitals on the basis of DRGs.

Figure 2.1 illustrates the DRG introduction process in different countries since the early 1980s. Every country took a different route at a different time to introduce a DRG-based system, often initially for the purpose of patient classification, and later also for payment purposes. Some countries used DRGs over an extended period of time exclusively for the purpose of patient classification and increasing transparency (for example, up to ten years in England), in order to become acquainted with the DRG grouping logic before they started paying hospitals on the basis of DRGs. Others introduced DRGs after a short period of conversion (for example, in Ireland DRGs were introduced in 1992 and first used for budgetary allocation in 1993).

The reason why the introduction of DRG systems was thought to improve transparency is that such systems condense the extremely large number of patients that all appear to be unique into a limited number of groups that have a set of certain characteristics in common (Fetter et al., 1980). By categorizing patients with similar resource utilization and clinical characteristics into groups, DRGs describe hospital activity in standardized units and enable analyses, which

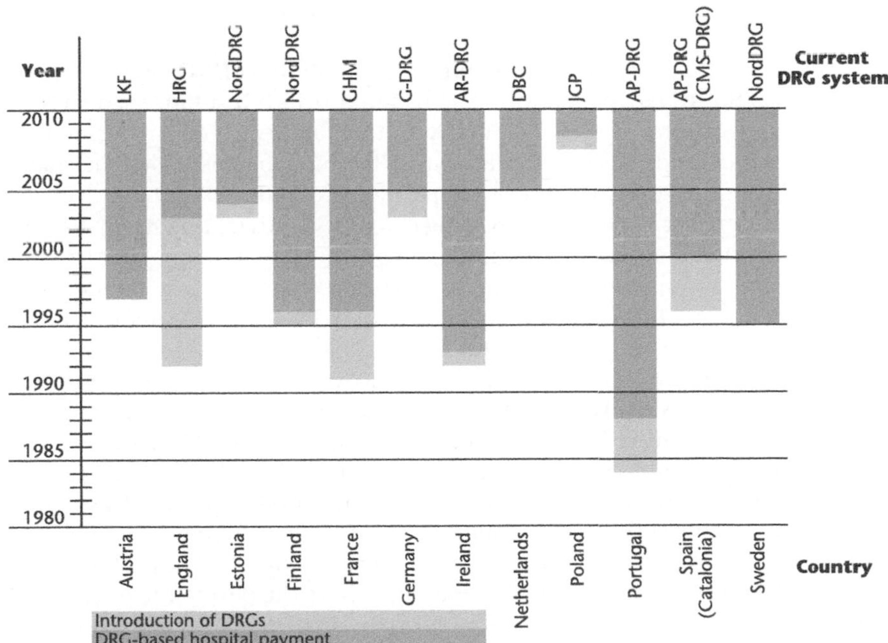

Figure 2.1 From DRG introduction to DRG-based budget allocation and payment

Source: Authors' own compilation based on information presented in the country-specific chapters of Part Two of this volume.

Note: Ireland started with HCFA-DRGs in 1992 and switched in 2003 to AR-DRGs.

otherwise would not be possible. For example, hospital managers and policy-makers can compare length of stay, costs, and quality of patients within the same DRG across different hospitals or across different hospital departments. In addition, DRGs offer a framework for an accurate assessment of the costs of treating a given patient, taking account of observable and measurable patient and service characteristics such as diagnoses and performed procedures. Consequently, DRGs facilitate performance comparisons and benchmarking, as well as contributing to increased transparency in an area of policy-making that previously was characterized by extreme agency problems. Especially in countries that traditionally used global budgets as their mode of hospital payment, the hospital management had very little information on what types of services were delivered and at what costs clinicians delivered these within their wards or departments.

The main purpose behind the introduction of DRGs in the countries that introduced them in the late 1990s and 2000s – namely, to use DRGs as a basis for hospital payment – was extremely ambitious. This is because the aim is not only to pay providers fairly, but also to discourage the provision of unnecessary services and to encourage the efficient delivery of appropriate care. In the context of the increasing health care costs in many European countries, DRG-based hospital payment systems fitted well with the paradigm of designing public policy according to general economic principles, in order to exert financial pressure and to incentivize efficient resource use (see Chapter 7) by mimicking product markets that produce at marginal costs (Shleifer, 1985).

In Europe, Portugal was the front-runner in operating a DRG-based hospital payment system for payments from occupational health insurance schemes in the late 1980s. More recently, in many other European countries (such as England, France and Germany) DRG-based hospital payment systems have evolved to become the main hospital payment system, with the objectives generally comprising, *inter alia*, increasing efficiency, activity and transparency; reducing waiting times and length of stay; supporting patient choice; enhancing quality of care; and encouraging competition between hospitals. In Sweden and Finland, however, DRGs are still primarily used to aid transparency in the planning and management of hospital services.

As illustrated in the top row of Figure 2.1, most countries are using country-specific DRG systems. Only Ireland, Portugal and Spain are operating DRG systems that were imported from Australia (Australian Refined (AR-)DRGs) or the United States (All Patient (AP-)DRGs, Centers for Medicare and Medicaid Services (CMS-)DRGs). However, many other countries also imported DRG systems from abroad and used these as the starting point for developing their own systems (see Chapter 4). The Nordic countries (Finland, Sweden and Estonia) are special, in that they decided to collaborate and share the development effort in order to create a common NordDRG system that is further adjustable to country-specific conditions (see Chapter 16), which may serve as an example for a pan-European model of coordinating DRG models or even developing a uniform system.

It is important to emphasize that countries introduced DRG-based payment systems irrespective of (1) which kind of hospital payment system was in place before (see section 2.3) and (2) their very different structural circumstances (see section 2.4).

2.3 Hospital payment systems and incentives

The move in most countries towards DRG-based hospital payment systems was driven by the objective of incentivizing hospitals to improve their performance (Langenbrunner & Wiley, 2002). Prior to the introduction of DRG-based hospital payment systems, countries used two basic mechanisms to pay for hospital care: fee-for-service payments and global budgets. These systems provide a specific set of incentives, which are different from the incentives of DRG-based systems. Therefore, in order to understand the international success of DRG-based systems, it is necessary to be aware of the incentives of theses alternative systems, and of the objectives that hospital payment systems are supposed to achieve. Hospital payment systems should motivate providers to treat patients in need of care and to deliver an adequate number of necessary services (level of activity), while taking into account the appropriateness of the services and patient outcomes (i.e. quality). Finally, a hospital payment system should balance activity and expenditure control incentives, thus contributing to increasing efficiency, while minimizing administrative effort and maximizing transparency. This demonstrates two things: (1) the design of 'good' payment systems needs to take into account various dimensions; namely, those of patients and of providers, of the provided services, of payers, and possibly of society at large; and (2) because of this complexity, it simply cannot be expected that any payment system is 'optimal' in all respects. Rather, all payment systems have their strengths and weaknesses in relation to the various objectives. Table 2.2 summarizes the advantages and disadvantages of the above-mentioned payment systems by evaluating their characteristics in relation to the requirements of modern hospital payment systems.

Table 2.2 Hospital payment systems and their theoretical advantages and disadvantages

Dimension / *System*	*Activity*						
	Number of cases	*Number of services/ case*	*Expenditure control*	*Technical efficiency*	*Quality*	*Administrative simplicity*	*Transparency*
Fee-for-service/ Cost reimbursement	+	+	–	0	0	–	0
DRG-based payment	+	–	0	+	0	–	+
Global budget	–	–	+	0	0	+	–

Sources: Authors' own compilation, based on Barnum et al. (1995) and WHO (2000).

Notes: +/–: increase/decrease; 0: neutral or unclear; for a definition of technical efficiency, see Chapter 7 of this volume.

2.3.1 Fee-for-service payments

In the United States and some European countries (such as Estonia), the ('retrospectively' determined) fee-for-service system was the principal means of allocating resources to hospitals prior to the use of – in comparison to fee-for-service payment – 'prospectively' determined DRG-based hospital payment systems. The sum of the fees in fee-for-service payment systems should ideally reflect the actual individual patient costs. This approach was often considered as fair or favourable by providers as long as fees covered at least their costs – preferably costs plus profit, of course. Fee-for-service payment provides strong incentives to be productive and to offer a large of number services per patient and therefore ensures that those hospitals treating more complex patients are adequately reimbursed. However, fee-for-service payment may lead to the provision of unnecessary services or may even encourage oversupply of inappropriate services, which negatively affects patient outcomes and the efficient delivery of services. In addition, providers under a pure fee-for-service regime (that is, without budget limitations) are incentivized to neglect expenditure considerations, which also contributes to an inefficient service delivery. Paying hospitals according to a fee-for-service scheme is administratively complex, as such systems require detailed and up-to-date price lists, as well as registration and billing of all service items provided. Furthermore, the only instrument for cost control is the specification of the price list, which details the unit payment for each item (Street et al., 2007).

2.3.2 Global budgets

In Europe global budgets were a common approach used for allocating financial resources to hospitals before the introduction of DRG-based hospital payment systems. In the context of global budgets a fixed payment for a certain activity level (typically determined in terms of number of cases or number of bed days) was negotiated and agreed between payers and hospitals, usually for the approaching year; namely, really 'prospectively'. In some countries global budgets were defined at or adjusted for specialty. Global budgets are administratively simple and can effectively contribute to cost-containment because of their expenditure cap characteristic. However, they run the risk of hospitals not producing sufficient services to meet patient or population needs, hence disregarding patient needs and therefore health outcomes. Some European countries were using target budgets blended with per diem payments as billing units (for example, Germany). Consequently, hospitals were provided with clear incentives to increase bed occupancy by prolonging the length of stay.

Fee-for-service systems and global budgets provide conflicting incentives for 'activity' and 'expenditure control' (see Table 2.2). Both are problematic in terms of ensuring high-quality care due to the inherent incentive to over-provide (fee-for-service) or to under-provide (global budgets) hospital services. Policy-makers (first in the United States and later in Europe) were therefore attracted by the idea of paying hospitals through DRGs, which to a certain extent provide incentives somewhere in between a fee-for-service system and global budgets.

2.3.3 DRG-based payments

The term DRGs is used here to highlight the theoretical incentives of DRG-based payments, which do not necessarily correspond to the actual incentives of the systems operated in the countries included in this book. Theoretically, DRG-based payments provide strong incentives to increase the number of cases treated and to reduce the number of services per case. In contrast to fee-for-service systems, DRGs incentivize hospitals to limit their activity to necessary services and – in contrast to global budgets – DRGs incentivize hospitals to treat more patients. In terms of expenditure control, the effect of DRG-based payments thus depends on which effect prevails: increasing the number of cases or reducing the number of services per case. In principle, this will also depend on the previous system in place; that is, moving from fee-for-service payment to DRGs can result in cost-containment, while moving from global budgets to DRGs does not.

If DRGs do not sufficiently control for differences between patient groups or for differences in provided services (within DRGs), payments for highly complex cases are too low, while payments for less-complex cases are too high. Consequently, hospitals could try to avoid the risk of treating more complex patients. Furthermore, DRG-based payment systems are administratively complex as they require detailed and standardized coding of diagnoses and procedures, as well as information on the average resource consumption (costs) per DRG.

However, as already outlined, each of the presented payment systems has certain advantages and disadvantages (see Table 2.2). Therefore, policy-makers across Europe have combined features of the different systems: current DRG-based hospital payment relies heavily on service characteristics to define DRGs. Consequently, hospitals are paid partly on the basis of the services that they provide, which introduces aspects of fee-for-service payment into DRG-based hospital payment. Furthermore, the systems are operated within global budgets and provide additional payments for specified services, high-cost drugs and patients with exceptionally long lengths of stay (see Figure 10.2). Interestingly, these payment reforms have been implemented in very diverse hospital environments, which are described in the following section (2.4).

2.4 The hospital landscape

For a long time, a hospital was seen simply as 'an institution which provides beds, meals, and constant nursing care for its patients while they undergo medical therapy at the hands of professional physicians. In carrying out these services, the hospital is striving to restore its patients to health' (Miller, 1997). Clearly, this definition describes very broadly the activities of a hospital and must therefore be constantly refined and extended by taking into account the key previous, ongoing and future changes in hospital care. Since the early 1980s, many European countries have shifted inpatient treatments towards outpatient settings in order to reduce and improve efficiency in the use of hospital resources. This development has led to enormous structural challenges for hospitals (McKee & Healy, 2002). Technological improvements and redesigned care pathways made it possible to extend the number of day cases and outpatient surgery cases treated outside the hospital or in specialized departments within the hospital. However, countries vary in terms of their level of integration between the ambulatory and inpatient sectors.

Table 2.3 provides an overview of these differences based on selected hospital-related indicators for the 12 countries included in Part Two of this book – for 1995 (that is, before DRGs were introduced for payment purposes) and 2008. The numbers and change rates (trends) indicate that different treatment patterns and organizational differences existed before DRGs were in use across Europe, and continue to exist.

All countries (except the United Kingdom) reduced to a different extent the amount of acute care hospitals and beds between the mid-1990s and 2008. However, the number of acute care hospitals and beds per capita differs by a factor of between 5 and 3 across the 12 countries for the year 2008, only slightly down from the sixfold and threefold differences seen in 1995. In terms of the trend in acute care hospital admissions, the picture is less clear: France and the United Kingdom show reduction rates between 1995 and 2008 of 18.1 per cent and 42.5 per cent, respectively, while the Nordic countries (Estonia, Finland and Sweden) and Ireland only slightly reduced the number of acute care admissions (from 2.6 per cent in Estonia up to 7.2 per cent in Ireland). In contrast, in Austria and the Netherlands the number of admissions to acute care hospitals increased by 22 per cent and 15 per cent, respectively.

The average length of stay (ALOS) in acute care hospitals decreased more (Estonia: 45 per cent) or less (France: 2 per cent) in each country except Sweden. However, as in 1995, in 2008 the ALOS still differed by up to a factor of 2 between countries (for example, Germany versus Finland). Unlike Estonia, Germany and the Netherlands, four countries (Austria, France, Spain and the United Kingdom) were able to increase the bed occupancy rates during 1995 and 2008. Nevertheless, in 2008 the bed occupancy rates varied by a factor of 1.6 between Ireland (89 per cent) and the Netherlands (56 per cent), a larger variation than in 1995.

In addition, comparing the inpatient expenditure as a share of the total health expenditure (which decreased in each country) – as a proxy for the relative importance of the hospital sector – shows that countries rely on different strategies to treat the same patients in different settings (namely, inpatient versus outpatient). This also becomes evident when comparing the number of hospital-based physicians across countries in 2008. Compared to Finland, only half as many physicians work in Dutch hospitals. Despite the fact that international comparisons are always accompanied by inconsistencies in the definition of variables (for example, acute care hospital beds were defined slightly differently across European countries), it becomes apparent that the range of services delivered in acute care hospitals is somehow different from one country to another.

Table 2.3 Key figures of the European acute care landscape in 1995 and 2008

Country	Austria			Estonia			Finland			France			Germany			Ireland			Factor minimum–maximum 2008
Data years	1995	2008	Change rate	1995	2008	Change rate	1995	2008	Change rate	1995	2008	Change rate	1995	2008	Change rate	1995	2008	Change rate	
Acute care hospitals per 100 000	1.8	1.6	–12.8	5.1	2.8	–45.7	n.a.	n.a.	n.a.	3.8[d]	*3.2*	–16.8	2.6	2.2	–14.9	1.7	1.2	–29.3	*5.0*
Acute care hospital beds per 1 000	6.5	5.6	–13.2	6.6	3.9	–41.9	3.0	*1.9*	–36.2	4.9[a]	3.6	–27.1	6.9	*5.7*	–18.2	3.1	2.7[j]	–13.1	*3.0*
Acute care hospital admissions per 100	21.9	*26.7*	22.0	17.2	16.8	–2.6	19.9	19.0	–4.7	20.3	16.7	–18.1	19.2	20.7	8.0	14.6	13.6	–7.2	*2.4*
ALOS, acute care hospitals only	9.7	6.8	–29.9	10.5	5.8	–45.2	5.4	*3.9*	–27.8	5.9	5.8	–2.2	10.8	*7.6*	–29.6	6.6	6.2	–5.8	*1.9*
Bed occupancy rate in %, acute care hospitals only	77.0	80.4	4.4	74.9	69.7	–7.0	74.0	n.a.	n.a.	75.3	76.4	1.5	81.8	76.2	–6.8	82.5	*88.9*	7.8	*1.6*
Total inpatient expenditure as % of total health expenditure	40.4	*40.0*	–1.0	35.7[c]	33.0	–7.6	42.1	35.0	–16.9	40.9	37.3	–8.8	36.4	34.1	–6.3	n.a.	n.a.	n.a.	*1.9*
Physicians per 1 000	3.5	*4.6*	32.4	3.2	3.3	4.9	2.2	2.7	24.1	3.3	3.4	4.5	3.1	3.6	16.1	2.1	3.1	48.2	*2.1*
% of physicians working in hospitals	56.2	55.1	–1.9	n.a.	67.1	n.a.	85.1	*81.2*[j]	–4.6	47.1	54.1	14.9	48.2	51.1	6.0	53.2	47.1	–11.4	*2.1*

Continued overleaf

Table 2.3 *Continued*

Country	Netherlands			Poland			Portugal			Spain			Sweden			United Kingdom			Factor minimum–maximum 2008
Data years	1995	2008	Change rate	1995	2008	Change rate	1995	2008	Change rate	1995	2008	Change rate	1995	2008	Change rate	1995	2008	Change rate	
Acute care hospitals per 100 000	0.8	*0.6*	–23.2	2.2[g]	2.0	–6.9	1.4	1.3	–7.1	1.5	1.2	–17.6	1.1	0.9[f]	–21.6	n.a.	n.a.	n.a.	*5.0*
Acute care hospital beds per 1 000	3.5	2.9	–19.2	5.8	4.4	–23.4	3.2	2.8	–13.6	3.0	2.5	–18.0	3.0	2.2[h]	–28.2	2.3	2.7	19.2	*3.0*
Acute care hospital admissions per 100	9.6	*11.1*	15.4	n.a.	n.a.	n.a.	11.1	11.2[j]	0.9	10.7	11.4	6.7	16.3	15.2[j]	–6.6	21.2	12.2	–42.5	*2.4*
ALOS, acute care hospitals only	9.9	5.9	–40.4	n.a.	n.a.	n.a.	7.9	6.8[j]	–13.9	8.2	6.5	–20.7	5.2	6.0[j]	15.4	8.5[d]	7.4	–12.8	*1.9*
Bed occupancy rate in %, acute care hospitals only	73.3	*55.7*	–24.0	n.a.	n.a.	n.a.	72.6	72.6[j]	0.0	76.4	77.7	1.7	75.9	n.a.	n.a.	82.3[d]	84.8	3.1	*1.6*
Total inpatient expenditure as % of total health expenditure	49.1	39.6[e]	–19.3	n.a.	32.0	n.a.	33.9	*20.8*[i]	–38.6	31.0	28.2	–9.0	54.7	29.6[j]	–45.9	n.a.	n.a.	n.a.	*1.9*
Physicians per 1 000	2.9[b]	3.7[j]	26.1	2.3	*2.2*	–6.7	2.9	3.7	25.2	2.7	3.5	30.1	2.9	3.6[i]	24.0	1.8	2.6	46.4	*2.1*
% of physicians working in hospitals	n.a.	*38.1*[j]	n.a.	n.a.	52.1	n.a.	60.2	54.1	–10.1	53.1	61.1	15.1	n.a.	n.a.	n.a.	n.a.	n.a.	n.a.	*2.1*

Key: [a]1993; [b]1997; [c]1999; [d]2000; [e]2001; [f]2003; [g]2004; [h]2005; [i]2006; [j]2007 due to lack of available data for 1995/2008.

Source: WHO Regional Office for Europe, 2011.

Notes: n/a not available; minimum and maximum values are prepared in italics.

Table 2.4 Share of ownership types across countries (% of acute care beds), 2008

Country	*Publically owned hospitals (%)*	*Non-profit-making, privately owned hospitals (%)*	*Profit-making, privately owned hospitals (%)*
Austria	73	19	9
Finland	89	0	11
France	66	9	25
Germany	49	36	15
Ireland	88	0	12
Netherlands	0	100	0
Poland	95	0	5
Portugal	86	7	8
Spain	74	17	9
Sweden	98	0	2
United Kingdom	96	4	0

Source: Paris et al., 2010.

Note: In Estonia all hospitals operate under private law and most of them are publically owned (see Chapter 17 of this volume).

The ownership structure of hospitals also varies widely. In some countries (such as France and Germany) private profit-making hospitals play an important role in the health system, but in many others, most hospital beds are operated under public or private non-profit-making ownership (Table 2.4).

In summary, DRGs were introduced in countries that were characterized by large structural differences in their hospital sectors. Furthermore, despite the introduction of DRG-based hospital payment systems, structural differences persist. Apparently, DRG-based hospital payment systems can be flexibly implemented in different settings and do not prescribe any clear development path. Therefore, the analysis of how these systems have been implemented in different health care contexts – as well as their impact on the efficiency and quality of service delivery – is the main aim of this book.

2.5 The book and its structure

Comparative information from different European countries regarding the specific characteristics of their DRG systems and how these characteristics contribute to achieving the aims of transparency, efficiency and quality in hospitals is largely absent. This book aims to contribute towards filling this gap.

This book is structured in two parts: **Part One** (up to and including Chapter 10) deals with the essential building blocks of DRG-based hospital payment systems and discusses the impact of these systems on quality and efficiency of service delivery, and on adoption and use of technological innovation. The aim of this first part is to highlight similarities and differences between different countries' systems, and to provide an overview of the key issues that need to be considered when developing and optimizing DRG-based hospital payment systems. At the same time, the discussion of these issues paves the way for considering the potential for harmonization of DRG systems and of DRG-based hospital payment across Europe. The 'building blocks' of DRG systems and of DRG-based hospital payment systems are described in detail in Chapter 3. The differences in DRG systems and similar patient classification systems (PCSs) across Europe are analysed in Chapter 4. The main challenges and differences in cost-accounting systems used in European countries are highlighted in Chapter 5. The intended and unintended consequences of using DRGs for hospital payment (rather than just patient classification) are discussed in Chapter 6. The available evidence of the impact of DRGs on the efficiency and quality of hospital care is discussed in chapters 7 and 8. Chapter 9 describes how the 12 countries included in this book attempt to overcome the potential problems relating to technological innovation that are associated with DRG-based hospital payment systems. Finally, the first part of the book closes in Chapter 10 with a summary of the main findings, and provides policy recommendations for further DRG developments.

Part Two of the book – that is, chapters 11 to 23 – provides clearly structured and detailed information about the most important DRG system characteristics in each of the 12 countries that participated in the EuroDRG project (Austria, England, Estonia, Finland, France, Germany, Ireland, Poland, Portugal, Spain, Sweden and the Netherlands). Each country has an interesting story to tell, which is contextualized within the prevailing health system. Part Two aims to overcome some of the difficulties that have existed for both researchers and policy-makers aiming to compare European DRG systems: information used to be mostly available only in national languages, and national descriptions of DRG systems often used country-specific terminology that complicated the task of making cross-border comparisons. Each country-specific chapter starts with a background section that provides an overview to hospital services and to the role of DRGs in the country (section 1). The developments and updates of the DRG systems are outlined in the second section. The current DRG system(s), which is (are) used to group patients into clinically meaningful and cost-homogeneous groups, is (are) described in section 3 of each country-specific chapter, while section 4 in each case deals with the countries' cost-accounting systems that are essential for determining DRG-based payments rates. The DRG-based hospital payment system of the country in question is described in section 5, and the countries' methods to integrate new and innovative treatments into their existing DRG-based payment systems are presented in section 6. Finally, each chapter closes with an assessment of the country's DRG system (section 7) and a summary of the outlook, in terms of future developments and reform (section 8).

2.6 References

Barnum, H., Kutzin, J., Saxenian, H. (1995). Incentives and provider payment methods. *International Journal of Health Planning and Management*, 10(1):23–45.

Busse, R., Schreyögg, J., Smith, P.C. (2006). Hospital case payment systems in Europe. *Health Care Management Science*, 9(3):211–13.

Fetter, J., Shin, Y., Freeman, J.L., Averill, R.F., Thompson, J.D. (1980). Casemix definition by diagnosis-related groups. *Medical Care*, 18(Suppl. 2):1–53.

Langenbrunner, J.C., Wiley, M. (2002). Hospital payment mechanisms: theory and practice in transition countries, in M. McKee, J.H. Healy, eds. *Hospitals in a Changing Europe*. Buckingham: Open University Press.

McKee, M., Healy, J.H. (2002). *Hospitals in a Changing Europe*. Buckingham: Open University Press.

Miller, T.S. (1997). *The Birth of the Hospital in the Byzantine Empire*. Baltimore, MD: Johns Hopkins University Press.

Paris, V., Devaux, M., Wei, L. (2010). *Health Systems Institutional Characteristics: A Survey of 29 OECD Countries*. Paris: Organisation for Economic Co-operation and Development (OECD Health Working Papers No. 50).

Schreyögg, J., Stargardt, T., Tiemann, O., Busse, R. (2006). Methods to determine reimbursement rates for diagnosis related groups (DRG): a comparison of nine European countries. *Health Care Management Science*, 9(3):215–23.

Shleifer, A. (1985). A theory of yard stick competition. *RAND Journal of Economics*, 16(3):319–27.

Street, A., Vitikainen, K., Bjorvatn, A., Hvenegaard, A. (2007). *Introducing Activity-Based Financing: A Review of Experience in Australia, Denmark, Norway and Sweden*. York: University of York Centre for Health Economics (CHE Research Paper 30).

WHO (2000). *The World Health Report 2000 – Health Systems: Improving Performance*. Geneva: World Health Organization.

WHO Regional Office for Europe (2011). *European Health for All Database* (HFA-DB) [online database]. Copenhagen: WHO Regional Office for Europe (http://data.euro.who.int/hfadb/, accessed 20 July 2011) (July 2011 update).

chapter three

Understanding DRGs and DRG-based hospital payment in Europe

Wilm Quentin, Alexander Geissler, David Scheller-Kreinsen and Reinhard Busse

3.1 Introduction

Despite the fact that diagnosis-related groups (DRGs) have been adopted in an increasingly large number of countries around the world (Kimberly et al., 2008), understanding of DRG systems and DRG-based hospital payment systems remains surprisingly limited. On the one hand, there is no good overview of alternative options for designing these systems because systematic comparisons of the specific system characteristics in different countries are extremely rare (France, 2003). Consequently, there is no agreed consensus on how best to design DRG systems and DRG-based hospital payment systems, because the differences between countries' systems remain poorly understood. On the other hand, despite the existence of numerous studies concerning the effects of DRG-based hospital payment systems on hospital efficiency, quality and technological innovation, these effects remain relatively unclear (Brügger, 2010) – also because the specific design features in different countries are rarely taken into account.

Nevertheless, a thorough understanding of international experiences with DRG systems and DRG-based hospital payment systems could inform countries when developing and optimizing their national systems. In addition, in a context of growing patient mobility facilitated by the European Union (EU) *Directive on the Application of Patients' Rights in Cross-Border Healthcare* (European Parliament and Council, 2011), an increasingly important issue relates to whether there is scope for harmonization of DRG systems within Europe. This is because if harmonization is not possible, it will remain difficult (or at least not transparent) to pay hospitals in one EU Member State for care provided to patients from another EU Member State. Furthermore, cross-border comparisons of hospital prices and performance – which are increasingly being conducted in attempts to improve the understanding of differences in terms of efficiency and costs (see, for example, Chapko et al., 2009 or Busse et al., 2008) – will continue to be complicated by the lack of a common basis for comparison.

The first part of this book aims to contribute to a better understanding of DRG systems and of how they are used for hospital payment in Europe by (1) systematically comparing DRG systems and DRG-based hospital payment systems across 12 European countries; and (2) by providing an overview of the effects of these systems on hospital efficiency, quality, and on the adoption and use of technological innovation. This chapter develops a framework for comparing DRG systems and DRG-based hospital payment systems in Europe. It presents the main building blocks of DRG-based hospital payment systems and introduces some of the assumed effects of these systems on hospital efficiency, quality and on the adoption and use of technological innovation. It highlights certain key concepts and raises a number of questions that should be considered when developing or optimizing DRG systems and DRG-based hospital payment systems. The six chapters that follow (chapters 4 to 9) develop these points in more detail. The scope for harmonization of DRG systems – or at least for more cooperation – in Europe is a cross-cutting issue that is discussed in several of the chapters. Chapter 10 picks up the questions raised here and draws conclusions from all the chapters in Part One.

3.2 How to understand DRG systems and DRG-based hospital payment systems in Europe

Trying to understand DRG systems and how they are used for hospital payment across countries requires a common framework. Without one, it is easy to get lost in the specificities of each country's system and confused by the diversity of terms that are used for describing similar things in different countries. Figure 3.1 presents a framework that we developed to guide the reader through the chapters of the first part of this book. All countries included in this book have a DRG system (Chapter 4), a system to collect cost information from hospitals (Chapter 5), and they use DRGs for hospital payment (Chapter 6). These building blocks are presented in more detail in subsection 3.2.1. Understanding each of these building blocks and how they interact is essential for understanding the effects of DRG-based hospital payment systems on efficiency (Chapter 7), quality (Chapter 8) and innovation (Chapter 9), which are introduced in subsection 3.2.2. The effect of DRG systems on transparency of service provision is not discussed in a separate chapter. However, increased transparency resulting from the use of DRGs is thought to contribute to both improved efficiency and quality of service provision.

3.2.1 Understanding the building blocks

DRG systems (Chapter 4)

A DRG system is a patient classification system (PCS) that has four main characteristics: (1) *routinely collected patient discharge data* (mostly concerning

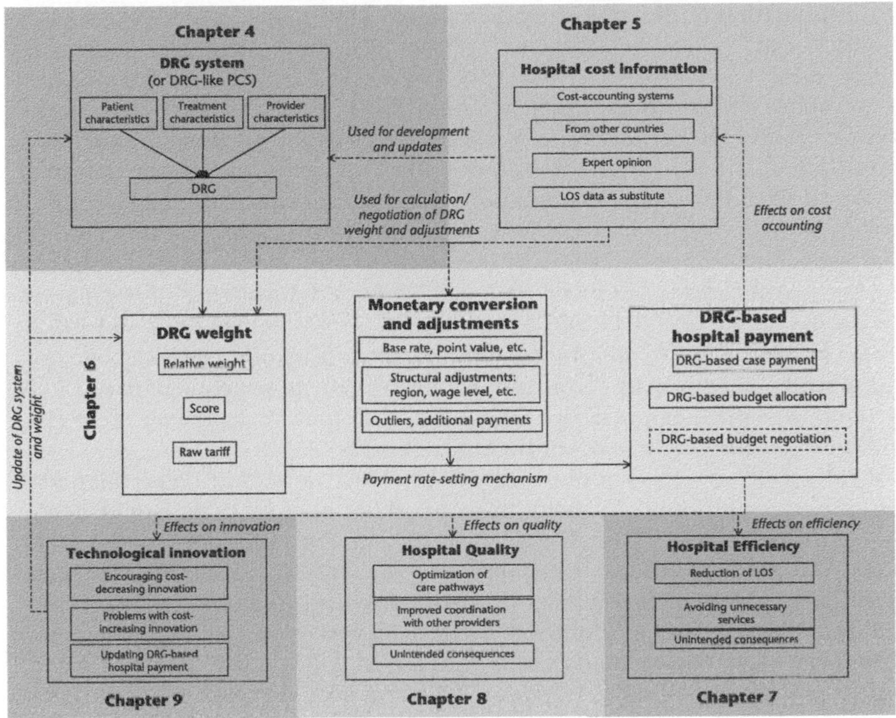

Figure 3.1 Framework for navigating through the book

patient, treatment and provider characteristics) are used to classify patients into (2) a *manageable number* of groups (that is, DRGs), which are intended to be (3) *clinically meaningful* and (4) *economically homogeneous*. DRGs summarize the confusingly large number of different (individual) patients treated by hospitals into a manageable number of clinically meaningful and economically homogeneous groups, thus providing a concise measure of hospital activity or, in other words, they define hospital products. Consequently, they facilitate comparisons of hospital costs, quality and efficiency, and contribute to increased transparency in hospitals.

When introducing DRG systems, two alternative options exist: DRG systems can either be adopted from abroad or they can be developed from scratch. Many countries originally adopted DRG systems from abroad and later used these systems as the basis for further developing their own systems (Chapter 4). Consequently, eight countries included in this book (Estonia, Finland, France, Germany, Ireland, Portugal, Spain and Sweden) use DRG systems that are at least remotely related to the Health Care Financing Administration (HCFA-) DRG system originally introduced in the United States in the early 1980s; two of them (Germany and Ireland) via the Australian Refined (AR-)DRG system. Austria, England, and the Netherlands have developed their own systems from scratch, while Poland used the English version to develop its own system. Although these self-developed systems do not define DRGs in the strictest sense of the word (that is, groups are not necessarily diagnosis-related), this book uses the term DRG system for all PCSs that share the above-mentioned four main characteristics.

The actual classification of patients into DRGs is almost always performed by computerized grouping software. Since diagnoses and procedures are the most important classification variables, an essential requirement for the operation of DRG systems is that diagnoses and procedures are coded in hospitals according to standardized classification systems, such as modifications of the International Classification of Diseases 10th revision (ICD-10) for diagnoses and country-specific classifications of procedures, such as the English Office of Population Censuses and Surveys (OPCS) Classification of Surgical Operations and Procedures. However, how this information is used for defining DRGs depends on the specific DRG grouping algorithm. While the general structure of many DRG systems is relatively similar (see Chapter 4), the precise definition of specific DRGs can be quite diverse (Quentin et al., in press).

Ideally, DRG systems should consider the most important determinants of resource consumption as classification variables; that is, they should define DRGs on the basis of those diagnoses, procedures or other classification variables that make treating one patient with (or without) a specific procedure more expensive than treating another patient with (or without) another procedure. Otherwise, if DRG systems fail to define economically homogeneous groups, performance comparisons on the basis of DRGs do not adequately control for differences of patients within DRGs. Further, DRG-based hospital payment may be inappropriate for a considerable number of patients – it can be either too high or too low. However, because hospitals may try to manipulate the classification of patients into DRGs by changing their coding or practice patterns (see Chapter 6), the selection of classification variables also needs to consider whether those variables are easy to manipulate or not.

In order to ensure that DRGs remain clinically meaningful and economically homogeneous, even when technological innovation or other factors lead to changes in practice patterns and costs, DRG systems need to be updated at regular intervals (see Chapter 9). Most countries use some kind of hospital cost information (see Chapter 5) to develop and update DRG systems, as illustrated by an arrow in Figure 3.1.

Furthermore, different alternatives exist in terms of the unit for which patients are classified into DRGs. For example, some DRG systems classify patients into one DRG per hospital admission; other systems classify patients into DRGs for every stay in a hospital department (see the Finnish system, described in Chapter 18); and still other systems classify patients into DRGs for a specific treatment related to a specific diagnosis, which may include several inpatient stays and outpatient visits (see Chapter 23 on the Netherlands). Finally, it is important to consider which patient groups are to be included in DRG systems. For some groups of patients, it may be more difficult to define clinically meaningful and economically homogeneous groups of patients. For example, psychiatric patients were originally excluded from DRG systems in most countries because it appeared to be more difficult to define economically homogeneous groups on the basis of diagnoses and procedures for this group of patients (Lave, 2003; McCrone & Phelan, 1994). However, several countries are now also in the process of developing or introducing DRGs for psychiatric patients (see Chapters 4 and 10).

Hospital cost information (Chapter 5)

As illustrated in Figure 3.1, hospital cost information is used to (1) define DRGs and (2) determine (adjust) payment rates. The availability of high-quality hospital cost information is essential for developing and updating DRG systems and for ensuring fair DRG-based hospital payment systems. If hospital cost information does not allow differences to be indentified between costs of individual patients, it is impossible to use a data-driven approach to develop economically homogeneous DRGs. In addition, if hospital cost information is imprecise, calculated weights for certain DRGs could be falsely estimated to be higher or lower than they really are and, consequently, hospitals will be over- or underpaid for specific DRGs. Therefore, the fairness of DRG-based hospital payment systems and the ability of these systems to encourage efficiency are to a large extent determined by the quality of the hospital cost information used to develop these systems and to calculate DRG weights.

Unfortunately, the availability of standardized and (therefore) comparable high-quality cost information is limited in many European countries. This is one of the reasons why some countries without high-quality patient-level cost information have imported DRG systems including weights from abroad (for example, Ireland, Portugal and Spain) and have only adjusted the imported DRG weights to the local cost context by using more aggregated cost-accounting figures, for example at the department level. Other countries have developed their own DRG systems on the basis of length-of-stay data as a proxy for costs, which makes it difficult to ensure that groups are economically homogeneous. Furthermore, hospital charges from fee-for-service payment systems (that in some countries existed prior to the introduction of DRGs), individual costing studies or even expert opinions have occasionally been used as a proxy for costs when calculating weights of DRGs (for example, in Estonia and Poland).

However, in many European countries, the introduction of DRGs has also encouraged changes in hospitals' cost-accounting systems. Following the introduction of DRGs for classification purposes – and even more so following the introduction of DRG-based hospital payment systems – standardized (sometimes mandatory) cost-accounting systems have been introduced in at least a sample of hospitals in most countries. Countries have often introduced national cost-accounting handbooks, which provide detailed rules and definitions concerning the types of cost centres and cost categories to be used, and which specify the allocation methods and allocation bases for distribution of costs to final cost centres and patients.

Yet, significant differences exist between countries in terms of (1) the number of hospitals that participate (voluntarily or not) in collecting standardized cost-accounting information; and (2) the level of detail required according to the national cost-accounting standards. In fact, there may be a trade-off between collecting detailed patient-level data using a bottom-up micro-costing approach (see Chapter 5) and the goal of having a large representative sample of hospitals contributing to a national cost database (Schreyögg et al., 2006). This is because a more complex cost-accounting system increases the costliness of the data-collection exercise, which may become prohibitively costly if data collection is extended to a large number of hospitals. In addition, as the importance of hospital cost information has increased, most countries have introduced regular data checks, with the aim of assuring the validity of reported hospital cost information.

While changes to cost-accounting systems resulting from regulations have been important, the introduction of DRG-based hospital payment systems has also increased the intrinsic motivation for hospital managers to introduce or optimize existing cost-accounting systems (see Berki, 1985). Without high-quality cost-accounting systems, hospital managers do not know whether hospitals are able to 'produce' DRGs at costs that are below the payment rate. Consequently, they do not know whether hospitals are making a profit or are incurring a loss by providing these DRGs. In addition, in order to be able to identify the cost drivers of hospital products (that is, of DRGs) and to manage the production of DRGs, hospital managers require detailed information about the costs of different inputs in the production process – an element that can be provided by high-quality cost-accounting systems. In summary, as illustrated by the arrows in Figure 3.1, hospital cost information is a necessary input for effective DRG-based hospital payment systems, and (ideally) improved hospital cost information is also an outcome of the changed incentive structure following the introduction of DRG-based hospital payment.

DRG-based hospital payment (Chapter 6)

While the use of DRGs for reporting purposes and for managing hospitals is important, most countries included in this book use DRGs primarily as the basis for hospital payment. In general, two main models of DRG-based hospital payment system can be distinguished. On the one hand, in DRG-based case payment systems, each discharged patient is grouped into the applicable DRG, and hospitals receive a payment per case that is determined by the weight of that DRG (after monetary conversion and relevant adjustments). On the other hand, in DRG-based budget allocation systems, the available regional or national hospital budget is distributed to individual hospitals on the basis of the number and type of DRGs that these hospitals produced during one of the previous years or that they are expected to produce in the next year. The casemix (that is, the sum of the weights of all DRGs produced by a hospital) and the casemix index (CMI) (that is, the casemix divided by the number of discharges) are usually the determining factors for distributing the budget. However, adjustments for structural indicators and for certain high-cost cases are also considered, and an implicit monetary conversion rate exists that can be used to estimate the implicit revenue contribution to the hospital budget of one patient in a specific DRG. In addition, some countries with DRG-based case payment systems, such as Germany or Finland, use DRGs to negotiate global hospital budgets, which limit (to a certain extent) the total amount of money that hospitals can earn from DRG-based case payments.

There are three main incentives for hospitals resulting from DRG-based hospital payment systems: (1) to reduce costs per treated patient, (2) to increase revenues per patient, and (3) to increase the number of patients. These incentives can have both intended and unintended consequences on efficiency, quality and technological innovation. However, the strength of these incentives is determined by the type of DRG-based hospital payment systems (case-based payment versus budget allocation), by the proportion of total hospital revenues related to DRG-based hospital payment, and by the degree to which DRG weights and monetary conversion rates are adjusted to reflect hospital-specific cost structures.

In all DRG-based hospital payment systems (except for that operating in the Netherlands), the actual payment rate is not the same as the DRG weight. As illustrated in Figure 3.1, three main approaches for expressing DRG weights exist in the countries included in this book: (1) relative weights, (2) raw tariffs, and (3) scores. Each of these approaches corresponds to a specific monetary conversion method. In countries using a relative weight approach, the relative weight provides a measure that relates the average costs of treating patients within one DRG to the average costs of treating all patients included in the DRG system in the country (see Chapter 6). Table 3.1 provides an example of how DRG weights for a hypothetical DRG determine hospital payment within the framework of the different approaches for expressing DRG weights. The idea of all three approaches is the same: the DRG weight (almost always) provides a measure of the average or expected costs of treating patients falling into that DRG. The actual hospital payment rate is calculated by multiplying the DRG weight with a country-specific monetary conversion/adjustment rate, which often takes into account structural, regional or hospital-specific differences in the costs of service provision.

Monetary conversion/adjustment rates may differ between types of hospitals, for example, by degree of specialization or geographic location, according to the country-specific choices for adjusting the DRG-based payment rate. Sometimes, monetary conversion rates are hospital specific, and are calculated in a way that shelters hospitals from budget cuts, which means that the incentives of DRG-based hospital payment are much reduced (see, for example, the Finnish system described in Chapter 18). In addition, DRG weights are generally adjusted in order to account for certain high-cost patients that stay in hospital much longer than the average case, or that receive additional services, which are not adequately reimbursed on the basis of the DRG-based payment system. Furthermore, most countries operating DRG-based case payment systems prevent an excessive increase in costs by applying macro-level price/volume

Table 3.1 DRG weights and monetary conversion example

	Hypothetical example				
DRG weight approach	*DRG weight (unit)*		*Monetary conversion/ adjustment (unit)*		*Hospital payment rate (€)*
Relative weight	1.95	×	2 000 €	=	3 900 €
Raw tariff	3 000 €	×	1.3	=	3 900 €
Score	130 points	×	30 €	=	3 900 €

control measures (such as global hospital budgets, sectoral budgets, or price reductions).

3.2.2 Understanding the effects of DRG-based hospital payment

Effects on hospital efficiency (Chapter 7)

In many countries, one of the most important purposes of introducing DRG-based hospital payment systems was to increase efficiency of hospital care. Because DRG-based hospital payment provides incentives to increase activity and to minimize costs, there is reason to believe that these systems contribute to improved efficiency. However, 'efficiency' is a widely used term that can have various meanings. Economists generally differentiate between technical efficiency – that is, maximizing outputs for a given level of inputs, or minimizing inputs for a given level of outputs; allocative efficiency – namely, ensuring the appropriate mix of inputs and outputs to maximize utility; and cost-efficiency – that is, minimizing costs for a given level of output.

DRG-based hospital payment systems are often discussed as representing a form of 'yard stick competition' (Shleifer, 1985). The idea of yard stick competition is that prices for a given product (for example, a specific DRG) are set at the level of average costs of other firms producing the same product (that is, the same DRG). With DRG-based hospital payment, if hospitals produce DRGs at costs that are below the average costs of other hospitals, they benefit directly by retaining the generated financial surplus; if they underperform, they generate deficits and, ultimately, risk bankruptcy. All hospitals, including the most efficient ones, are incentivized to continually reduce costs. In practice, numerous options exist for hospitals to increase (technical and cost-) efficiency: care pathways can be optimized to reduce the length of stay; duplicate and unnecessary tests can be avoided; and costly treatments can be replaced by similarly effective but less costly alternatives.

However, unfortunately, if the incentives for cost reduction are too strong, and if regulatory authorities do not have sufficient capacity to monitor adequately the quality of care, DRG-based hospital payment can lead to unintended consequences (see Chapter 6). For example, hospitals could discharge patients inappropriately early, and service intensity could be reduced to a level at which necessary services are withheld from patients – thus leading to cost reductions but not to improvements in efficiency. Consequently, the effects of DRG-based hospital payment systems on efficiency have been highly controversial.

Although improving hospital efficiency is generally a key motivation for introducing DRG-based hospital payment, relatively few studies have explicitly identified and quantified its impact using established methods, such as data envelopment analyses (DEAs) or stochastic frontier analyses (Jacobs et al., 2006). Rather, most research has concentrated on indicators of efficiency – such as activity, length of stay and costs – which are more easily measured, but by definition provide only a partial picture. Given the challenges inherent in undertaking cross-country efficiency comparisons, most available studies have adopted a longitudinal perspective, comparing hospital efficiency before and after the introduction of DRG-based hospital payment. Chapter 7 reviews both types of studies, efficiency analyses and studies of indicators of efficiency.

When interpreting the results of these (longitudinal) studies, it is important to consider the difficulties that often arise in clearly separating the effect of the introduction of DRG-based hospital payment from other concurrent influences, such as changes in medical technology or new legislation. Furthermore, in longitudinal studies, the measured effect of introducing DRG-based hospital payment depends on the hospital payment system that existed prior to the introduction of the system. In the United States, where DRG-based hospital payment replaced a fee-for-service system, the DRG-based hospital payment system provided strong incentives to reduce costs (Berki, 1985). In contrast, in Europe, where DRG-based hospital payment systems often replaced global hospital budgets, the incentives of DRG-based hospital payment would be expected to lead to an increase in hospital activity, which could also result in increased costs.

Effects on hospital quality (Chapter 8)

The effect of DRGs on hospital quality is not straightforward (Davis & Rhodes, 1988; Farrar et al., 2009). On the one hand, because DRGs provide a concise and meaningful measure of hospital activity and thus facilitate monitoring and comparisons of hospital quality, they could contribute to better quality of care. In addition, cost-reduction incentives of DRG-based hospital payment systems could lead to increased efforts to improve quality, if quality contributes to reduced costs. For example, improved coordination between hospitals, outpatient providers and long-term care facilities would reduce costs but could also contribute to better quality of care. However, on the other hand, and this has been a reason for continuous concern (Rogers et al., 1990), hospitals may be tempted to reduce costs by reducing quality, if DRG-based payments do not depend on quality. For example, because DRGs do not specify which services must be provided when treating a specific patient, hospitals can 'skimp' on quality by avoiding certain diagnostic tests, disregarding hygiene standards, or by lowering staffing ratios per bed.

Assessments of the effect of DRGs on hospital quality are often complicated by the fact that the notion of quality is rather diffuse (Legido-Quigley et al., 2008). This book defines quality as any aspect of hospital services that benefits patients during the process of treatment or improves health outcome after treatment (Chalkley & Malcomson, 1998). To measure 'quality', a common framework developed by Donabedian (1966) differentiates between structural, process and outcome indicators of quality. Structural indicators, such as qualification(s) of medical staff or available equipment are easy to measure and are relevant to quality if they represent conditions for the delivery of a given quality of health care. Process indicators can also be measured relatively easily, but should be based on the available evidence of what constitutes 'good' quality of care in the treatment of a specific patient and in a specific situation (Smith et al., 2010). Thus, they usually provide clear pathways for action. Outcome indicators assess what is most meaningful for policy-makers and patients (for example, mortality), but it is not always possible to determine the contribution of health care to health outcomes because outcomes are also influenced by (unobserved) patient-level factors. Therefore, careful risk adjustment is necessary if outcome indicators are to be used.

The effect of DRGs and of DRG-based hospital payment systems on the quality of hospital care has been assessed in numerous studies from the United States and several studies from Europe, using a range of indicators. Again, when interpreting the results, which are presented in Chapter 8, it is important to consider that the effects of the introduction of DRGs and of DRG-based hospital payment on quality may be different depending on the hospital payment system previously in existence.

In theory, DRG-based hospital payment systems could be modified to explicitly consider quality of care. However, basic information on the quality of services provided is still lacking in most countries in which DRGs are used for hospital payment. Yet, the availability of information regarding the quality of services (in terms of structure, process or outcomes) is a prerequisite for any attempts to explicitly integrate financial incentives for quality into DRG-based hospital payment systems (see Chapter 8).

Effects on technological innovation (Chapter 9)

Since the introduction of DRG-based hospital payment systems, there have been concerns that these systems may not provide sufficient incentives to encourage the desired adoption and use of technological innovations in health care (OTA, 1983; MedPAC, 2003; Shih & Berliner, 2008). However, the effect of DRG-based hospital payment systems on any specific technological innovation depends on how the technological innovation influences total hospital costs (both capital and operating costs) per admission.

Technological innovations may increase or decrease capital costs, operating costs or both. DRG-based hospital payment systems encourage hospitals to invest in technological innovations that reduce total costs per patient and discourage hospitals from introducing technological innovations that lead to higher costs per patient. Yet, whether this effect of DRG-based hospital payment on technological innovation is socially desirable or not depends on whether the innovations in question really improve the quality of care. In cases in which technological innovation is more costly but does not improve quality of care, the effect of DRG-based hospital payment (namely, preventing hospitals from adopting these innovations) is in line with societal objectives. However, when technological innovations increase quality of care and are associated with higher costs, DRG-based hospital payment becomes problematic.

The problem is that hospitals are paid on the basis of cost information that was collected in hospitals in the past. Consequently, when technological innovations first enter the market, the higher costs of those innovations are not yet accounted for in current DRG weights. Only once hospitals have started using these technological innovations, and when data relating to the costs of using these innovations in routine practice have been collected, can DRG systems and DRG weights be updated to account for the change in practice patterns and costs. Therefore, the ability of DRG-based hospital payment systems to respond to technological innovation is determined by (1) the frequency of updates of DRG systems and of DRG weights, and (2) the time-lag to data used for these updates (see Chapter 9).

Furthermore, most countries included in this book have developed additional payment incentives to encourage the use of quality-increasing technological innovations that also increase costs, within the time period during which the DRG-based hospital payment system does not yet account for the innovation. Because the available evidence relating to the effects of DRGs on technological innovation is virtually non-existent, Chapter 9 is less focused on reviewing the limited available literature than on providing an overview regarding how European countries deal with technological innovation.

3.3 In summary: What do we want to understand?

This chapter provides a framework for understanding and comparing DRG systems and DRG-based hospital payment systems in Europe. It introduces the building blocks of DRG-based hospital payment systems and highlights their likely effects on efficiency, quality and technological innovation. The chapter also outlines some alternative options that exist when designing DRG-based hospital payment systems, indicating that the specific design features will influence the effects of those systems.

Table 3.2 summarizes key questions that are raised in this chapter and that are addressed within the chapters that follow (Part One of this book). The concluding chapter of Part One (Chapter 10) draws on the findings of chapters 4–9: (1) in order to make specific recommendations for policy-makers regarding how best to design DRG-based hospital payment systems given country-specific aims and objectives; and (2) to explore the potential for harmonization of DRG systems and DRG-based hospital payment systems across Europe.

Table 3.2 Key questions to be answered by this book

Chapter	*Key questions*
Chapter 4: DRG systems and similar patient classification systems in Europe	1. What are the advantages and disadvantages of importing DRG systems? 2. How are diagnoses and procedures coded? 3. Which classification variables can be used? 4. What should be the scope of included services? 5. How many groups are justified?
Chapter 5: DRGs and cost accounting: Which is driving which?	1. Why is cost accounting important? 2. How many hospitals should be included in the data sample? 3. What incentives exist for hospitals to calculate their costs? 4. What cost-accounting methods should be used? 5. Which cost categories should be included?

Continued overleaf

Table 3.2 *Continued*

Chapter	*Key questions*
Chapter 6: DRG-based hospital payment: Intended and unintended consequences	1. How can hospitals be paid using DRGs? 2. What are the incentives of DRG-based hospital payment? 3. What determines the strength of these incentives? 4. How can unintended consequences be avoided? 5. How can DRG-based hospital payment be adjusted?
Chapter 7: DRG-based hospital payment and efficiency: Theory, evidence and challenges	1. Why should DRG-based hospital payment improve efficiency of hospitals? 2. How has the effect of DRG-based hospital payment on efficiency been measured? 3. Does DRG-based hospital payment improve efficiency? 4. What challenges need to be overcome?
Chapter 8: DRGs and quality: For better or worse?	1. Why should DRGs and DRG-based hospital payment influence the quality of hospital care? 2. How has the effect of DRG-based hospital payment on quality been measured? 3. Does DRG-based hospital payment lead to better or worse quality of care? 4. How can DRG-based hospital payment be modified to improve quality of care?
Chapter 9: Technological innovation in DRG-based hospital payment systems across Europe	1. Why should DRG-based hospital payment influence the adoption of technological innovation? 2. How do countries in Europe encourage technological innovation? 3. How does technological innovation become incorporated into DRG-based hospital payment? 4. How could innovation management be improved in DRG-based hospital payment systems?

3.4 References

Berki, S.E. (1985). DRGs, incentives, hospitals, and physicians. *Health Affairs (Millwood)*, 4(4):70–6.

Brügger, U. (2010). *Impact of DRGs: Introducing a DRG Reimbursement System. A Literature Review*. Zurich: SGGP (Schriftenreihe der SGGP, Vol. 98).

Busse, R., Schreyögg, J., Smith, P.C. (2008). Variability in healthcare treatment costs amongst nine EU countries – results from the HealthBASKET project. *Health Economics*, 17(Suppl. 1):1–8.

Chalkley, M., Malcomson, J.M. (1998). Contracting for health services when patient demand does not reflect quality. *Journal of Health Economics*, 17(1):1–19.

Chapko, M.K., Liu, C., Perkins, M. et al. (2009). Equivalence of two healthcare costing methods: bottom-up and top-down. *Health Economics*, 18(10):1188–201.

Davis, C., Rhodes, D.J. (1988). The impact of DRGs on the cost and quality of health care in the United States. *Health Policy*, 9(2):117–31.

Donabedian, A. (1966). Evaluating the quality of medical care. *The Milbank Memorial Fund Quarterly*, 44(3)2:166–203.

European Parliament and Council (2011). *Directive 2011/24/EU on the Application of Patients' Rights in Cross-Border Healthcare*. Brussels: Official Journal of the European Union (L88/45–L88/65).

Farrar, S., Yi, D., Sutton, M. et al. (2009). Has payment by results affected the way that English hospitals provide care? Difference-in-differences analysis. *British Medical Journal*, 339:b3047.

France, F.H.R. (2003). Casemix use in 25 countries: a migration success but international comparisons failure. *International Journal of Medical Informatics*, 70(2–3):215–19.

Jacobs, R., Smith, P., Street, A. (2006). *Measuring Efficiency in Health Care*. Cambridge: Cambridge University Press.

Kimberly, J.R., de Pouvourville, G., D'Aunno, T., eds (2008). *The Globalization of Managerial Innovation in Health Care*. Cambridge: Cambridge University Press.

Lave, J.R. (2003). Developing a Medicare prospective payment system for inpatient psychiatric care. *Health Affairs (Millwood)*, 22(5):97–109.

Legido-Quigley, H., McKee, M., Nolte, E., Glinos, I.A. (2008). *Assuring the Quality of Health Care in the European Union: A Case for Action*. Copenhagen: WHO Regional Office for Europe on behalf of the European Observatory on Health Systems and Policies.

McCrone, P., Phelan, M. (1994). Diagnosis and length of psychiatric inpatient stay. *Psychological Medicine*, 24(4):1025–30.

MedPAC (2003). Payment for new technologies in Medicare's prospective payment system, in MedPAC. *Report to the Congress: Medicare Payment Policy*. Washington, DC: Medicare Payment Advisory Commission.

OTA (1983). *Diagnosis-Related Groups (DRGs) and the Medicare Program: Implications for Medical Technology – A Technical Memorandum*. Washington, DC: Office of Technology Assessment.

Quentin, W., Scheller-Kreinsen, D., Geissler, A., Busse, R. (in press). Appendectomy and diagnosis-related groups (DRGs): patient classification and hospital reimbursement in 11 European countries. *Langenbeck's Archives of Surgery* (in press).

Rogers, W.H., Draper, D., Kahn, K.L. et al. (1990). Quality of care before and after implementation of the DRG-based prospective payment system. A summary of effects. *Journal of the American Medical Association*, 264(15):1989–94.

Schreyögg, J., Stargardt, T., Tiemann, O., Busse, R. (2006). Methods to determine reimbursement rates for diagnosis related groups (DRG): a comparison of nine European countries. *Health Care Management Science*, 9(3):215–23.

Shih, C., Berliner, E. (2008). Diffusion of new technology and payment policies: coronary stents. *Health Affairs (Millwood)*, 27(6):1566–76.

Shleifer, A (1985). A theory of yard stick competition. *The RAND Journal of Economics*, 16(3):319–27.

Smith, P.C., Mossialos, E., Papanicolas, I., Leatherman, S. (2010). Conclusions, in P.C. Smith, ed. *Performance Measurement for Health System Improvement*. Cambridge: Cambridge University Press.

chapter four

DRG systems and similar patient classification systems in Europe

Conrad Kobel, Josselin Thuilliez, Martine Bellanger and Karl-Peter Pfeiffer

4.1 Introduction

The idea of any patient classification system(s) (PCSs) is to combine the confusingly large number of different patients, all appearing to be unique, into a limited number of groups with roughly similar features. Diagnosis-related group (DRG) systems are PCSs that have four main characteristics: (1) *routinely collected data* on patient discharge are used to classify patients into (2) a *manageable number* of groups that are (3) *clinically meaningful* and (4) *economically homogeneous*. In addition, all DRG systems are at least remotely related to the original DRG system that was developed by a group of researchers including Robert Fetter at Yale University during the 1970s (Fetter et al., 1980; Fetter, 1999).

Today, DRG systems are the most widely employed PCS in Europe. They are used in eight countries (Estonia, Finland, France, Germany, Ireland, Portugal, Spain and Sweden) out of the 12 countries covered in this book. Only Austria, England, the Netherlands and Poland have introduced PCSs that do not originate from the original United States Health Care Financing Administration (HCFA-)DRG system (Fischer, 2008). However, most of the self-developed systems are similar to DRG systems in that they share the basic characteristics. Only the Dutch PCS differs to a great extent from the DRG approach (see Chapter 23 of this volume). All PCSs of countries included in this book are referred to as 'DRG-like patient classification systems'.

Yet, in spite of many similarities in the basic characteristics of different DRG-like PCSs, each country's system is unique, and thus defines patient groups or hospital products in a different way. On the one hand, it is very likely that this ability to adapt DRG systems to country-specific needs was one of the reasons for their success and their widespread application in European countries. On the other hand, in a context of increasing patient mobility and growing interest in cross-border comparisons of hospital performance, the lack of a common definition of hospital products is starting to become problematic (European Parliament and Council, 2011). Therefore, this chapter intends to provide a systematic overview of the similarities and differences between DRG-like PCSs in Europe.

The chapter is organized as follows: the next section (4.2) first describes the historical origins of DRG-like PCSs in the countries included in this book. Section 4.3 provides an overview of some of the main characteristics of these systems and compares major diagnostic categories (MDCs) or similar categories that play an important role in most systems across the countries concerned. Section 4.4 presents the coding systems for diagnoses and procedures that form the basis of all PCSs. Subsequently, section 4.5 describes the classification algorithms of the systems, before section 4.6 looks in more detail at the specific classification variables used. Section 4.7 describes current trends in European DRG-like PCSs and last, but not least, the final section (4.8) concludes the chapter with a discussion of the opportunities and requirements for the harmonization of DRG-like PCSs in Europe.

4.2 Historical origins of DRG-like PCSs in Europe

Figure 4.1 illustrates the historical origins of DRG-like PCSs used in the European countries included in this book. It shows that all currently existing DRG systems are at least remotely related to the original HCFA-DRGs, while this is not true for the other '*DRG-like*' PCSs (shown at the far right of Figure 4.1) (Fischer, 2008). The first DRG system, Yale DRG, developed at Yale University and introduced in the late 1970s was initially intended as a tool to measure hospital resource utilization. However, recognizing the potential of a system that enabled assessment of hospital production, the United States' HCFA adapted the system for the purpose of monitoring and reimbursing hospital care delivered to elderly patients insured under Medicare (the federal tax-funded old-age insurance in the United States) (Fischer, 1997; Chilingerian, 2008).

In 1986, France modified the HCFA-DRG system and developed its own national DRG system called *groupes homogènes des malades* (GHMs) (ATIH, 2010), translated as 'homogeneous groups of patients'. Later, in 1988, 3M™ Health Information Systems adapted and extended HCFA-DRGs in order to better reflect the pathologies of non-elderly populations (3M, 2005). The resulting All Patients (AP-)DRG system was widely applied in the United States and, subsequently, updated versions of AP-DRGs were adopted in various European countries, such as Spain and Portugal, as well as influencing the development of national DRG systems, such as those of France and Australia. AP-DRGs were later refined by changing the determination of severity levels in order to respond to demands for more accurate assessment of case severity and differences in resource intensity, thus leading to the All Patient Refined (APR-) DRGs (3M, 2003). Together, AP-DRGs and APR-DRGs formed the basis for the

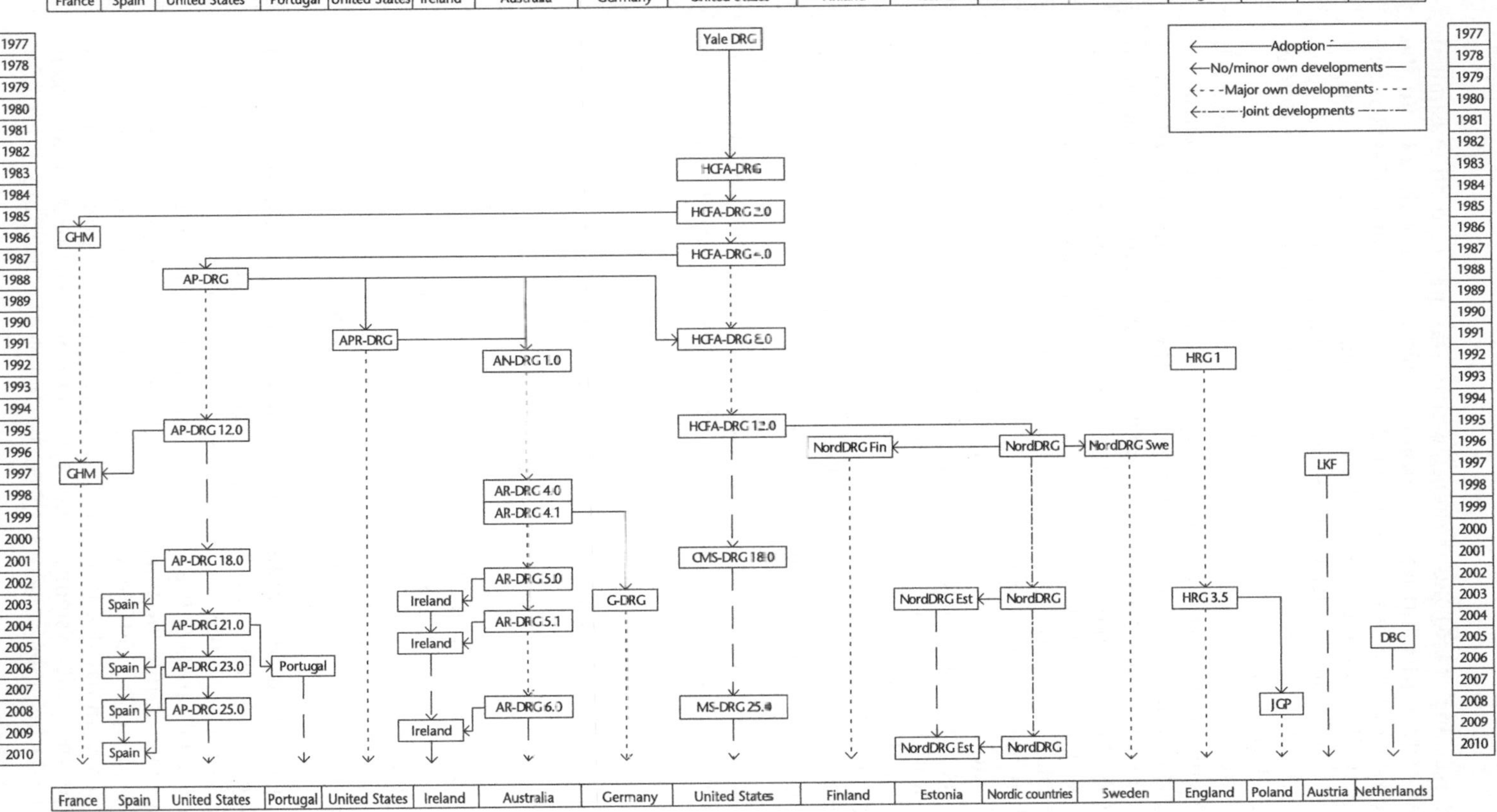

Figure 4.1 Historical development

Sources: Authors' own compilation, based on Fischer, 2008; Schreyögg et al., 2006; and information provided in ATIH, 2010; 3M, 2005; Australian Government, 2004; InEK, 2009; NHS Information Centre for Health and Social Care, 2010; and the relevant country-specific chapters in Part Two of this volume.

* Discontinued developments are not shown, such as the use of HCFA-DRGs in Ireland and Portugal or the flat-rate/additional payment (*Fallpauschale/ Sonderentgelt*) approach in Germany.

Australian National (AN-)DRG system, which was renamed to Australian Refined (AR-)DRGs after further modifications had been introduced into the system (Australian Government, 2004). In 2003, Ireland adopted AR-DRGs (see Chapter 15 of this volume), while Germany used AR-DRGs as the basis for developing its own German (G-)DRG system (see Chapter 14).

The Nordic countries are special in that they started to collaborate in 1996 in order to develop a common Nordic DRG system, called NordDRG – a PCS based on HCFA-DRGs. NordDRGs are jointly updated and then imported by each country before country-specific modifications are added to each new version of NordDRGs (see Chapter 16 of this volume). Of the countries covered in this book, Sweden and Finland are using NordDRGs. In addition, Estonia adopted NordDRGs in 2003 and has continued to use the same version of the system until the first update in 2010 (see Chapter 17). Unless otherwise explained, the term 'NordDRG' refers to the common Full NordDRG system that is jointly developed among the Nordic countries.

England, Austria and the Netherlands decided to develop their own PCSs. In 1992, the English Healthcare Resource Group (HRG) system was developed, and was later adopted by Poland, with a number of modifications. This led to the emergence of the *Jednorodne Grupy Pacjentów* (JGP), which can be translated (like the French GHMs) as 'homogeneous groups of patients'. In Austria a national self-developed PCS, described as a performance-oriented hospital financing system (*Leistungsorientierte Krankenanstaltenfinanzierung*; LKF) has been used since 1997 (see Chapter 11 of this volume). The Netherlands developed its own – very special – system of diagnosis–treatment combinations (*Diagnose Behandeling Combinaties*; DBCs), which has been in use since 2005 (see Chapter 23).

4.3 DRG-like PCSs in Europe: Overview

As illustrated by the historical origins of DRG-like PCSs in Europe, current PCSs are either self-developed or have their (remote) origins in various successors of the original Yale DRG system. Table 4.1 describes some basic characteristics of nine DRG-like PCSs. First, the systems differ in the number of groups they define: most systems contain between 650 and 2300 groups. The Polish JGP system defines fewer groups than all other systems (only 518), while the Dutch DBC system is an extreme outlier, comprising about 30 000 DBCs in the 2010 version.

In all HCFA-derived DRG systems, DRGs are organized within MDCs. Even the DRG-like PCSs – HRGs and JGPs – categorize their groups into 'chapters'; only in LKF and DBC is this technique of subdivision not used. The chapters/MDCs cover certain parts of the body or certain disease entities and are similar across all systems. While the total number of DRGs differs greatly across PCSs, the number of chapters/MDCs is around 25 for all systems, except the JGP system, which eliminated a number of chapters when adopting the English HRGs. Since in most systems, each MDC/chapter represents one organ system, the MDC/chapter structure of PCSs parallels the structure of medical specialties.

Table 4.1 Basic characteristics of DRG-like PCSs in Europe (based on 2008)

	AP-DRG	*AR-DRG*	*G-DRG*	*GHM*	*Nord-DRG*	*HRG*	*JGP*	*LKF*	*DBC*
Groups	679	665	1 200	2 297	794	1 389	518	979	≈30 000
MDCs/Chapters	25	24	26	28	28	23	16	–	–
Partitions	2	3	3	4	2	2*	2*	2*	–

Source: Authors' own compilation based on data provided by the Nordic Casemix Centre (2011), as well as information contained in the relevant chapters of Part Two of this volume.

* HRG, JGP, and LKF do not define partitions per se, but distinguish between treatment- and diagnosis-driven episodes.

Furthermore, all DRG-like PCSs except the DBC system define 'partitions' to further divide cases into more homogeneous groups. These partitions are defined by the kind of treatment, namely 'surgical' (or 'operating room' (OR)) versus 'medical' treatment. In addition, in some systems, partitions distinguish between OR procedures and non-OR procedures. Only the French GHM contains a fourth partition in certain MDCs, whereby the classification process does not check for the type of procedure (ATIH, 2010).

Figure 4.2 presents a graphical illustration of the distribution of DRG-like groups into MDCs (or chapters). On the left-hand side of the figure is a list of the MDCs as currently used in Medicare Severity (MS-)DRGs (the successor to HCFA-DRGs), which served as the reference for this comparison. Since MDCs are not used in the LKF system, LKF groups were mapped to MS-DRGs on the basis of the LKF group names. The Dutch DBC system was excluded from this comparison, since no mapping seemed feasible. Each cell represents one MDC in a PCS. The letters within the cells are the codes that are used in the different PCSs as names for each category. The ordering of the codes demonstrates that in all countries almost exactly the same categories are used to form MDCs, and that they follow in almost exactly the same order. Even the self-developed HRG system uses similar categories in a similar order. However, some MDCs are only used by a specific PCS. This is the case for 'Vascular disease' (JGPs), 'Breast problems' (NordDRGs) and 'HIV infection' (AP-DRGs, G-DRGs, GHMs). These are highlighted in Figure 4.2.

Figure 4.2 can be interpreted thus: the wider a column is, the higher the total number of groups of this DRG-like PCS in comparison to the others. The higher a cell is, the higher the share of groups in this system's MDC. For example, the column representing the GHM system is more than four times wider than the column representing the JGP system. Comparing the height of the cells shows that the distribution of DRGs into MDCs/chapters is similar across all DRG-like PCSs. This illustrates that all systems need similar shares of their total groups to describe cases within a specific category of diseases. However, some minor differences exist: for example, the MDC 'Circulatory system' represents around 10 per cent of the total number of groups in most PCSs, but only 4.5 per cent of all groups in the HRG system. Furthermore, the category 'Pre-MDC' is defined either explicitly or only implicitly (for example, as 'Organ transplants' in the GHM system). However, as this analysis does not assess the specific groups

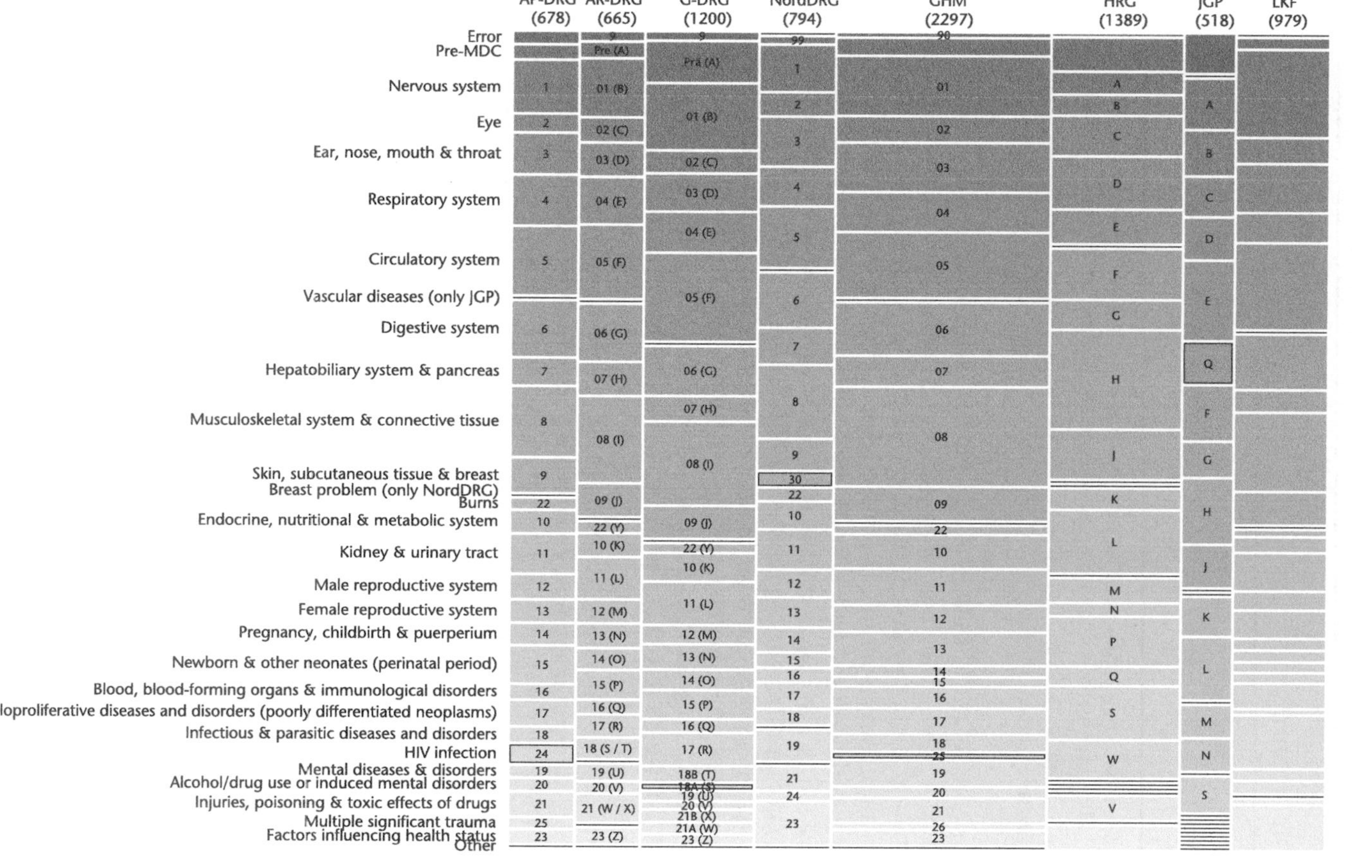

Figure 4.2 Comparison of MDCs across eight DRG systems and similar PCSs

Sources: Authors' own compilation based on information available in BMG, 2009; NHS Information Centre for Health and Social Care, 2010; ATIH, 2010; InEK, 2009; Australian Government, 2004; 3M, 2005; data provided by the Nordic Casemix Centre (2011); and information contained in Chapter 20 (Poland) of this volume.

included within MDCs/chapters in different PCSs, it cannot be ignored that differences in the distribution of groups might be either greater or smaller than they appear.

4.4 Data requirements: Coding of diagnoses and procedures

In all DRG-like PCSs, the coding of diagnoses and procedures is important, since this information forms the basis for the definition of patient groups. For coding of diagnoses, an international standard exists: most countries use the 10th revision of the WHO's International Classification of Diseases (ICD-10). Only in Spain and Portugal is the previous version of the ICD system (ICD-9) still in use because the AP-DRG system requires ICD-9 codes. However, even within the group of countries using the ICD-10 version, significant differences exist, since almost all countries are using ICD-10 codes with country-specific modifications (see Table 4.2). Country-specific modifications usually add a fifth digit to the general structure of ICD-10 codes, which allows for more detailed specification of certain conditions. However, sometimes country-specific modifications even deviate from the ICD-10 logic for specific conditions. For example, the German Modification ICD-10-GM does not contain the O84 code for multiple deliveries. Instead, Z37 codes are used, which specify the outcome of delivery (for example single birth, multiple births). Furthermore, each country has its own coding standards and guidelines.

Table 4.2 Coding of diagnoses and procedures

Country	*Diagnoses coding*	*Procedure coding*
Austria	ICD-10-BMSG-2001	Leistungskatalog
England	ICD-10	OPCS
Estonia	ICD-10	NCSP
Finland	ICD-10-FI	NCSP-FI
France	CIM-10	CCAM Classification Commune des Actes Médicaux
Germany	ICD-10-GM	OPS Operationen- und Prozedurenschlüssel
Ireland	ICD-10-AM	ACHI Australian Classification of Health Interventions
The Netherlands	ICD-10	Elektronische DBC Typeringslijst
Poland	ICD-10	ICD-9-CM
Portugal	ICD-9-CM	ICD-9-CM
Spain	ICD-9-CM	ICD-9-CM
Sweden	ICD-10-SE	KVÅ Klassifikation av vårdåtgärder (Swedish adaption of NCSP)
NordDRG	ICD-10	NCSP Nomesco Classification of Surgical Procedures

Sources: Authors' own compilation based on data provided by the Nordic Casemix Centre (2011), as well as information contained in the relevant country-specific chapters of Part Two of this volume.

For procedure coding, the differences between countries are even greater, since no similar international standard exists. Almost every country has developed its own procedure coding system tailored to its needs. Consequently, these systems are very heterogeneous. They range from sequential numbered lists, such as the Australian Classification of Health Interventions (ACHI) to multi-axial procedure classifications, such as the French classification of procedures (*classification commune des actes médicaux*, CCAM), or the Austrian *Leistungskatalog*. In addition, granularity differs to a great extent. The LKF system includes only selected procedures and therefore contains only 1500 items. At the other end of the scale, the German procedure classification codes (*Operationen- und Prozedurenschlüssel*, OPS) – designed to include all procedures – contain more than 30 000 items; 20 times more than the Austrian system.

4.5 The classification algorithm in European DRG-like PCSs

DRG-like PCSs group patients into a manageable number of groups. In order to do so, they follow a certain classification algorithm. This is similar across all the DRG systems that are based on different modifications of the original HCFA-DRGs. In particular, diagnoses are the predominating classification criteria. The classification algorithm in other DRG-like PCSs (for example in England, Poland and Austria) differs in that procedures become more important at an earlier stage and diagnoses only play a subordinate role (NHS Information Centre for Health and Social Care, 2010; BMG, 2009). In the Netherlands, the medical specialty department forms the first step in the grouping process (see Chapter 23 of this volume).

The following subsections contain descriptions of classification algorithms in PCSs derived from the HCFA-DRG system and other DRG-like PCSs, and they describe both similarities and differences within and between these groups of classification systems.

4.5.1 PCSs derived from HCFA-DRGs

Figure 4.3 shows the general grouping algorithm of PCSs derived from HCFA-DRGs and DRG system-specific modifications of the basic algorithm. The Nord-DRG system is not mentioned explicitly in the diagram because its developments do not change the general grouping algorithm.

There are six major steps common to all systems. Before the actual classification starts, the data are (1) checked to exclude cases with incorrect or missing information. Then, (2) very high-cost cases (for example, cases with transplantations) are isolated from all other cases into a special category of groups called 'Pre-MDCs'. Subsequently, (3) cases are allocated to mutually exclusive MDCs based on the principal diagnosis (although some systems sporadically use other variables, such as age, to assign cases to a neonatal MDC).

In the next step, (4) the grouping algorithm checks whether or not an OR procedure was performed and separates patients into a 'surgical' or into a 'medical' partition. In addition, the AR-DRG, the (derived) G-DRG, and the GHM

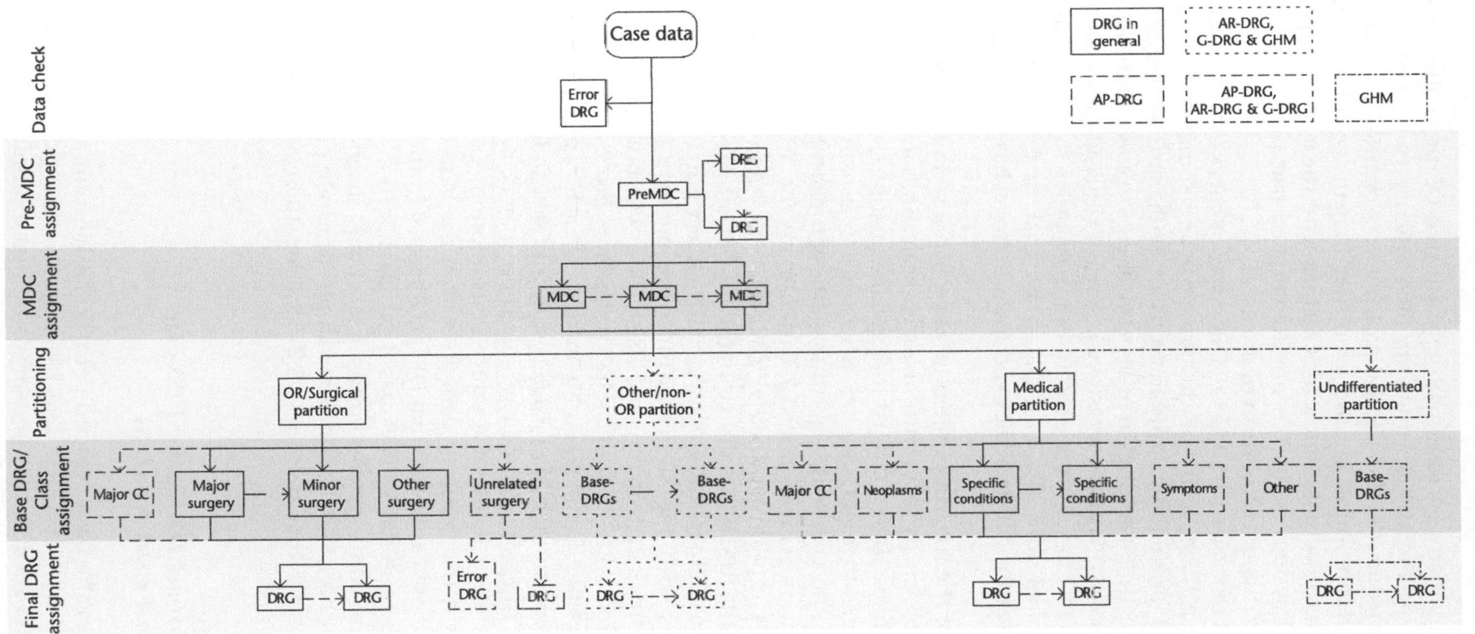

Figure 4.3 Classification algorithm of different HCFA-DRG derived PCSs, including system-specific modifications

Sources: Authors' own compilation based on information provided available in ATIH, 2010; InEK, 2009; Australian Government, 2004; 3M, 2005; and information contained in chapters 13 (France), 14 (Germany) and 15 (Ireland) of this volume.

systems differentiate between cases with relevant non-OR procedures (that is, relevant within a specific MDC), which are then assigned to the 'other'/'non-OR' partition. Consequently, the medical partition in NordDRG countries may contain cases which are found in other countries' systems within the 'other'/ 'non-OR' partition; the actual name varies according to the system. A particularity of the GHM system is that an undifferentiated partition exists within certain MDCs (see Chapter 13 of this volume).

After assignment of the partition, (5) all DRG systems check for further characteristics of the case (complexity of the principal and sometimes secondary diagnoses, type of procedures, combinations of both, and sometimes age, length of stay or treatment setting) in order to assign it to a class (in the AP-DRG system) or to a 'base-DRG' (in other systems). The algorithm usually checks first for more complicated procedures or conditions in order to make sure that patients are classified into the base-DRG/class that best reflects resource consumption of the case (illustrated by the arrow between base-DRGs/classes in Figure 4.3).

A particularity of the AP-DRG system is that a list of secondary diagnoses is checked in order to identify cases with major complications and co-morbidities (major CCs), which are then collected in a specific major-CC class (3M, 2005). This is different from other DRG systems, where CCs are usually only considered in the last step of the grouping algorithm (although exceptions to this rule exist, for example in the G-DRG system). Furthermore, the AP-DRG system has explicit classes for symptoms and 'other' conditions that do not exist in other DRG systems. Yet, the AP-DRG is similar to the AR-DRG and G-DRG systems, in terms of their approach to identifying cases with surgery unrelated to the MDC. For example, cases with hip surgery within the nervous system MDC are classified into the unrelated surgery class/base-DRG, which will determine an Error DRG in the final AR-DRG and G-DRG assignment process.

In the last step of the classification algorithm, (6) each case is grouped into the final DRG. Often, the class/base-DRG is split into several DRGs (the arrows between the DRGs in Figure 4.3 indicate that there may be more than two) in order to reflect different levels of resource consumption. Other classes/base-DRGs are not split if the group of patients within the base-DRG is relatively homogeneous. In these cases, the final DRG is identical to the base-DRG/class. The assignment to the final DRG is based on classification variables, which differ across systems. Most systems consider secondary diagnoses, procedures, age, and type of discharge (including, for example, death) in order to assign the final DRG. The section that follows (4.5.2) explores these variables in more detail.

4.5.2 Self-developed DRG-like PCSs in England, Poland and Austria

Figure 4.4 illustrates the basic structure of the classification algorithm for the self-developed DRG-like HRG, JGP and LKF systems. Since JGPs were derived from an earlier HRG version, it is not surprising that a number of similarities exist between these two systems (see Chapter 20 of this volume). The grouping

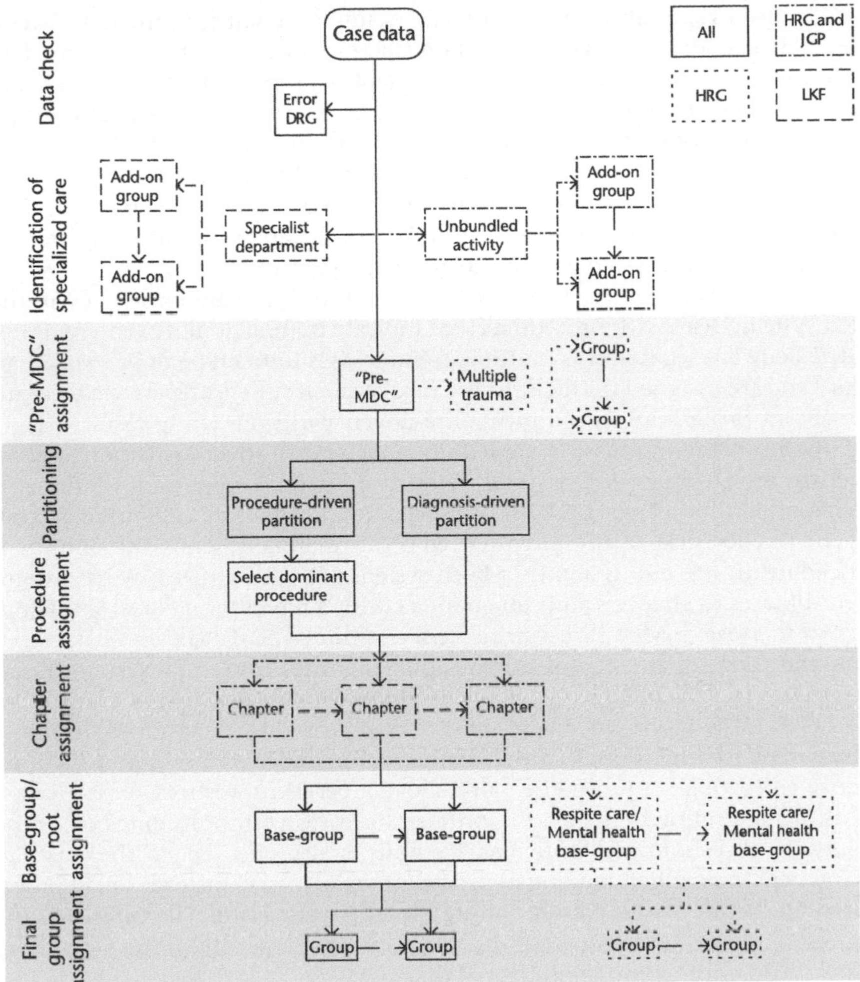

Figure 4.4 Classification algorithm in self-developed DRG-like PCSs (HRG, JGP and LKF)

Sources: Authors' own compilation based on information available in BMG, 2009; NHS Information Centre for Health and Social Care, 2010; and information contained in chapters 12 (England) and 20 (Poland) of this volume.

algorithm of all three systems consists of between five and seven consecutive steps, similar to those shown in Figure 4.4. However, the steps do not necessarily coincide, and the most important difference in comparison to the PCSs derived from HCFA-DRGs is that procedures play the dominant role in the grouping algorithm, while diagnoses are less important.

In the first step, all three systems identify whether the patients in each case received certain well-defined specialized services, for example computerized tomography (CT) scans, intensive care unit (ICU) treatment or chemotherapy. If patients received specific procedures (in the HRG and JGP systems), or if they were treated in specialist departments (for example, geriatrics in the LKF system) the PCSs classify patients into certain add-on groups that are assigned in addition to the final groups. The idea is to separate services that are provided to heterogeneous groups of patients (but not necessarily to all patients within these groups) from all other services, in order to increase the ability to define homogeneous groups of patients. In PCSs derived from HCFA-DRGs, similar mechanisms exist to identify certain well-defined specialized services and to reimburse them separately (see section 4.8 and Chapter 6), but these are not always directly integrated within the grouping algorithm.

The second step, which is similar to Pre-MDC assignment, exists only in the HRG system: cases with procedures that indicate trauma of more than two sites of the body are separated as multiple trauma cases into a type of Pre-MDC category and are assigned to HRGs. In the next step, all systems separate cases with significant procedures into a procedure-driven partition, while cases with no significant procedures are assigned to a diagnosis-driven partition. Subsequently, the HRG and JGP systems determine the most important (dominant) procedure, either using a rank list of procedures (in the HRG system) or according to the decision of the provider, who can manually select the dominant procedure (in the JGP system). In both systems, this is followed by the assignment of cases to chapters and sub-chapters, which represent medical specialties similar to those of MDCs in systems derived from HCFA-DRGs.

In the penultimate step of the grouping algorithm, the LKF system differs again from the HRG and JGP systems. Within the procedure-driven partition in the HRG and JGP systems, the highest ranked procedure determines the 'base-group'/root to which each case is assigned. For major procedures, which are identified through a procedure rank above a certain threshold, base-groups/roots are determined directly. In contrast, for cases with procedures of a rank below the threshold, the principal diagnosis is also checked. In the Austrian LKF system, no explicit ranking of procedures takes place. Instead, for all procedures, the score of the corresponding group is calculated. The one with the highest score is then selected. In the diagnosis-driven partition, the base-group is always determined by the principal diagnosis.

In the final step of the grouping algorithm, which is similar to that of PCSs derived from the HCFA-DRG system, patients are classified into the final group. Base-groups are either split into several final groups, in order to differentiate between different levels of resource consumption, or they remain unsplit. In the HRG and JGP systems, it depends on the chapter as to whether specific CCs are considered to be relevant in the grouping algorithm or not. In the LKF system, age is used most often to separate groups.

4.5.3 The Dutch DBC classification

The DBC classification system is very different from all the other systems. In most cases it consists of four dimensions: (1) the first dimension specifies one of 27 medical specialties, under which the patient was treated. Then (2) one of five types of care is determined (for example, regular inpatient care or ICU treatment). Subsequently (3) the diagnosis of the patient is considered, before finally (4) the treatment dimension differentiates between the treatment setting (inpatient versus outpatient) and the type of care (conservative treatment, type of surgery). For certain medical specialties, a fifth dimension exists, which identifies whether certain conditions existed that are expected to result in higher-than-average resource consumption (such as age < 11 years or requirement for a second surgeon). Any specification can be chosen for each dimension, resulting in a very high number of groups (Warners, 2008; see also Chapter 23 of this volume).

4.6 Classification variables and severity levels in European DRG-like PCSs

This section provides more details regarding the variables considered in the classification process, with an emphasis on the final split into DRGs or DRG-like groups. In addition, differences in the number of severity/complexity levels per base-group are explored and the approaches to using CCs are explained.

4.6.1 Classification variables

All DRG-like PCSs in Europe use routinely collected patient discharge data in order to classify patients. Table 4.3 provides an overview of clinical, demographic/administrative and resource-consumption variables used in European DRG-like PCSs. Clinical information (relating to diagnoses and procedures) is used as classification variables in all systems. In addition, all PCSs except the Netherlands' DBC system use the concept of one principal diagnosis as the highest ranked diagnosis for hospital discharge. However, the definition of what constitutes the principal diagnosis differs. In some countries the principal diagnosis is defined as the 'main reason' for a hospital stay (in, for example, the AR-DRG, G-DRG and LKF systems). In other countries, where the hospital discharge is aggregated based on several departmental discharges (the GHM or HRG systems, for example), a diagnosis hierarchy is used to determine the most important diagnosis. Procedures are also used, in all systems, but their importance in the classification algorithm varies – even between similar systems. For example, procedures play a more prominent role in the classification algorithm in the G-DRG system than in the AR-DRG system, on which the German system was originally based (InEK, 2009). In the self-developed HRG, JGP and LKF systems, information about procedures actually dominates information about diagnoses (see section 4.5.2).

Demographic and administrative variables, especially age and discharge type (for example, death or transfer) are frequently used variables in all systems, except the DBC system. Gender is a relevant classification variable only in the NordDRG system, although many systems use it to verify consistency of data (for example, where obstetric diagnosis codes are accepted only for female patients).

Similarly, resource-consumption variables are used in many DRG-like PCSs. Length of stay is the most frequently used explicit resource-consumption variable. However, even if systems do not explicitly include resource-consumption

Table 4.3 Classification variables and severity levels in European DRG-like PCSs

Systems	*AP-DRG*	*AR-DRG*	*G-DRG*	*GHM*	*NordDRG*	*HRG*	*JGP*	*LKF*	*DBC*
Classification variables									
Clinical variables									
Diagnoses	×	×	×	×	×	×	×	×	×
Procedures	×	×	×	×	×	×	×	×	×
Neoplasms/Malignancy	×	×	×	–	–	–	–	–	–
Type of care	–	–	–	–	–	–	–	–	×
Administrative/demographic variables									
Admission type		–	–	–	–	×	×	–	–
Age	×	×	×	×	×	×	×	×	–
Birth weight (newborn)	×	×	×	×	–	–	–	–	
Discharge type	×	×	×	×	×	×	×	–	–
Gender	–	–	–	–	×	–	–	–	–
Mental health legal status	–	×	×	–	–	–	–	–	–
Resource consumption variables									
LOS/Same-day status	–	×	×	×	×	×	×	–	–
Mechanical ventilation	–	–	×	–	–	–	–	–	–
Setting	–	–	–	×	–	–	–	–	×
Stay at specialist departments	–	–	–	–	–	–	–	×	–
Medical specialty	–	–	–	–	–	–	–	–	×
Demands for care	–	–	–	–	–	–	–	–	×
Severity/complexity levels	3*	4	not limited	5**	2	3	3	not limited	–
Aggregate case complexity measure	–	PCC	PCC	×	–	–	–	–	–

Sources: Authors' own compilation based on ATIH, 2010; InEK, 2009; Australian Government, 2004; 3M, 2005; BMG, 2009; NHS Information Centre for Health and Social Care, 2010; Warners, 2008; data provided by the Nordic Casemix Centre (2011), as well as information contained in the relevant country-specific chapters of Part Two of this volume.

*Not explicitly mentioned (major CCs at MDC level plus 2 levels of severity at DRG level)
** 4 levels of severity plus one GHM for short stays or outpatient care

variables, such as mechanical ventilation, these variables are regularly considered in the classification algorithms by other means. For example, while the G-DRG system explicitly considers duration of mechanical ventilation, other systems use procedure codes for tracheostomy in order to identify cases with mechanical ventilation.

4.6.2 Severity levels

Table 4.3 also shows the number of severity levels in different DRG-like PCSs. Most countries limit the number of possible severity levels. For example, the number of severity levels is restricted to only two in NordDRG systems and to three in the HRG system. The same logic of splitting base-groups only when necessary is also used in other systems (AR-DRG and HRG systems). However, in GHM, if a base-group is split, it is almost always split into four levels, plus one additional group for short stays or day cases. At the other end of the scale, the G-DRG and LKF systems do not limit the number of severity levels. They subdivide base-groups into as many final groups as necessary in order to achieve relative homogeneity of resource consumption within each group. The DBC system is the only system that does not split base-groups during the final step of the grouping algorithm.

4.6.3 Dealing with CCs

In all systems, except for the DBC and LKF PCSs, secondary diagnoses determine to a large degree the classification of cases into the appropriate level of severity or complexity. In most DRG-like PCSs, lists of secondary diagnoses are defined that represent CCs. The same CC list usually applies to all cases, except in the HRG system, which has one specific CC list for each chapter. However, even systems with global CC lists always define certain exclusion criteria – mostly usually principal diagnosis, for which specific secondary diagnoses are not considered a CC. Depending on the number of severity/complexity levels of the PCS, CC lists specify different levels of severity for each CC.

Furthermore, a number of approaches to dealing with multiple secondary diagnoses exist. While in the AR-DRG and G-DRG systems a cumulative measure (called Patient Clinical Complexity Level (PCCL)) of all secondary diagnoses is applied, in most other DRG systems it is the highest ranked secondary diagnosis that defines the severity. In the GHM system, another cumulative approach is used: the highest ranked secondary diagnosis together with age, length of stay and death during admission define the severity for a number of DRGs. In the Netherlands' DBC system, secondary diagnoses are not taken into account. Instead, a new DBC is allocated if patients are treated for additional diagnoses.

4.7 Trends

When analysing the developments of DRG-like PCSs over time, three main developments come to light: (1) DRG-like PCSs are progressively being applied to settings that are beyond the acute care hospital inpatient sector for which they were originally developed; (2) the number of groups has continued to increase in all systems; and (3) systems increasingly develop measures to ensure that specific complicated, high-cost services are adequately reflected.

4.7.1 Coverage of services

Since the early 1990s, researchers have tried to expand the concept of DRGs into settings other than inpatient acute hospital care (Goldfield, 2010.) Table 4.4 shows that the majority of countries are also using DRG-like PCSs for day care – or they are planning to do so. In order to use DRG-like PCSs for day care, countries have either extended their PCS (for example Finland, France and Sweden) or assigned different weights for DRGs in different settings.

Countries using the same PCS for inpatients and day cases should introduce additional algorithms into their classification systems in order to identify day cases. For example, the French GHM system splits base-DRGs according to the length of stay (LOS) in order to identify day cases as cases with a LOS = 0 (ATIH, 2010). In the Swedish and Finnish versions of the NordDRG system, a split is used in the grouping algorithm in order to separate day cases from inpatients according to the treatment setting (see Chapter 19 of this volume). In Austria, England and Germany, day cases are not identified explicitly as part of the grouping process. For reimbursement purposes, LKF groups, HRGs, and G-DRGs are adjusted for cases with a LOS = 0. In addition, the English HRG system identifies certain procedures as being only applicable to day cases (NHS Information Centre for Health and Social Care, 2010).

Furthermore, many countries are planning to develop DRG-like PCSs for psychiatric and rehabilitation care (see Table 4.4). For rehabilitation care, several PCSs have been proposed but heterogeneous duration and resource consumption – as well as the absence of dominant procedures – make it difficult to define homogeneous groups of patients. However, in contrast to acute hospital care, grouping can be used to classify cases or days (or weeks). The German Rehabilitation Treatment Groups (RBG) system (Neubauer & Pfister, 2008) or the American Inpatient Rehabilitation Facility Prospective Payment System (IRF-PPS) (MedPAC, 2009) classify cases. These systems take into account scores relating to impairment, possible co-morbidities and age. The French *Groupes homogène de journées* (Homogeneous groups of days, GHJ) (Metral et al., 2008) and the Swiss *Leistungsorientiertes Tarifmodell Rehabilitation* (Performance-oriented payment system for rehabilitation, LTR) (Fischer et al., 2010) classify days or weeks.

4.7.2 Number of groups

Figure 4.5 illustrates changes in the number of groups in different DRG-like PCSs in Europe over time. It shows that the number of groups has continued to increase in all systems. In most cases, there are only minor changes from year to year. However, in France (GHMs) and England (HRGs), major revisions of the

Table 4.4 Trends in coverage of services in DRG-like PCSs in Europe

Country	*Inpatient*	*Day cases*	*Psychiatry*	*Rehabilitation*
Austria	X	X[a]	–	–
England	X	X	in the process of extension	
Estonia	X	X[e]	–	–
Finland	X	X	X[b]	X[b]
France	X	X	in the process of extension	
Germany	X	X[a]	planned for 2013	–
The Netherlands	X	X	X	X
Ireland	X	X	–	–
Poland	X	X[a]	in the process of extension	
Portugal	X	X[a]	–[c]	–[c]
Spain	X	–[d]	–	–
Sweden	X	X	X	X

Source: Authors' own compilation based on information contained in the relevant country-specific chapters of Part Two of this volume.

Notes: [a] Not explicitly part of the grouping algorithm but day-case status is explicitly considered for payment purposes; [b] The DRG system is designed to cover such cases, but 'in all hospitals, psychiatric patients and patients requiring long-term intensive treatment (such as patients suffering from respiratory arrest) are excluded' from DRG billing (see Chapter 18 of this volume, subsection 18.5.1); [c] Studies have been undertaken regarding the possibility of including psychiatry and rehabilitation, but nothing concrete has come of this research; [d] Surgical day cases are grouped and financed using AP-DRGs in the same way as for inpatient care; Ongoing research is taking place regarding International Refined (IR-)DRGs; [e] Only surgical day cases are grouped and financed using DRGs.

grouping algorithm have taken place in recent years, and consequently the number of groups has more than doubled in both countries. The G-DRG system is the only PCS with large increases in the number of groups every year before 2010, when this trend was stopped.

There are several reasons for which the number of groups in DRG-like PCSs is increasing: first, most systems have tried to improve their ability to reflect differences in the complexity of treating different patients. In the G-DRG system, the number of final DRGs per base-DRG (reflecting case complexity) has continuously increased over time. In France, the recent revision of the coding algorithm introduced four severity levels for most base-DRGs; and in England, the increase in the number of groups can be mostly attributed to the introduction of more severity levels. Second, countries are increasingly moving to incorporating day care into their DRG-like PCSs. If day care is included within the same classification system, this may necessitate the creation of new groups to specifically reflect resource consumption of day cases. Third, new medical devices, drugs and medical knowledge become available, influence treatment patterns, and may necessitate separating certain cases of one group of patients into a new group, in order to assure medical and economic homogeneity of groups (see Chapter 9 of this volume). In addition, the underlying coding systems (for both diagnoses and procedures) are regularly updated in most countries. If the accuracy (granularity) of the coding systems is improved, this enables the creation of patient groups that better reflect specific characteristics of procedures or patients, and are thus more homogeneous. Finally, improved cost accounting

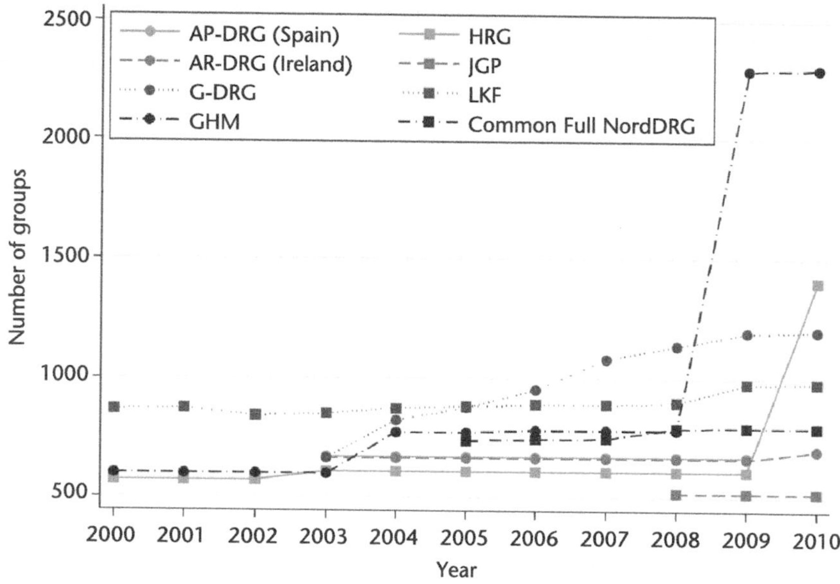

Figure 4.5 Trends in the number of groups in DRG-like PCSs in Europe

Sources: Authors' own compilation based on data provided by the Nordic Casemix Centre (2011), as well as information contained in the relevant country-specific chapters of Part Two of this volume and complemented by personal communications with the authors of those chapters.

in hospitals increases the ability of regulators to identify determinants of the costs of treating patients and to adapt the PCS accordingly (see Chapter 5).

The Dutch DBC system is not included in Figure 4.5, since the number of DBCs differs greatly from the number of groups in all other systems. However, it is interesting to note that the DBC system is reducing the number of groups with each revision of the system. Having started with about 100 000 DBCs in 2005, the number of groups was reduced to about 30 000 by 2010, and the intention is to define about 3000 DBCs, including severity levels similar to DRGs (Warners, 2008).

4.7.3 Specific high-cost services: Unbundling, séances, and supplementary payments

All DRG-like PCSs are faced with the problem of how to ensure that certain specific high-cost services required by heterogeneous patients belonging to different DRG-like groups are adequately reflected in the grouping process. In order to do so, the English HRG system has developed the concept of 'unbundling'. This separates a set of certain services, such as chemotherapy, radiotherapy, diagnostic imaging, renal dialysis, and high-cost drugs, from the core HRGs (NHS Information Centre for Health and Social Care, 2009). By separating these services, the economic homogeneity of core HRGs is improved and, at the same time, adequate reimbursement through supplementary payments can be guaranteed (see Chapter 6 of this volume). In the French GHM system, there is a category called 'sessions' (*séances*), which fulfils a similar purpose, also separating renal dialysis, chemotherapy and radiotherapy from other services. In Germany, an increasingly large number of supplementary payments exist (see Chapter 14), which are not directly part of the grouping process but still fulfil the same purpose as unbundling or *séances*.

Another trend in DRG-like PCSs internationally is that attempts are being made to differentiate better between co-morbidities on the one hand, and complications attributable to poor-quality care, on the other. However, until now only the United States MS-DRG system differentiates in this way, by requiring providers to assign codes revealing whether diagnoses were present on admission. If certain diagnoses that should not occur during hospitalization were not identified (coded) on admission, they are considered to reflect poor quality of care. How this information is used to adjust payment rates is discussed by Or and Häkkinen in Chapter 8 of this volume.

4.8 Conclusions: Likelihood of a common Euro-DRG system?

In the context of an emerging European hospital market, a common definition of hospital products through a common DRG-like PCS could be a major catalyst to facilitate cross-border movements of patients and payments. Therefore, establishing the likelihood of harmonization of DRG-like PCSs or, alternatively, the development of a common European DRG-like system is of high relevance for politicians and patients. In the introduction to this chapter, DRG-like PCSs were defined as systems that have four main characteristics. (1) *routinely collected data* on patient discharge are used to classify patients into (2) a *manageable number* of groups that are (3) *clinically meaningful* and (4) *economically homogeneous*. These points can also be used to guide discussion about the possibility of a common 'Euro-DRG' PCS.

Regarding the availability of routine data, section 4.6 discussed the fact that similar information is used to classify patients in all systems, and is readily available from hospital discharge summaries, while section 4.4 demonstrated that information is often coded in different ways. Therefore, an initial requirement for a common European DRG-like system would be to harmonize coding of diagnoses and procedures or to develop a mapping system that would allow the translation of codes from different coding systems into a common European coding system. The Hospital Data Project as part of the European Union (EU)'s Health Monitoring Programme has suggested a common format for hospital activity data, to improve comparability (Magee, 2003). For the coding of diagnoses, an agreement on a coding system should be relatively unproblematic, since the WHO ICD-10 system is already used for cause-of-death statistics in all countries and the next revision, ICD-11 is currently being developed.

A question that is changing over time relates to what is regarded as a manageable number of groups. Current developments of European DRG-like PCSs seem to indicate that a number of between 1000 and 1500 groups is necessary to describe the activity of hospitals. Since all countries use software tools to classify patients into groups, the manageability of a system depends mostly on the ability to reliably calculate average costs of patients within each group. In a European DRG-based system, the population basis for calculating average costs of patients within each group would be much larger. Therefore, it would be possible to develop a more detailed DRG system than currently exists in each individual Member State.

In order to define economically homogeneous groups of patients, the grouping algorithm of the DRG-like PCS needs to reflect the most important determinants of costs. If the determinants of costs are the same across European countries, it should be possible to classify patients using the same DRG-like PCS. Current research projects – such as the EU-funded EuroDRG project – aim to identify the most important determinants of costs in 11 European countries. The results of this project should be able to inform decisions about the feasibility of developing a common European DRG-based system. However, if such a system is to be developed, detailed cost-accounting information from a sufficiently large and representative sample of hospitals is essential (see Chapter 5 of this volume). In addition, mechanisms to ensure that the system is regularly updated must be developed (see Chapter 9).

As shown in section 4.2, all currently existing DRG systems originate from the original HCFA-DRG system, and even the self-developed DRG-like PCSs share many elements of these systems. The most likely scenario for developing a Euro-DRG system according to European needs seems to be that the existing systems will form the basis for this work. In order to ensure that these modifications do not change the principal of clinically meaningful groups, a process would need to be set up to incorporate consultation with medical professionals in developing and refining the DRG system.

In conclusion, while a European DRG system is unlikely to emerge within a medium- to short-term time frame, the development of such a system does not appear to be impossible. On the one hand, a number of requirements would need to be fulfilled, such as the development of common coding systems, cost-accounting systems, and consultation mechanisms. On the other hand, over a decade of experience using DRG-like PCSs in most countries has resulted in several highly refined DRG-like PCSs that could serve as the starting point for developing a new Euro-DRG system. Empirical analyses will be needed to identify the system that best reflects resource-consumption patterns in European hospitals. However, similar to the historical emergence of DRG-like PCSs as a result of political decisions, a common European PCS is only likely to emerge if there is sufficiently strong political will to support the emergence of a common European hospital market.

4.9 Note

1 The authors thank Wilm Quentin for his efforts in revising this chapter and Caroline Linhart for her work on the graphical representations.

4.10 References

3M (2005). *All Patient DRG Definitions Manual (Version 23.0)*. St. Paul, MN: 3M Health Information Systems.

3M (2003). *All Patient Refined DRGs (Version 20.0) Methodology Overview*. St. Paul, MN: 3M Health Information Systems.

ATIH (2010). *Manuel des GHM, Version 11b*. Lyon: Agence Technique de l'Information sur l'Hospitalisation (http://www.atih.sante.fr/index.php?id=000250002DFF, accessed 10 August 2010).

Australian Government (2004). *Australian Refined Diagnosis Related Groups Version 5.1. Definitions Manual Volume One (DRGs A01Z-I78B)*. Canberra: Commonwealth of Australia Department of Health and Ageing.

BMG (2009). *Leistungsorientierte Krankenanstaltenfinanzierung – LKF – Modell 2010*. Vienna: Bundesministerium für Gesundheit.

Chilingerian, J. (2008). Origins of DRGs in the United States: A technical, political and cultural story, in J. Kimberly, G. de Pouvourville, T. D'Aunno, eds. *The Globalization of Managerial Innovation in Health Care*. Cambridge: Cambridge Universtiy Press.

European Parliament and Council (2011). *Directive 2011/24/EU of the European Parliament and of the Council of 9 March 2011 on the Application of Patients' Rights in Cross-Border Health Care*. Brussels: Official Journal of the European Union.

Fetter, R.B. (1999). Casemix classification systems. *Australian Health Review*, 22(2): 16–34.

Fetter, R.B., Shin, Y., Freeman, J., Averill, R.F., Thompson, J.D. (1980). Casemix definition by diagnosis-related groups. *Medical Care*, 18(2):i–53.

Fischer, W. (1997). *Patientenklassifikationssysteme zur Bildung von Behandlungsfallgruppen im stationären Bereich – Prinzipien und Beispiele*. Wolfertswil: Zentrum für Informatik und wirtschaftliche Medizin (ZIM).

Fischer, W. (2008). *Die DRG-Familie*. Wolfertswil: Zentrum für Informatik und wirtschaftliche Medizin (ZIM) (http://www.fischer-zim.ch/textk-pcs/index.htm, accessed 10 July 2011).

Fischer, W., Blanco, J., Butt, M., Hund, M., Boldt, C. (2010). Leistungsorientiertes Tarifmodell Rehabilitation (LTR). *Neurologie & Rehabilitation*, (16)3:1–18.

Goldfield, N. (2010). The evolution of diagnosis-related groups (DRGs): from its beginnings in casemix and resource-use theory, to its implementation for payment and now for its current utilization for quality within and outside the hospital. *Quality Management in Healthcare*, 19(1):1–16.

InEK (2009). *German Diagnosis-Related Groups Version 2010. Definitionshandbuch Kompaktversion Band 1 (DRGs A01A-I98Z)*. Siegburg: Institut für das Entgeltsystem im Krankenhaus gGmbH.

Magee, H.F. (2003). The hospital data project: comparing hospital activity within Europe. *European Journal of Public Health*, 13(Suppl. 1):73–9.

MedPAC (2009). *Rehabilitation Facilities (Inpatient) Payment System: Payment Basics*. Washington, DC: Medicare Payment Advisory Commission (http://www.medpac.gov/documents/MedPAC_Payment_Basics_09_IRF.pdf, accessed 20 July 2010).

Metral, P., Ducret, N., Patris, A., Steunou, P. (2008). Improving casemix for description and funding in rehabilitation in France: additive model is better than tree-classification. *BMC Health Services Research*, 8(Suppl. 1):A2.

Neubauer, G., Pfister, F. (2008). *Entwicklung einer leistungsorientierten, fallgruppenspezifischen Vergütung in der Rehabilitation: Abschlussbericht*. Munich: Institut für Gesundheitsökonomik (http://www.bdpk.de/media/file/358.Abschlussbericht_Prof._Neubauer_Februar%202008.pdf, accessed 20 July 2010).

NHS Information Centre for Health and Social Care (2009). *The Casemix Service HRG4, Guide to Unbundling*. Leeds: NHS Information Centre for Health and Social Care.

NHS Information Centre for Health and Social Care (2010). *The Casemix Service HRG4 Design Concepts*. Leeds: NHS Information Centre for Health and Social Care.

Nordic Casemix Centre (2011). *Nordic Common Version (based on NCSP+)* (NordDRG manuals). Helsinki: Nordic Casemix Centre (http://www.nordcase.org/eng/norddrg_manuals/versions/common/, accessed 26 July 2011).

Schreyögg, J., Stargardt, T., Tiemann, O., Busse, R (2006). Methods to determine reimbursement rates for diagnosis related groups (DRG): a comparison of nine European countries. *Health Care Management Science*, 9(3):215–23.

Warners, J. (2008). Redesigning the Dutch DBC-system; towards increased transparency. From ideas and directions for improvement to implementation. *Patient Classification Systems International: 2008 Case Mix Conference, Lisbon, 8–11 October.*

chapter five

DRGs and cost accounting: Which is driving which?

Siok Swan Tan, Lisbeth Serdén, Alexander Geissler, Martin van Ineveld, Ken Redekop, Mona Heurgren and Leona Hakkaart-van Roijen

5.1 Introduction

Cost-accounting systems could enable hospital managers to collect, summarize, analyse and control the most relevant information regarding the allocation of resources and reimbursement of hospital services (Finkler et al., 2007; Horngren et al., 2006). Comprehensive cost-accounting systems are able to identify the costs which are generated by some unit of analysis (such as by a diagnosis-related group (DRG)) and could support the development of DRG-based payment rate-setting mechanisms based on standardized cost data (Nathanson, 1984).

In the past, cost accounting has not been of high priority to hospitals in conventional payment systems, such as fee-for-service reimbursement and global budgets. With respect to fee-for-service reimbursement, prices charged for typical conditions linked with standard services (that is, charges/bills invoiced to payers) did not necessarily represent a good estimate of the cost of individual services (Cohen et al., 1993; Ott, 1996). However, costs were, if at all, likely to be registered in decentralized and mutually incompatible information systems (Feyrer et al., 2005). Global budgets used to be the common funding model in most European health care systems. One of the key advantages of global budget arrangements was cost control; a fixed payment was agreed in advance for a target level of activity and hospitals' level of reimbursement was not directly related to the costs per patient (see Chapter 6 of this volume). The inability of prospective budgeting to provide insight into hospital activity restricted the planning – and possibly also the control – of the ever-growing hospital costs.

With the aim of improving the efficiency of hospital care, DRG-based hospital payment systems have been introduced in many European countries since 1983 (see Chapter 2). This development fundamentally changed hospital services from being sources of incremental revenue (revenue centres) to being sources of incremental costs (cost centres) (Berki, 1985).

Figure 5.1 provides an overview of the relevance of cost-accounting systems in the DRG era. Regulatory authorities throughout Europe came to realize that DRGs could not serve as payment rate-setting mechanisms without a functioning cost-accounting system (Feyrer et al., 2005); that is, effective and fair DRG-based hospital payment systems to a large extent depend on high-quality and accurate cost-accounting systems within hospitals (see Chapter 6 of this volume). Therefore, many countries started to routinely collect cost-accounting data from a representative sample of hospitals in order to calculate and continuously update national DRG weights (for example, England, France and Germany). Other countries have imported relative weights from abroad. In any case, the use of DRGs as a payment mechanism increased the awareness of the importance of accurate cost accounting in all hospitals, including those which did not collect data for calculating national DRG prices, since erroneous cost information would lead to inadequate relative weights and, ultimately, unintended incentives for the delivery of services. However, the collection of hospital cost information has led to greater transparency. Moreover, hospital managers recognized that cost accounting could support other purposes than simply payment rate-setting, such as systematic benchmarking and managed competition (Schuster et al., 2006; van de Ven & Schut, 2009). Precise cost information enabled hospital managers to detect sources of resource consumption in order to redesign treatment processes more efficiently.

The aims of this chapter are to give a short introduction to cost accounting in health care (section 5.2), to provide an overview of the different cost-accounting methods across Europe (section 5.3) and to examine the interaction between DRGs and cost accounting (section 5.4). The final section (5.5) contains some conclusions regarding the interdependency of DRGs and cost accounting, and the prospects for harmonizing cost-accounting systems across Europe. The 12

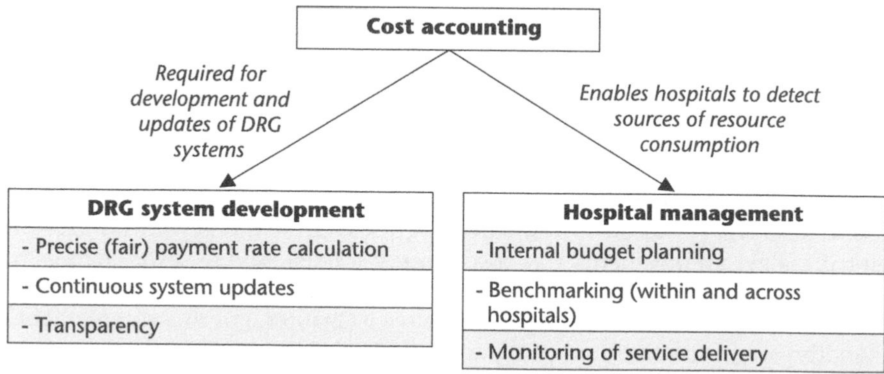

Figure 5.1 Cost accounting in the DRG era

countries considered were Austria, England, Estonia, Finland, France, Germany, Ireland, the Netherlands, Poland, Portugal, Spain and Sweden.

5.2 Cost accounting in health care

In theory, there are three subsequent steps involved in allocating hospital costs either to individual patients or groups of patient cases that are both medically coherent and cost-homogeneous (St-Hilaire & Crepeau, 2000; Tan et al., 2009c):

1. *overhead cost allocation*: allocation of hospital overhead costs to medical departments (subsection 5.2.1);
2. *indirect cost allocation*: allocation of department overhead costs to patients (subsection 5.2.2)
3. *direct cost allocation*: allocation of department direct costs to patients (subsection 5.2.3).

5.2.1 Overhead allocation

The available literature describes different frameworks for allocating hospital overhead costs to medical departments (Drummond et al., 2005; Williams et al., 1982). The most commonly used framework is cost-centre allocation (Finkler et al., 2007; St-Hilaire & Crepeau, 2000). In cost-centre allocation, a distinction is made between medical departments and overhead departments. Medical departments provide patient care and may involve in- and outpatient clinics, laboratories, operating rooms (ORs) and radiology departments. Overhead departments do not provide patient care and may include departments for administration, facility management, logistics and security. Overhead costs from such departments may be assigned to medical departments by means of various allocation bases, such as the number of inpatient days or the amount of direct costs (Finkler et al., 2007; Horngren et al., 2006).

An alternative, very similar framework is 'activity-based costing'. Activity-based costing does not refer to a separate allocation methodology, but instead emphasizes the importance of identifying the most accurate allocation base; an allocation base should most closely reflect a cause-and-effect relationship between the overhead costs and the medical department (Cooper & Kaplan, 1988). Hospital overhead costs are allocated to medical departments based on the activities which drive them (for example, the area (m^2) to allocate costs of accommodation, and the number of full-time equivalents to allocate administration costs), instead of using a more generic allocation base for all overhead departments, such as inpatient days or direct costs (Drummond et al., 2005).

Within either cost-centre allocation or activity-based costing, the available literature describes three methods for allocating hospital overhead costs to medical departments. The simplest method is 'direct allocation', in which overhead costs are allocated to medical departments without interaction between overhead departments (Figure 5.2).

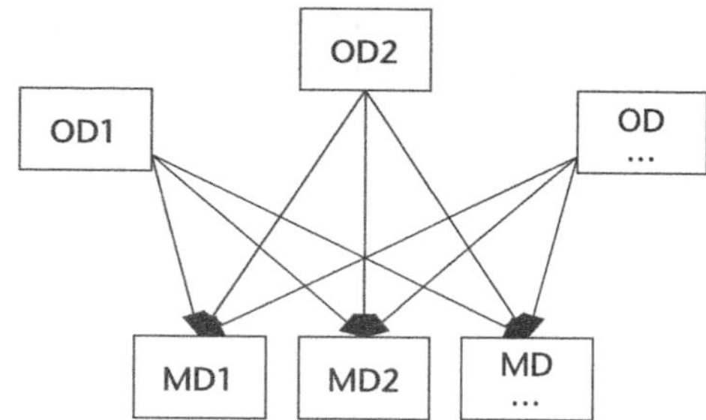

Figure 5.2 Direct method for overhead allocation

Notes: OD: overhead department; MD: medical department.

A second method, 'step-down allocation', partially adjusts for interaction between overhead departments. The method appoints overhead costs to both the medical departments and the remaining overhead departments in a stepwise fashion. The step-down method accounts for unilateral deliveries between overhead departments. This means that the sequence in which overhead departments allocate their costs is important (Figure 5.3); that is, costs of the second overhead department cannot be allocated to the first one.

A final method for allocating costs to medical departments is the 'reciprocal' method in which overhead costs are appointed to both the medical departments and to all other overhead departments. The reciprocal method takes into account bilateral deliveries between overhead departments. This means that the procedure should be repeated a number of times to eliminate residual unallocated amounts (Figure 5.4).

5.2.2 Indirect cost allocation

Department overhead costs (indirect costs) are those costs incurred by medical departments that are not directly related to patients, such as the personnel costs of non-medical staff and inventory. Cost-centre allocation and activity-based costing are not applicable to the allocation of costs to patients, because they assume a cause-and-effect relationship with the medical department, rather

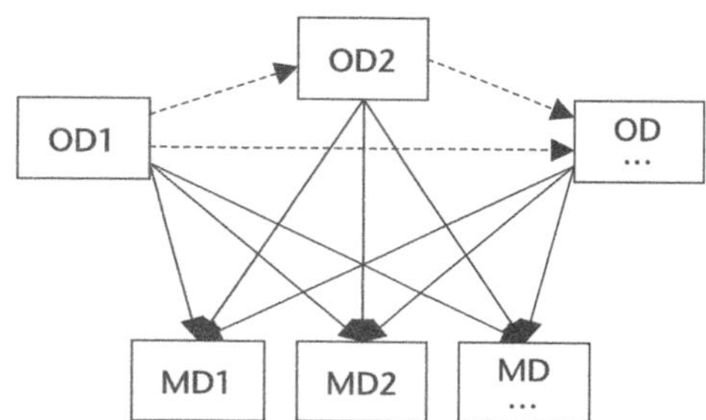

Figure 5.3 Step-down method for overhead allocation

Notes: OD: overhead department; MD: medical department.

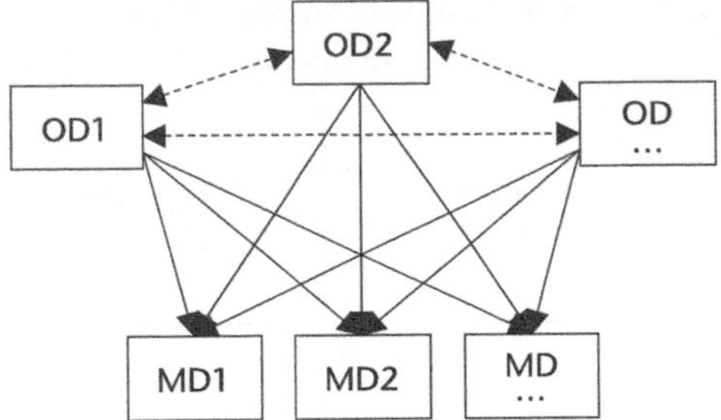

Figure 5.4 Reciprocal method for overhead allocation

Notes: OD: overhead department; MD: medical department.

than with patients. Instead, department overhead costs may be assigned to patients using the following methods (Finkler et al., 2007; Tan et al., 2009c):

- marginal mark-up percentages: indirect costs distributed to direct costs by raising the direct costs with a mark-up percentage;
- weighting statistics: service time, for example, used as a proxy for resource consumption, yielding a cost per treatment minute or inpatient day;
- relative value units: establish the relative cost of each patient by assigning a base value to the base-line resource use of the hospital service and adding relative values to this base value when the patient uses additional resources.

5.2.3 Direct cost allocation

Direct costs refer to the costs incurred by medical departments which are directly linked to patients, such as the personnel costs of medical staff (especially if clearly involved with a particular procedure), medications and materials.

Direct costs per patient are calculated by subsequently identifying the quantities of hospital services a patient consumed and valuing these hospital services with their unit costs (Drummond et al., 2005; Jackson, 2000). Overall, there are four methodologies to calculate the direct costs per patient (Figure 5.5). These methodologies differ in terms of the level of accuracy with which they identify hospital services ('gross-costing' versus 'micro-costing') and value hospital services (the 'top-down' versus 'bottom-up' approaches) (Tan et al., 2009b; Tan, 2009).

Gross-costing identifies hospital services at a highly aggregated level; often inpatient days are defined as the only hospital service (Jackson, 2000; Tan et al., 2009b). Top-down gross-costing values inpatient days per *average* patient, whereas bottom-up gross-costing values inpatient days per *individual* patient.

Top-down micro-costing identifies all relevant hospital services at the most detailed level, but values each hospital service per *average* patient (Tan et al., 2009b; Wordsworth et al., 2005). Hospital services may comprise staff time, laboratory services, medical imaging services, medications, medical materials and (surgical) procedures. As the methodology does not require patient-level data, statistical analyses of costs cannot be carried out, and differences between patients cannot be detected (Clement Nee Shrive et al., 2009).

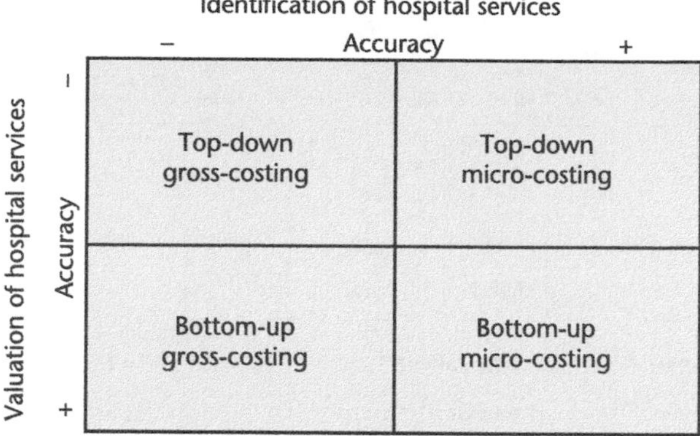

Figure 5.5 Methodology matrix: Level of accuracy of the identification and valuation of hospital services

Sources: Tan, 2009; Tan et al., 2009b.

Bottom-up micro-costing identifies and values all relevant hospital services at the most detailed level. Because the methodology values hospital services per *individual* patient, bottom-up micro-costing enables statistical analyses to determine whether there are cost differences between patients for each single hospital service and combinations of hospital services (Tan et al., 2009b; Wordsworth et al., 2005).

5.3 Costing approaches across Europe

5.3.1 Ascertaining cost data across Europe

Nearly every European country has a unique approach to collecting cost data in order to further develop their DRG-based system(s).

Mandatory cost-accounting systems

Most countries allow their hospitals to use a cost-accounting system which best fulfils their own needs, but some countries require their hospitals to have mandatory cost-accounting systems (such as England and Portugal). However, despite the presence of mandatory cost-accounting systems, some variations between systems may still exist within countries.

Presence of national costing guidelines

In addition, the absence of mandatory cost-accounting systems does not prevent some countries from encouraging systematic cost accounting by means of national costing guidelines. For example, hospitals in France are recommended to apply the hospital cost-accounting model 'analytical accounting'. In Ireland, regulation relating to the collection of cost data is enforced centrally, using a national costing manual and auditing. In Sweden, national guidelines have been developed for cost-per-case calculations.

Cost-accounting data used for calculating DRG prices

The majority of countries use nationally collected cost-accounting data to calculate DRG prices (Austria, England, Estonia, Finland, France, Germany, the Netherlands and Sweden). Other countries have imported DRG weights from abroad (Ireland, Poland, Portugal and Spain), but each of these countries uses at least some cost-accounting data to adjust imported DRG weights to their local situation. Ireland initially adopted a slightly modified version of the Victorian Cost Weights methodology for casemix modelling. These relative cost weights have been refreshed, adjusted to the local context and updated for the Irish health care system in subsequent years. Poland only calculates DRG weights for specific procedures; costs for the remaining procedures are determined relative to the costs of the United Kingdom Healthcare Resource Groups (HRG) system (Version 3.5). Portugal allocates inpatient costs to DRGs based on the cost weights of Maryland in the United States and on the lengths of stay in Portuguese hospitals. Spain also uses relative weights from the United States, adjusting them to the Spanish context. Table 5.1 presents an overview of the different approaches to collecting cost data in 12 European countries.

5.3.2 Cost-accounting methods across Europe

Number (share) of cost-collecting hospitals

In most of the countries that use national cost-accounting data for calculating DRG weights, the calculation is based on a selected number of hospitals from which reliable cost-accounting data are collected and pooled. Selected hospitals typically use comparable cost-accounting systems meeting predefined quality standards (for example, Finland, Germany, the Netherlands and Sweden) (Schreyögg et al., 2006). DRG weights may also be based on cost-accounting data from a sample of hospitals which have contracts with the country's national health insurance fund (such as the EHIF in Estonia), or which participate in ongoing projects (for example, in France). Other countries require all

Table 5.1 Different approaches to collecting cost data in Europe

	Mandatory cost-accounting system	*National costing guidelines*	*Cost-accounting data used for developing DRG prices*
Austria	–	–	×
England	×	×	×
Estonia	–	–	×
Finland	–	–	×
France	–	×	×
Germany	–	×	×
Ireland	–	×	–
Poland	–	–	–
Portugal	×	×	–
Netherlands	×	×	×
Spain	–	–	–
Sweden	–	×	×

hospitals to report their activity and unit costs annually to their regulatory authority (as is the case in England).

For example, the subset of 15–25 cost-collecting hospitals in the Netherlands were required to implement cost-accounting systems that were able to capture patient-level data for the allocation of costs to the individual patient and to support the maintenance, registration and validation of the 30 000 diagnosis–treatment combinations (*Diagnose Behandeling Combinaties*, DBCs).

The regulatory authorities in some countries started to provide special monetary incentives to hospitals which complied with predefined standards for cost accounting. In France, the regional health authorities award the yearly salary for a financial controller, by means of the 'payment for general interest missions' (MiGAC)[1] to each of the hospitals providing cost-accounting data. After having calculated relative weights without using monetary incentives for participating hospitals in the years 2003 and 2004, Germany introduced such payments in 2005. Currently, the Institute for the Hospital Remuneration System (InEK) reimburses hospitals with an additional fee for voluntarily collecting patient-level cost-accounting data. This consists of a lump sum and a variable amount related to the number of delivered cases and their data quality. In 2008, the InEK spent €9 million to compensate hospitals for their additional efforts (InEK, 2009).

There is a trade-off between ensuring high-quality data standards and obtaining a representative number of cost-collecting hospitals. A large number of hospitals may provide a clearer picture of differences in the severity of cases, or in the structure of hospitals in a particular country, insofar as these factors have already not been adjusted for separately. However, a small number of cost-collecting hospitals – with comparable, high-quality cost-accounting systems – may allow the data quality obtained to be higher, but with the disadvantage that data on rare treatments (for multiple trauma patients, for example) might not be available (Schreyögg et al., 2006).

Overhead allocation

For the allocation of overhead costs to the medical departments, European countries either use the direct method (England, Estonia, Finland, the Netherlands and Sweden) or the step-down method (France). Germany intends to use the step-down method in the hospitals from which cost-accounting data are collected. If this is not feasible, however, a combination of the step-down cost-accounting method and other methods (such as the direct method) can be used. In the Netherlands, hospitals are free to choose the method to be used for the allocation of hospital costs. As the allocation method was found to have only a minor impact on individual patients' costs, hospitals commonly use the simple method of direct allocation.

Indirect and direct cost allocation

Most countries require their cost-collecting hospitals to report minimum datasets containing patient and/or hospital characteristics, some clinical parameters (such as diagnoses, status at discharge) as well as cost-accounting data. Minimum datasets containing cost-accounting data are fairly similar across European countries. For example, Finland collects resource-use and unit cost data relating to inpatient days, outpatient visits, laboratory services, medical imaging services, medications, blood products, surgical procedures and pathological services for each treated patient.

In Austria, hospitals can implement cost-accounting systems to suit their needs. However, hospitals financed by State Health Funds report highly aggregated and standardized data (113 out of 264 hospitals). In contrast, most countries apply various weighting statistics in combination with the micro-costing methodology to allocate costs from the medical department to patients. Countries recording data on itemized resource consumption apply the bottom-up approach to allocate hospital costs to *individual* patients (or hospital services) (Finland, Germany, the Netherlands and Sweden). Countries in which patient-level data are not available apply the top-down approach to allocate hospital costs to *average* patients (inpatient admissions) (England, Estonia and France). In England, a working group of costing experts has been established to support the implementation of Patient-Level Information and Costing Systems (PLICS) within the National Health Service (NHS). As of yet, the implementation of PLICS is not mandatory and the number of hospitals that have introduced patient-level costing is not known. In Estonia and France, the calculation of DRG costs is a combination of the top-down accounting model with a (small) proportion of costs being identified at the patient level.

Data checks on reported cost data

In most countries, data checks on reported cost-accounting data initially take place internally at the hospitals. In addition, data checks are commonly carried out annually either by the national authority (in England, Estonia, Germany and the Netherlands) or by the regional authority (in Austria and France). In Finland, ensuring data quality is the sole responsibility of the hospitals, as no official data quality and plausibility checks are undertaken at the national or regional levels. In Sweden, the National Board of Health and Welfare publishes reports on coding activity and quality based on information from the National Patient Register (NPR) but it is the county councils' responsibility to check the quality of data through case record audits.

In most countries, national/regional data checks on reported cost-accounting data primarily focus on resource-use information, in terms of technical and clinical validity; that is, coded hospital services are held against certain patient and/or hospital characteristics. For example, a check is performed to establish whether a procedure is allowed/plausible for a specific hospital or patient. In some countries, data checks are additionally performed on unit cost information (Germany, the Netherlands and Sweden). In Germany, unit costs are compared to minimum and maximum values, to unit cost ratios between hospital services, and to corresponding resource-use information; for example, costs for a hip replacement must reflect the material cost of implants. Cost-accounting data are either checked for all hospitals (in Germany, the Netherlands and Sweden) or for random samples (in Austria, England, Estonia and France).

Table 5.2 presents some characteristics of the cost-accounting methods in eight European countries, using their own cost-accounting data for calculating DRG prices.

Table 5.2 Different characteristics of the cost-accounting methods in eight European countries

	Overhead cost allocation to medical departments	*Indirect cost allocation to patients*	*Direct cost allocation to patients*	*Number (share) of cost-collecting hospitals*	*Data checks (regularity)*
Austria	Varying by hospital	Varying by hospital	Gross-costing	20 reference hospitals (~ 8% of all hospitals)	Regional authority (irregularly)
England	Direct	Weighting statistics	Top-down micro-costing	All hospitals	National authority (annually)
Estonia	Direct	Mark-up percentage	Top-down micro-costing	Hospitals contracted with the EHIF	National authority (annually)
Finland	Direct	Weighting statistics	Bottom-up micro-costing	5 reference hospitals meeting particular cost-accounting standards (~ 30% of specialized care)	No, responsibility of hospitals
France	Step down	Weighting statistics	Top-down micro-costing	99 volunteering hospitals participating in the ENCC (~ 13% of inpatient admissions)	Regional authority (annually)
Germany	Step down (preferably)	Weighting statistics	Bottom-up micro-costing	125 volunteering hospitals meeting InEK cost-accounting standards (~ 6% of all hospitals)	National authority (annually)
Netherlands	Direct	Weighting statistics	Bottom-up micro-costing	Unit costs: 15–25 volunteering general hospitals (~ 24% of all hospitals)	National authority (annually)
Sweden	Direct	Weighting statistics	Bottom-up micro-costing	Hospitals with case costing systems (~ 62% of inpatients admissions)	National and regional authorities (annually)

5.3.3 Breadth of costs covered by European DRG-based payments

The relative importance of any DRG-based hospital payment system is determined by the share of hospital costs that are covered by DRG-based payments (see Chapter 6, section 6.3, Table 6.2). DRG payment is the principal means of reimbursing hospitals in the majority of European countries. For example, inpatient care funding through DRGs represents 75–85 per cent of hospital costs in Germany and Portugal. However, most countries exclude some (medical) specialties and/or hospital services due to (Schreyögg et al., 2006):

- the usual incentive set by the DRG system to shorten the patient's length of stay, which is considered harmful in these specialties (for example, intensive care);
- coding problems in hospital services for which DRG prices cannot be reliably calculated because they are rarely provided (for example, for multiple trauma care);
- circumstances involving specialties in which a diagnosis seems to be a bad predictor for costs (for example, psychiatric care).

Some countries therefore exclude the costs for rehabilitation (France, Germany, Ireland and Sweden), psychiatric services (England, Finland, France, Germany and Ireland), and intensive and emergency care (Finland, France and Poland). Other costs excluded from the system may involve primary care services, community services and ambulance services (England); neonatology, dialysis and radiotherapy performed during hospitalization (France); geriatric services (Ireland); and burn treatment (Sweden). Costs for excluded hospital services are mostly reimbursed via supplementary fees, fee-for-service reimbursement and/or surcharges (see Chapter 6 of this volume).

In addition, the costs for expensive drugs (in France, Germany, the Netherlands, Poland and Sweden) and/or expensive materials (in France, Spain and Sweden) are not commonly reimbursed using DRGs.

With respect to specialties, the costs for education and research are not commonly funded through DRGs. Some countries also exclude capital costs and interest (for example Austria, Finland, Germany and Ireland) and allowance for debts (for example Germany and Ireland). Other disregarded costs may relate to taxes, charges and insurance (in Germany), pensions (in Ireland) and accreditation (in Sweden).

5.4 Developing DRG systems with cost data

5.4.1 Relevance of cost-accounting systems

Cost-accounting data play an important role in calculating DRG weights (Nathanson, 1984). If the data given by cost-accounting systems are imprecise, hospitals are likely to be over- or underpaid for specific DRGs. In practice, profitable DRGs may compensate for less-profitable DRGs (cross-subsidizing). However, if cost-accounting data lead to an overestimated payment for a specific

DRG, hospitals are disincentivized to reorganize treatment processes in order to improve efficiency for certain groups of patients. On the other hand, if cost-accounting data lead to an underestimated payment for a specific DRG, hospitals are disincentivized to provide high-quality care as this may lead to costs above the payment level. These hospitals may start to compromise quality in order to reduce their costs (or losses). Consequently, the appropriate level of hospital payment to a large extent determines the effectiveness and fairness of DRG-based hospital payment systems. Hospital managers, as well as regulating authorities, should consider whether the benefits of more reliable cost data justify the additional costs and complexity incurred in improving the cost-accounting systems to obtain accurate and detailed information. The choice that they make between costing methods should reflect the importance of accurate cost estimates, feasibility and the costs associated with introducing the system (Clement Nee Shrive et al., 2009).

Several previous studies have demonstrated that DRG-based hospital payments do not always adequately reflect costs (Busse et al., 2008; Heerey et al., 2002; Skeie et al., 2002; Tan et al., 2009a). This may be explained by inaccuracies in the patient classification and cost-accounting systems.

Inaccuracies in the patient classification

Although health care providers have long contended that every patient is unique, the reality of DRG-based hospital payment systems is that patients are grouped together, and that some groups represent a mixture of diagnoses to a greater extent than others. Countries with itemized resource use per patient commonly use cost accounting to support adequate resource allocation, to assess the homogeneity of resource consumption within each DRG, to calculate separate DRG payments for patients requiring more complex resource use (for example, due to complications and co-morbidities (CCs)) and/or to test the effect of changes in the PCS (for example France, Germany, the Netherlands and Sweden). For instance, medical DRGs were found to be less homogeneous than surgical DRGs in France, but the creation of new DRGs was restricted by the small number of cases which would be affected in different medical stays. Cost accounting has shown that the dispersion around the mean costs varies greatly between DRGs, with highly variable DRGs most likely to comprise a wide variety of different diagnoses and treatments (Jackson, 2000).

Inaccuracies in cost-accounting systems

The extent to which cost-accounting systems could support the efficient and fair use of DRG systems as a reimbursement tool relies on:

- the number and composition (sample characteristics) of hospitals from which cost-accounting data are collected and the quality of data delivered by these hospitals;
- the accuracy of the cost-accounting method (see subsection 5.4.2);
- the ability to maintain/update the cost-accounting data in a timely manner.

5.4.2 The accuracy of the cost-accounting method

The extent to which cost-accounting systems could support the effective and fair development of DRG-based hospital payment systems as a reimbursement tool is determined by the accuracy of the cost-accounting method used in the respective country or region. However, the nature of costs is such that the more refined the analysis, the more costly it generally is. The reciprocal method theoretically allocates hospital costs to medical departments most precisely. At the same time, it is more time-consuming than the methods used across Europe ('step-down' and 'direct' methods). Earlier studies have revealed no statistically significant relationship between alternative cost-accounting methods and the unit costs produced (St-Hilaire & Crepeau, 2000; Zuurbier & Krabbe-Alkemade, 2007). Likewise, relative value units are believed to most closely reflect actual resource consumption for the allocation of hospital costs to patients, but their calculation requires more detailed data than operational methods require (weighting statistics and marginal mark-up percentages). Weighting statistics have been shown to provide reasonably similar cost estimates, while marginal mark-up percentages result in substantially different cost estimates compared to those based on relative value units (Tan et al., 2009c).

Bottom-up micro-costing may be the preferred methodology for calculating DRG weights because it helps hospital managers to understand whether cost differences between and within DRGs arise from variation in resource-use intensity or from variations in the costs of hospital services; it can also help to understand the distributional form of the cost-accounting data on which DRG payments are based (Jackson, 2000; Tan et al., 2009b). Unlike the alternative methodologies, bottom-up micro-costing allows for insight into the costs directly employed for *individual* patients, cost homogeneities and high-cost outliers. However, countries need to rely on top-down micro-costing (or gross-costing) if their hospitals' cost-accounting systems do not collect itemized resource-use data for each individual patient (as is the case in England, for example). Top-down micro-costing has proven to be a strong alternative to bottom-up micro-costing in terms of accuracy, and the approach is fairly feasible with respect to data availability, costs and complexity (Tan et al., 2009b). In contrast, both economic theory and empirical studies support the notion that gross-costing results in rather inaccurate cost estimates. For example, the patient's diagnosis has an important effect on the use of resources, and this is something which is not generally reflected by gross-costing methods (Jackson, 2000; Swindle et al., 1999).

5.5 Impact of cost accounting on hospitals

Currently, cost-accounting systems certainly represent an improvement over the information that was formerly available in many institutions. Cost-accounting systems offer an efficient and clinically sound approach for describing and managing hospital activity, in order to offer greater transparency in the financing of health care. Hospitals across Europe recognized that cost-accounting data are fundamental for systematic benchmarking and for managed competition approaches that can improve the efficiency of hospital service delivery (Schuster et al., 2006; van de Ven & Schut, 2009). First, cost-accounting systems facilitate the comparison of performance indicators, along with productivity and efficiency parameters. Benchmarking has also helped hospitals to manage and control operating processes and thus improves their performance; for example, it encouraged the use of DRGs in assessing the budgetary impact of anticipated changes in the volume and casemix of patients and in monitoring actual expenditure versus expected levels (for example in England, France and Estonia). Second, managed competition has allowed authorities in many European countries to provide powerful incentives to other actors in the system, such as health insurers/sickness funds (Busse et al., 2006). It led to the use of DRGs to negotiate on service quality and access, as well as on detailed cost- and volume-based financial components (for example in England, Estonia, the Netherlands and Spain). Finally, cost-accounting data enable regulatory authorities to monitor unintended incentives that are supposed to accompany DRG-based payments, such as treatment of patients whose expected costs are lower than the associated reimbursement, up-coding of expensive DRGs to increase revenue, cost minimization or shifting of treatment costs onto other parties, and compromising quality of care (see Chapter 6 of this volume).

5.6 Conclusions: Which is driving which?

One may argue that cost accounting is driving the further development of DRGs. The introduction of DRG-based hospital payment systems in Europe partly originated from the absence, or inadequacy, of information relating to cost data (Feyrer et al., 2005). Cost-accounting data made it possible to validate cost homogeneities and to detect cost-outliers in the patient population. This led to revisions and refinements of the existing DRG systems. However, one could also argue that DRGs are driving cost accounting. The introduction of comprehensive and standardized cost-accounting systems was encouraged by the need to collect data for calculating DRG weights as well as supporting hospital management and auditing. Revisions of existing cost-accounting systems are undertaken to improve the effectiveness and fairness of DRG-based hospital payment systems. Regardless of which argument one chooses, the following observations cannot be disputed: (1) DRG systems cannot function well without accurate cost accounting; and (2) the necessity of cost-accounting systems to use costs based on a unit of analysis is met by DRGs. However, it is crucial to note that DRG and cost-accounting systems should be developed independently of each other; otherwise it will be impossible to validate the systems' performance individually.

The way in which cost-accounting data are collected for developing DRG-based hospital payment systems and the way in which DRG weights are calculated differ substantially among the European countries concerned. Two observations are important in this regard. First, the characteristics of the DRG and cost-accounting systems reflect the current situation but are, in effect, subject to (rapid) change based on the dynamics of the systems they represent.

Second, there is no 'best' cost-accounting system in general, because the choice of the system must be made based on the characteristics of the cost-collecting hospitals and the national health systems concerned, as well as on the objective that health policy-makers intend to fulfil by using DRG systems. However, the only way to truly evaluate DRGs in terms of medical coherence and cost homogeneity is to define costs at the *individual* patient level. Cost-accounting systems may not be sufficiently meaningful to measure, compare and improve efficiency of hospital care if DRG costs are not defined according to bottom-up micro-costing.

Each DRG-based hospital payment system has similar aims (for example, to increase transparency, to ensure adequate hospital reimbursement) but reaching these is to be achieved within different nation-specific health system contexts (see Chapter 2). Therefore, it is unlikely that cost-accounting systems across Europe will be harmonized in the near future. However, European countries are likely to deal with many of the same issues concerning the ongoing process of developing and updating DRGs and cost-accounting systems in the years to come. An overall similarity in terms of the problems they encounter may in time lead to greater interest in finding common solutions that are adjustable for each country.

5.7 Note

1 *Missions d'intérêt général et de l'aide à la contractualisation*: Missions of general interest and assistance with contracting, including payments for education, research and public health programmes.

5.8 References

Berki, S.E. (1985). DRGs, incentives, hospitals, and physicians. *Health Affairs (Millwood)*, 4:70–6.

Busse, R., Schreyögg, J., Smith, P.C. (2006). Hospital case payment systems in Europe. *Health Care Management Science*, 9:211–13.

Busse, R., Schreyögg, J., Smith, P.C. (2008). Variability in healthcare treatment costs amongst nine EU countries – Results from the HealthBASKET project. *Health Economics*, 17:1–8.

Clement Nee Shrive, F.M., Ghali, W.A., Donaldson, C., Manns, B.J. (2009). The impact of using different costing methods on the results of an economic evaluation of cardiac care: micro-costing vs gross-costing approaches. *Health Economics*, 18:377–88.

Cohen, D.J., Breall, J.A., Ho, K.K. et al. (1993). Economics of elective coronary revascularization. Comparison of costs and charges for conventional angioplasty, directional atherectomy, stenting and bypass surgery. *Journal of the American College of Cardiology*, 22:1052–9.

Cooper, R., Kaplan, R.S. (1988). Measure costs right. Make the right decisions. *Harvard Business Review*, Sep/Oct:96–103.

Drummond, M.F., Sculpher, M.J., Torrance, G.W., O'Brien, B.J., Stoddart, G.L. (2005). *Methods for the Economic Evaluation of Health Care Programmes*. Oxford: Oxford University Press.

Feyrer, R., Rosch, J., Weyand, M., Kunzmann, U. (2005). Cost unit accounting based on a clinical pathway: a practical tool for DRG implementation. *The Thoracic and cardiovascular surgeon*, 53:261–6.

Finkler, S.A., Ward, D.M., Baker, J.J. (2007). *Essentials of Cost Accounting for Health Care Organizations*. New York, NY: Aspen Publishers.

Heerey, A., McGowan, B., Ryan, M., Barry, M. (2002). Micro-costing versus DRGs in the provision of cost estimates for use in pharmacoeconomic evaluation. *Expert Review of Pharmacoeconomics and Outcomes Research*, 2:29–33.

Horngren, C.T., Datar, S.M., Foster, G. (2006). *Cost Accounting: A Managerial Emphasis*. Upper Saddle River, NJ: Pearson Prentice Hall.

InEK (2009). *Abschlussbericht zur Weiterentwicklung des G-DRG-Systems für das Jahr 2010*. Siegburg: Institut für das Entgeltsystem im Krankenhaus gGmbH.

Jackson, T. (2000). Cost estimates for hospital inpatient care in Australia: evaluation of alternative sources. *Australian and New Zealand Journal of Public Health*, 24:234–41.

Nathanson, M. (1984). DRG cost-per-case management. Comprehensive cost accounting systems give chains an edge. *Modern Healthcare*, 14(3):122, 124, 128.

Ott, K. (1996). A comparison of craniotomy and Gamma Knife charges in a community-based Gamma Knife Center. *Stereotactic and Functional Neurosurgery*, 66(Suppl 1.):357–64.

Schreyögg, J., Stargardt, T., Tiemann, O., Busse, R. (2006). Methods to determine reimbursement rates for diagnosis related groups (DRG): a comparison of nine European countries. *Health Care Management Science*, 9:215–23.

Schuster, M., Kuntz, L., Hermening, D. et al. (2006). The use of diagnosis-related-groups data for external benchmarking of anesthesia and intensive care services. *Anaesthesist*, 55(1):26–32.

Skeie, B., Mishra, V., Vaaler, S., Amlie, E. (2002). A comparison of actual cost, DRG-based cost, and hospital reimbursement for liver transplant patients. *Transplant International*, 15:439–45.

St-Hilaire, C., Crepeau, P.K. (2000). Hospital and unit cost-allocation methods. *Healthcare Management Forum*, 13:12–32.

Swindle, R., Lukas, C.V., Meyer, D.A., Barnett, P.G., Hendricks, A.M. (1999). Cost analysis in the department of veterans affairs: consensus and future directions. *Medical Care*, 37:AS3–8.

Tan, S.S. (2009). *Micro-costing in Economic Evaluations: Issues of Accuracy, Feasibility, Consistency and Generalizability*. Rotterdam: Erasmus Universiteit Rotterdam.

Tan, S.S., Oppe, M., Zoet-Nugteren, S.K. et al. (2009a). A micro-costing study of diagnostic tests for the detection of coronary artery disease in the Netherlands. *European Journal of Radiology*, 72:98–103.

Tan, S.S., Rutten, F.F., van Ineveld, B.M., Redekop, W.K., Hakkaart-van Roijen, L. (2009b). Comparing methodologies for the cost estimation of hospital services. *European Journal of Health Economics*, 10:39–45.

Tan, S.S., van Ineveld, B.M., Redekop, W.K., Hakkaart-van Roijen, L. (2009c). Comparing methodologies for the allocation of overhead and capital costs to hospital services. *Value in Health*, 12:530–5.

Van de Ven, W.P., Schut, F.T. (2009). Managed competition in the Netherlands: still work-in-progress. *Health Economics*, 18:253–5.

Williams, S.V., Finkler, S.A., Murphy, C.M., Eisenberg, J.M. (1982). Improved cost allocation in casemix accounting. *Medical Care*, 20:450–9.

Wordsworth, S., Ludbrook, A., Caskey, F., Macleod, A. (2005). Collecting unit cost data in multicentre studies. Creating comparable methods. *European Journal of Health Economics*, 6:38–44.

Zuurbier, J., Krabbe-Alkemade, Y. (2007). *Onderhandelen Over DBC's [Negotiating on DBCs]*. Maarssen: Elsevier Gezondheidszorg.

chapter six

DRG-based hospital payment: Intended and unintended consequences

Francesc Cots, Pietro Chiarello, Xavier Salvador, Xavier Castells and Wilm Quentin[1]

6.1 Introduction

Almost 30 years after the first introduction of a diagnosis-related group (DRG)-based hospital payment system in the United States in 1983 (Fetter, 1991), DRG systems have become the basis for hospital payment in most European countries, and in many other countries around the world (Kimberly et al., 2008). In fact, as illustrated in Chapter 2, one of the main purposes of the use of DRG systems in all countries discussed in this volume is to enable DRG-based hospital payment. Figure 6.1 illustrates the basic set-up of DRG-based hospital payment systems: (1) a patient classification system (PCS) is used to group patients with similar clinical characteristics and relatively homogeneous resource consumption into DRGs (see Chapter 4); (2) some kind of hospital cost information is used to determine DRG weight levels, usually at (about) the average treatment costs of patients falling within a specific DRG (see Chapter 5); (3) DRG weights are converted into monetary values and the payment rate may be adjusted for structural (teaching status, region) and further resource-consumption variables (length of stay, utilization of high-cost drugs or services); before (4) hospitals are paid on the basis of the number and type of DRGs that they produce.

DRG-based hospital payment systems provide a specific set of incentives that is different from other hospital payment systems, and the popularity of DRG-based systems is related to the fact that they are thought to have a number of (predominantly desirable) effects on quality and efficiency, which are discussed

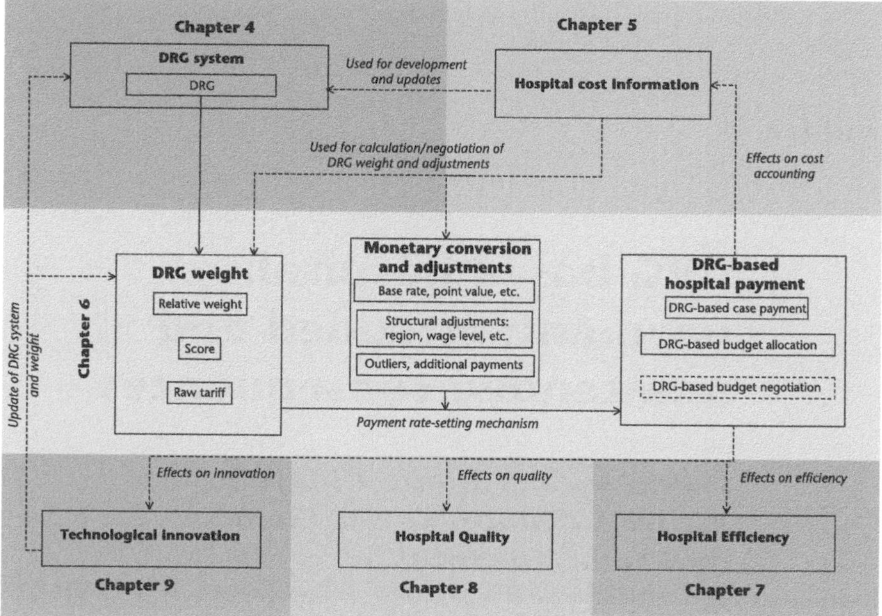

Figure 6.1 DRG-based hospital payment within the framework of this book

in Chapters 7 and 8 of this volume. Yet, since the introduction of the first DRG-based hospital payment system, discussions regarding negative or 'unintended' consequences of these systems have persisted in the United States (Lave, 1989; Ellis, 1998) as well as in Europe, following the adoption of DRGs for hospital payment (Böcking et al., 2005; Steinbusch et al., 2007; Farrar et al., 2009).

This chapter focuses on DRG-based hospital payment systems in the 12 countries included in this book, and on the main incentives generally attributed to these systems, which may generate both intended and unintended consequences. The chapter starts with an overview of how the payment rate is determined in DRG-based hospital payment systems (section 6.2). This is followed in section 6.3 by an introduction to the two main models of DRG-based hospital payment; namely, DRG-based case payment and DRG-based budget allocation. Section 6.4 provides a theoretical discussion of the main incentives attributed to the most basic model of DRG-based hospital payment and the related potential intended and unintended consequences. In section 6.5 we discuss how the countries analysed attempt to overcome some of the unintended consequences by modifying the basic model of DRG-based payment. Section 6.6 summarizes the findings and concludes that the incentives related to DRG-based payment systems have the potential to contribute to achieving the intended consequences, as long as they succeed at avoiding the unintended ones by implementing adequate control measures.

6.2 Paying hospitals on the basis of DRGs: Determining the payment rate

As illustrated in Figure 6.1, the hospital payment rate in DRG-based hospital payment systems is determined on the basis of the DRG weights and their conversion into monetary values. In general, the aim is that DRG weights are set at about the average costs of treating patients within a DRG. However, countries differ in terms of how they express DRG weights, usually calculated on the basis of information about average costs (see Chapter 5), or alternatively, a 'best practice' approach (see Chapter 7). Table 6.1 shows the distribution of the three main approaches that prevail in the 12 countries included in this book: (1) relative weights, (2) raw tariffs, and (3) scores. Each of these approaches corresponds to a specific monetary conversion method. The applicability of DRG weights and monetary conversion factors differs between countries and allows for adjusting hospital payments according to structural factors and/or national or regional priorities.

6.2.1 DRG weights and their applicability in 12 European countries

Most countries calculate DRG relative weights or use imported and adapted relative weights from other countries. The idea behind using DRG relative weights is that the weight of a DRG is expressed in relation to the average treatment costs of all cases in a country. In greatly simplified terms, DRG relative weights are computed by dividing the average costs of cases falling within a DRG through the average treatment costs of all cases in a country. Consequently, a DRG with a relative weight of one implies that average treatment costs of patients falling into that DRG are equal to the average treatment costs of all cases within the country. If relative weights are imported from abroad, DRG relative weights do not necessarily reflect national practice patterns. However, by adapting relative weights to national cost data (as in Ireland and Portugal, for example), countries aim to ensure that the adapted relative weights are linked to national resource-consumption patterns and that DRG weights can be interpreted in terms of above/below-average treatment costs.

England, France, the Netherlands and Spain calculate raw tariffs. These differ from relative weights in that they are expressed in monetary terms. In general, raw tariffs are calculated directly from the average treatment costs of patients within a DRG, even though they may be adjusted for inflation (as in England) or for national global budget control purposes (as in France). In Spain, raw tariffs are calculated on the basis of imported internal relative weights and national cost-accounting data. Interestingly, although the raw tariff is already expressed in monetary terms, it is not necessarily equal to the actual hospital payment, which is determined after further adjustments (discussed in more detail in the sections that follow).

Austria and Poland are the only two countries that express DRG weights as scores. The difference between scores and raw tariffs is that the score is not expressed in monetary terms but as a number of points. At the same time, and

Table 6.1 DRG weights, monetary conversion and their applicability in 12 European countries

Country	*DRG weight (unit)*	*Applicability of DRG weight*	*Monetary conversion*	*Applicability of conversion rate*
Austria	Score	Nationwide	(Implicit) Point value	Depending on state
England	Raw tariff	Nationwide (separate tariffs for emergencies, elective cases, day cases, children, orthopaedic activity)	Market forces factor	Hospital-specific
Estonia	Relative weight	Nationwide	Base rate	Nationwide
Finland	Relative weight	National (8 districts), District-specific (5 districts)	Base rate	Hospital-specific
France	Raw tariff	Nationwide (separate tariffs for public and private hospitals)	(1) Regional adjustment (2) Transition coefficient (until 2012)	(1) Region-specific (2) Hospital-specific
Germany	Relative weight	Nationwide	Base rate	State-wide
Ireland	(Adapted) Relative weight (locally referred to as relative value)	Nationwide (separate weights for paediatric hospitals)	Base rates	(1) Specific to one of four hospital peer groups (2) Hospital-specific
Netherlands	Raw tariff	Nationwide (67% of DRGs), hospital-specific (33% of DRGs)	Direct (no conversion)	Not applicable
Poland	Score	Nationwide (separate tariffs for emergencies, elective cases, day cases)	Point value	Nationwide
Portugal	(Adapted) Relative weight	Nationwide	Base rate	Hospital peer group
Spain (Catalonia)	(1) (Adapted) Raw tariff (AP-DRGs); (2) (Imported) Relative weight (CMS-DRGs)	(1) Nationwide (AP-DRGs) (2) Region-wide (CMS-DRGs)	(1) Direct (no conversion) (2) Base rate	(1) Not applicable (2) Region-wide (CMS-DRGs)
Sweden	Relative weight	Nationwide, county-specific (some counties)	Base rate	County-specific

Source: Based on the country-specific chapters in Part Two of this volume (most recent information available).

in contrast to relative weights, the score does not relate the DRG weight of one DRG to the average treatment costs of all cases within a country. Therefore, unlike relative weights, scores and raw tariffs do not facilitate the calculation of the casemix indices (CMIs) of hospitals, which are frequently used in countries using a relative/weight approach to comparing differences in patient populations across hospitals.

In the majority of countries, the same DRG weights apply to all hospitals and regions, nationwide. However, in Ireland, a separate set of relative weights is calculated for paediatric hospitals, and in England, different tariffs exist for (amongst others) day cases, emergencies, elective cases, children, and orthopaedic activity. In Finland and Sweden, national relative weights exist as well as district- or county-specific relative weights, and districts or counties are free to choose the set of relative weights that best suits their needs. In France, separate tariffs are calculated for public and private hospitals, as physicians' salaries are included only in DRG-based payments for public hospitals. In the Netherlands, national tariffs apply only for 67 per cent of DRGs, while 33 per cent of tariffs are the result of negotiations between hospitals and insurers. In Spain, raw tariffs for All Patient (AP-)DRGs apply only for patients treated in regions in which they are not ordinarily resident, while relative weights of Centers for Medicare and Medicaid Services (CMS-)DRGs apply only to the autonomous community of Catalonia. Furthermore, even if the DRG weight is the same for all hospitals and regions within the country, monetary conversion and adjustments may result in different payments for hospitals in different regions (see subsection 6.2.2).

6.2.2 Monetary conversion and structural adjustments

Table 6.1 also shows that all countries except for the Netherlands and Spain (AP-DRGs) multiply DRG weights with some sort of monetary conversion factor in order to determine actual DRG-based hospital payments. All countries that use a 'relative weight' approach multiply the relative weight with a so-called 'base rate'. However, significant differences exist between countries in terms of the applicability of the base rate to different hospitals. Estonia is the only country in which the same base rate is applied to all hospitals, nationwide. In Finland and Sweden, base rates are calculated specifically for every hospital according to predetermined global budgets and the expected hospital activity. In Germany, different base rates are negotiated between the self-governmental bodies (most importantly the social health insurance associations and the hospitals) for every *Land* (federal state). In Ireland, an increasing share of the DRG-based budgets is determined on the basis of a hospital peer-group (for example, major teaching hospitals, other hospitals, paediatric hospitals) base rate, which ensures that similar hospitals are grouped together for payment purposes; the hospital-specific base rate, which sheltered hospitals from excessive budget cuts during the introduction period, currently determines only 20 per cent of hospitals' budgets. In Portugal, a similar approach is taken, as hospitals are also paid on the basis of a base rate that is specific to the hospitals' peer group. In Catalonia, the base rate is the same for the entire region.

In England and France, raw tariffs are multiplied by adjustment factors, which ensure that certain structural characteristics (such as higher salary levels), are taken into account in DRG-based payments. In addition, DRG weights in France are still adjusted for a transition coefficient, reflecting historical cost patterns of hospitals in order to shelter them from excessive budget cuts, which is similar to the approach used in Ireland and other countries during the introduction period of DRG-based payments. In the Netherlands and Spain (for nation-wide use of AP-DRGs) raw tariffs are not adjusted but are directly used for payment.

In Poland, DRG scores are multiplied by a point value that is the same for the entire country. In Austria, the point value is implicit and state specific, as point values are not published and hospital budget allocations are determined on the basis of state-specific rules. For example, some states inflate the scores of teaching hospitals or hospitals located in areas with higher salary levels. The implicit point value is then determined by dividing the entire inpatient budget available for DRG-based payment within a state through the total (adjusted) scores produced by all hospitals. In Poland, the point value depends on the available national hospital budget and is determined through negotiations between the National Health Fund (NFZ), the Ministry of Health and representatives of associations of medical professionals.

6.3 DRG-based hospital payment

After monetary conversion and structural adjustments, hospitals in all 12 countries are paid – to at least some extent – on the basis of DRGs. Table 6.2 shows the distribution of DRG-based case payment and DRG-based budget allocation systems across countries. It also indicates the percentage of hospital revenues related to DRGs in acute care hospitals, and specifies further payment components of the hospital payment system in each country.

Most countries included in this book use a variant of DRG-based case payment systems, whereby each discharged patient is grouped into an applicable DRG, and hospitals receive a payment per case that is determined by the weight of that DRG (after monetary conversion and relevant adjustments). Several other countries use some kind of a DRG-based budget allocation system, whereby the available regional or national hospital budget is distributed to individual hospitals on the basis of the DRGs that they produced during one of the previous years, or that they are expected to produce in the next year. In these cases, the casemix (that is, the sum of the weights of all DRGs produced by a hospital) and the CMI (the casemix divided by the number of discharges) are usually the determining factors. In addition, some countries with DRG-based case payment systems – such as Germany or Finland – use DRGs to negotiate global hospital budgets, which limit (to a certain degree) the total amount of money that hospitals can earn from DRG-based case payments.

Table 6.2 shows that DRG-based hospital payment accounts for the majority of hospital revenues in all countries except for Spain (that is, Catalonia) and Estonia. Consequently, the incentives related to these payment systems are particularly important. However, it should be borne in mind that in most countries, psychiatric, rehabilitation and long-term care hospitals are not financed on the basis of DRGs, although several countries plan to extend their DRG systems beyond the acute care hospital sector (see Chapter 4). In addition, the hospital payment system in almost all countries includes other payment components aside from DRG-based hospital payment, such as global budgets and additional payments for certain activities or cost categories. For example, in some countries, DRG-based payments do not include capital costs (see Chapter 5), and almost all countries have additional payments for certain innovative and high-cost services (see Chapters 4 and Chapter 9 of this volume), as well as additional budgets for teaching and research or availability of emergency care.

To appreciate fully the discussion that follows regarding the incentives associated with DRG-based payment systems, it is important to be aware of the differences between and within the two basic models of DRG-based hospital payment. First, in theory, DRG-based case payment systems could provide stronger incentives to hospitals than DRG-based budget allocation systems

Table 6.2 DRG-based hospital payment for acute care hospitals

Country	*DRG-based hospital payment model*	*% of hospital revenues related to DRGs*	*Other payment components*
Austria	DRG-based budget allocation	≈ 96	Per diems
England	DRG-based case payments	≈ 60	GB, additional payments
Estonia	DRG-based case payments	≈ 39	FFS (33%), per diem (28%)
Finland	In 13 out of 21 districts: DRG-based case payments (within GB)	Varies	Varies
France	DRG-based case payments, MLPC	≈ 80	GB, additional payments
Germany	DRG-based case payments (within GB)	≈ 80	GB, additional payments
Ireland	DRG-based budget allocation	≈ 80	GB, additional payments
Netherlands	DRG-based case payments (within GB for 67% of DRGs)	≈ 84	GB, additional payments
Poland	DRG-based case payments, MLPC	≥ 60	GB, additional payments
Portugal	(1) DRG-based budget allocation (NHS) (2) DRG-based case payments (health insurance)	≈ 80	Additional payments
Spain (Catalonia)	DRG-based budget allocation (Catalonia)	≈ 20	GB (based on structural index), FFS, additional payments
Sweden	DRG-based case payments with volume ceilings or GBs (region-specific allocation methods)	Varies	Varies

Source: Based on the country-specific chapters in Part Two of this volume (most recent information available).

Notes: FFS: fee-for-service (payment); GB: global budget; MLPC: macro-level price control.

because the link between hospital service provision and payment is more direct and transparent: hospitals know how much money they can expect if providing a specific set of services to a specific patient. In contrast, in DRG-based budget allocation systems, hospitals only know that the provision of a specific set of services to a specific patient in one year will increase the DRG-based budget for one of the following years, but the exact size of the payment remains unknown: it depends on the number of DRGs produced by other hospitals and on the available budget in the following year. Consequently, it is more difficult for hospitals to predict whether the provision of certain DRGs is profitable or not.

Second, incentives relating to DRG-based case payment systems can be more or less intensive, depending on country-specific modifications. For example, in Germany or the Netherlands, where DRG-based case payment systems are operated within global budgets, the incentives to increase hospital activity are less strong than in England, where hospital activity is not (yet) limited by global budgets or volume thresholds. Furthermore, the situation in countries with DRG-based case payment systems that operate within global budgets differs depending on whether or not hospitals are allowed to exceed the budgets. For example, in Germany, hospitals are allowed to exceed the budget but are paid at a reduced rate for those cases that are treated in addition to the negotiated budget. In the Netherlands, however, hospitals must pay back at the end of the year all revenue from DRG-based case payments that they received in excess of the global budget.

Third, independent of the model of DRG-based hospital payment, the strength of the theoretical incentives (see section 6.4) depends on how the monetary conversion rate is determined. For example, on the one hand, in Poland, where a nationally uniform monetary conversion rate is used, hospitals face strong incentives to reduce their treatment costs to below the DRG payment rate. On the other hand, in Finland, hospitals are paid according to a hospital-specific payment rate, as the base rate is determined by dividing the negotiated hospital budget by the predicted activity. Consequently, there are no incentives for Finnish hospitals to lower their costs to the level of treatment costs in other hospitals – and even less so since any potential deficits accruing to hospitals are compensated by the municipalities, which are both the purchasers and providers of hospital care.

6.4 DRG-based hospital payment in theory: Incentives and their consequences

As already mentioned, the principal reason for the popularity of DRG-based hospital payment systems is that they are thought to have predominantly desirable effects on hospital efficiency and quality. In general, there are three main incentives attributed to DRG-based hospital payment systems (Lave, 1989). Hospitals are incentivized (1) to reduce costs per treated patient, (2) to increase revenues per patient, and (3) to increase the number of patients. Table 6.3 summarizes these basic incentives of DRG-based hospital payment systems, presents the most important response strategies of hospitals, and indicates whether these imply positive or negative effects on efficiency and quality.

Table 6.3 Incentives of DRG-based hospital payment systems and their effects on quality and efficiency

Incentives of DRG-based hospital payment	*Strategies of hospitals*	*Effects*
1. Reduce costs per patient	**a) Reduce length of stay**	
	• optimize internal care pathways	• quality ↑, efficiency ↑
	• transfer to other providers	
	– improve coordination/integration with other providers	• quality ↑, efficiency ↑
	– transfer/avoidance of unprofitable cases ('dumping' or 'cost-shifting')	• quality ↓
	• inappropriate early discharge ('bloody discharge')	• quality ↓
	b) Reduce intensity of provided services	
	• avoid delivering unnecessary services	• efficiency ↑
	• substitute high-cost services with low-cost alternatives (labour/capital)	• efficiency ↑
	• withhold necessary services ('skimping/undertreatment')	• quality ↓
	c) Select patients	
	• specialize in treating patients for which the hospital has a competitive advantage	• efficiency ↑, quality ↑
	• select low-cost patients within DRGs ('cream skimming')	• efficiency ↓
2. Increase revenue per patient	**a) Change coding practice**	
	• improve coding of diagnoses and procedures	• quality↑
	• fraudulent reclassification of patients, e.g. by adding inexistent secondary diagnoses ('up-coding')	• efficiency ↓
	b) Change practice patterns	
	• provide services that lead to reclassification of patients into higher paying DRGs ('gaming/ overtreatment')	• efficiency ↓, quality ↓
3. Increase number of patients	**a) Change admission rules**	
	• reduce waiting list	• efficiency ↑
	• split care episodes into multiple admissions	• efficiency ↓↑, quality ↓↑
	• admit patients for unnecessary services ('supplier-induced demand')	• efficiency ↓
	b) Improve reputation of hospital	
	• improve quality of services	quality ↑
	• focus efforts exclusively on measurable areas	quality ↓↑

Taking a step back: how are these incentives generated? The first main incentive (that is, to reduce costs per case) is generated because, in mathematical terms, the most basic DRG-based hospital (case) payment system is one in which hospital revenue for treating a patient falling into a specific DRG (R^1) is determined by the fixed payment rate per DRG_1 ($\hat{p}_1$) (Ellis & McGuire, 1986):

$$R^1 = \hat{p}_1 \quad (1)$$

Figure 6.2 provides a simplified graphical illustration of the relationship between costs, length of stay, revenue of hospitals, and the incentives related to this basic DRG-based hospital payment system for a hypothetical standard patient in DRG_1. As hospital revenue (R^1) per patient in DRG_1 does not depend on the costs of service provision, hospitals are strongly incentivized to reduce their costs below the payment rate ($\hat{p}_1$).

The three most important response strategies for hospitals trying to reduce costs per case are (Berki, 1985; Miraldo et al., 2006): (1a) to reduce the length of stay, (1b) to reduce the intensity of the services provided, and (1c) to select patients for whom hospitals can provide care at costs that are below the DRG payment rate (not shown in Figure 6.2). On the one hand, reducing the length of stay and the intensity of services are intended effects of DRG-based hospital payment systems because both can contribute to increased efficiency of hospital care. For example, length of stay can be reduced by optimizing internal care pathways (Kahn et al., 1990); and intensity of services may be reduced by not providing unnecessary services. However, on the other hand, reducing length of stay could result in inappropriately early ('bloody') discharges and service intensity could be reduced to a level at which necessary services begin to be withheld from patients ('skimping'; Ellis, 1998), both leading to reductions in quality (see Table 6.3). Similarly, the selection of patients can have intended and unintended consequences. On the one hand, hospitals could specialize in treating those patients for whom they have a competitive advantage (for example, better qualified personnel or better care pathways), which could lead

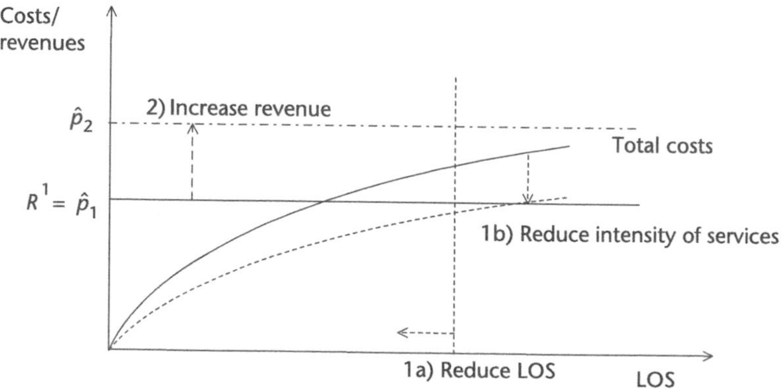

Figure 6.2 Selected incentives of DRG-based hospital payment for a hypothetical standard patient

to greater efficiency and higher quality. However, on the other hand, there is also the danger that hospitals engage in 'cream-skimming' (Levaggi & Montefiori, 2003; Martinussen & Hagen, 2009); that is, they attempt to admit only those patients within each DRG that can be expected to have costs below the payment rate (for example, by selecting patients without co-morbidities, if these are not adequately accounted for in the DRG system) or that they 'dump' unprofitable patients by transferring them to other providers or avoiding them altogether (Ellis, 1998; Newhouse & Byrne, 1988).

The second main incentive of basic DRG-based hospital payment systems – that is, to increase revenues per case (see Table 6.3) – can be achieved by hospitals through one of two strategies: (2a) changing coding practices, or (2b) changing practice patterns. As illustrated in Figure 6.2, the aim of both strategies is to reclassify patients into a different DRG (DRG_2) with an associated higher payment rate ($\hat{p}_2$). While more thorough coding of secondary diagnoses and procedures is an intended effect of the introduction of DRG-based hospital payment systems, the attempt by hospitals to increase revenues through fraudulent coding practices – such as adding inexistent secondary diagnoses or inverting primary and secondary diagnoses (known as 'up-coding' or 'DRG creep'; Simborg, 1981; Steinbusch et al., 2007; Silverman & Skinner, 2004) – is not intended because it leads to unjustified payments to hospitals. Furthermore, changed practice patterns would be an unintended consequence if hospitals provide additional (unnecessary) procedures that lead to the reclassification of patients into higher paying DRGs ('gaming/overtreatment'). However, this should be relevant only if these procedures can be performed at marginal costs that are below the level of the additional obtainable revenue as a result of the reclassification.

Finally, because hospital revenue in basic DRG-based hospital payment systems is determined simply by multiplying activity in each DRG by the fixed payment per DRG, the third main incentive for hospitals is to increase the number of admitted patients. Again, an increase in activity can be both an intended and an unintended consequence of the introduction of this type of hospital payment. On the one hand, if waiting lists existed under the old hospital payment system, an increase in hospital activity is an intended consequence that can contribute to increasing efficiency of hospitals. On the other hand, if activity is increased by admitting patients for services that could be provided in outpatient settings, efficiency is reduced. Furthermore, in competitive environments, hospitals' efforts to attract more patients may result in strategies to improve the reputation of hospitals by providing higher quality services, but could also lead to strategies that focus all efforts on improving only those services that are visible to patients or measurable by quality assurance programmes.

In summary, the intended and unintended consequences of DRG-based hospital payment systems are deeply intertwined. Most importantly, they are related to the fact that payment in these systems is independent of the costs of care provided to a specific patient. This becomes particularly problematic in the context of health care markets, in which information asymmetries are highly prevalent and make it difficult for payers to monitor and control providers' activity or behaviour (Lave, 1989). Furthermore, unintended consequences are related to the fact that DRG-based hospital payment systems can be interpreted as providing highly powerful incentives (Frant, 1996) because hospital payment depends directly on provider behaviour.

6.5 DRG-based hospital payment in practice: Modifications and instruments to avoid unintended consequences

In practice, DRG-based hospital payment systems in the 12 countries included in this book are far more complicated than the basic model of DRG-based hospital payment presented in the previous section. As already mentioned, different models of DRG-based hospital payment systems, selective applicability of DRG weights and monetary conversion and adjustment factors, and structural payment adjustments modify the basic incentives of DRG-based payments. This section focuses more closely on the explicit attempts of the 12 countries to avoid and control unintended consequences.

6.5.1 Fairness of payment: assuring adequate payment for outliers and high-cost services

While DRG-based hospital payment systems can be considered to provide adequate reimbursement for the average patient within each DRG, they overpay hospitals for patients with below-average resource consumption and underpay for patients with above-average costs. In general, most of these differences are compensated automatically, as relatively more expensive cases within a DRG are compensated by cheaper cases within the same DRG, and even unprofitable DRGs may be compensated by highly profitable DRGs within the same hospital. However, ensuring that DRGs comprise cases with relatively homogeneous costs has been a major concern in all countries, as evidenced by the increasingly large number of DRGs in all systems (see Chapter 2). On the one hand, if DRG systems adequately account for differences between patients (by considering all relevant secondary diagnoses) and necessary treatments (by considering all relevant procedures), the incentives for certain unintended consequences, such as cream-skimming and skimping/undertreatment, could be greatly reduced. On the other hand, refined DRG systems with more narrowly defined DRGs also increase the scope for other unintended consequences, such as up-coding (if DRGs are defined on the basis of classification criteria that are easy to manipulate) and gaming/overtreatment (if procedural classification criteria introduce strong incentives to deliver certain services) (Hafsteinsdottir & Siciliani, 2010).

Yet, in spite of the continuous refinement of DRG systems, DRGs in all systems incorporate patients that require much more resources than most patients belonging to the same DRG. These high-cost 'outlier' cases often account for a sizeable share of total hospital costs and consequently have a strong influence on the average costs of cases within a DRG (Cots et al., 2003). If DRG weights were calculated based on the average costs of patients within a DRG, including the outlier cases, this would lead to hospitals being overpaid for the majority of patients. Furthermore, if outlier cases were not paid for separately, hospitals would experience particularly strong incentives to avoid these high-cost cases ('dumping'), or to discharge them inappropriately early ('bloody' discharge).

Consequently, most of the countries analysed in this book have developed mechanisms to identify outlier cases and to pay hospitals separately for the extra costs of treating such patients. Table 6.4 shows that most countries define outlier cases on the basis of a length-of-stay threshold (a certain number of days beyond which cases are considered outliers), as cost data are usually available only for a sample of patients across the country (see Chapter 5). The Nordic countries (Estonia, Finland, and Sweden) are an exception as they define outlier cases on the basis of costs. However, while all countries (except for the Netherlands) define outliers, the trimming methods determining the outlier threshold differ. They are either based on a variant of the interquartile method or the parametric method (Schreyögg et al., 2006), leading to varying percentages of all cases being considered outliers.

Figure 6.3 illustrates how hospital payment systems in most countries ensure adequate payment for outlier patients. Most often, the DRG-based payment rate is increased for long-stay outlier cases by a surcharge that depends on the number of days that patients were in hospital beyond the specified threshold. In Estonia and Finland, where outliers are defined on the basis of costs, the extra costs of outlier patients are reimbursed directly through a fee-for-service system. In Catalonia and the Netherlands, hospitals do not receive surcharges

Table 6.4 Definition of outliers and associated deductions/surcharges

	Definition of outliers (trimming method)	*Outliers as % of total cases*	*Outlier payment*	
			Deductions/ payments	*Surcharges*
Austria	LOS (interquartile)	~ 12–15	Per day	Per day
England	LOS (interquartile)	7	No (but short-stay tariff)	Per day
Estonia	Cost (parametric)	9	?	FFS
Finland	Cost (parametric)	5	No	FFS
France	LOS (interquartile)	0.4 (public hospitals)	Per day	Per day
Germany	LOS (parametric)	22	Per day	Per day
Ireland	LOS (parametric)	6	Per day	Per day
Netherlands	–	–	Not applicable	Not applicable
Poland	LOS (interquartile)	~ 2	No (but short-stay tariff)	Per day
Portugal	LOS (interquartile)	–	Per day	Per day
Spain (Catalonia)	LOS (interquartile)	5	No	No
Sweden	Cost/LOS (parametric)	5	Varies	varies

Source: Based on the country-specific chapters in Part Two of this volume (most recent information available).

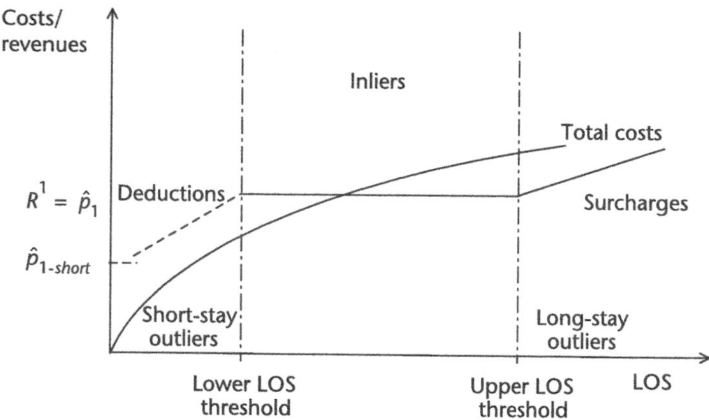

Figure 6.3 Trimming and reimbursement for outliers

for outlier cases. In Catalonia, the extra costs of outlier cases are supposed to be taken into account in the structural adjustments that determine the majority of hospital budgets.

In the Netherlands, the problem of outlier cases is dealt with very differently: if a patient has more than one diagnosis requiring treatment, this additional 'diagnosis–treatment combination' (the Dutch equivalent of a DRG, known as a DBC) triggers an additional DRG-based payment to the hospital. Interestingly, in Finland (and, prior to the recent update, also in England), a similar approach exists, whereby hospitals can assign more than one DRG for patients that were treated in several departments during one hospital stay.

Furthermore, several countries also determine lower length-of-stay outlier thresholds, which are sometimes an explicit attempt at avoiding inappropriately early ('bloody') discharges. These countries calculate a reduced payment rate for patients that are discharged prior to the lower length-of-stay threshold, either by deducting a certain amount from the standard DRG rate for each day that patients are discharged before the lower length-of-stay threshold, or by calculating the sum of a minimum payment plus a certain daily rate. England and Poland do not determine lower length-of-stay thresholds but have specific short-stay (one-day) weights ($\hat{p}_{1\text{–}short}$) for certain DRGs. In the Finnish and Swedish versions of the NordDRG system, specific DRGs exist for day-care patients.

Aside from the issue of outlier cases, all DRG systems are confronted with the problem that certain high-cost services are provided to a heterogeneous group of patients that fall into different DRGs. As discussed in Chapter 3, most DRG systems have instituted additional payment mechanisms for certain services that cannot be assigned to a specific DRG. Consequently, these services are exempt from the incentives that tend to apply to DRG-based hospital payment, and this can therefore be interpreted as an attempt to avoid skimping/under-treatment relating to these services. In addition, most countries have developed similar payment mechanisms for certain innovative drugs and treatments that are not adequately accounted for by their DRG systems (see Chapter 9).

6.5.2 Asymmetry of information: Monitoring and controlling unintended consequences

The asymmetry of information between providers and payers gives rise to several unintended consequences of DRG-based hospital payment systems: for example, payers do not necessarily know whether a specific patient was in need of a specific procedure; whether the patient really needed to be admitted as an inpatient; whether non-existing secondary diagnoses were coded; and whether certain secondary diagnoses resulted from medical errors. Consequently, providers can perform procedures that lead to the reclassification of patients into higher paying DRGs (gaming/overtreatment); they can increase the volume of admitted patients; they can up-code their patients; and they may receive higher payments for providing services of poorer quality (see Chapter 8).

In order to control some of these unintended consequences, several countries have implemented auditing systems that aim to reduce the asymmetry of information. For example, in Germany, the regional medical review boards of the sickness funds send teams to randomly selected hospitals to evaluate the coding and treatment of patients by auditing patients' medical records (MDS, 2011). In 2009, 12 per cent of all hospital cases were audited by the sickness funds, resulting in average costs of around €800 per audited case being recovered. In France, 1 per cent of hospital discharges were audited by the Regional Hospitalization Agencies (ARH) in 2006, which found that 60 per cent of evaluated records had some kind of coding error.

Other control mechanisms aim to limit the ability of hospitals to exploit the asymmetry of information by determining global budgets or volume thresholds (see Table 6.2), which ensure that hospitals do not increase their activity beyond predetermined limits. Furthermore, in order to control frequent readmissions, Germany and England financially penalize hospitals if patients are readmitted for the same problem within 30 days after initial discharge: for these patients, hospitals do not receive a second DRG-based payment. In addition, if countries in Europe were to follow the example of the United States in obligating hospitals to specify whether secondary diagnoses were present on admission (see Chapter 8), they would be able to differentiate between hospital-acquired (potentially avoidable) conditions, and those that were beyond the control of hospitals.

Finally, the regular recalculation of DRG weights and monetary conversion factors (see Chapter 9) reduces the ability of hospitals to benefit from up-coding: if all hospitals engage in up-coding, the recalculation of DRG weights and monetary conversion factors will lead to reduced payment rates for previously higher paying DRGs. However, if some hospitals engage in up-coding and others do not, the honest hospitals are likely to be penalized by reduced payment rates. Therefore, the readjustment of payment rates is useful as an effective mechanism for cost control, but it does not replace the need for thorough auditing of hospital coding activities.

6.5.3 The power of incentives: Reducing the share of DRG-based payment in total hospital revenues

As illustrated in Table 6.2, DRG-based hospital payment systems never determine the entirety of hospital revenues.[2] These other sources of revenue contribute to reducing the power of the incentives related to DRG-based hospital payment, as hospitals can focus their efforts on maximizing revenues through other strategies.

For example, in Spain (Catalonia), where DRG-based hospital payment accounts for only 20 per cent of hospital revenues, the power of the incentives related to DRG-based hospital payment are relatively weak. As pointed out by Cots and colleagues (see Chapter 22, subsection 22.7.2, p. 420), 'since hospital revenues are mostly determined by their SRI [structural relative index], hospitals are more likely to focus on introducing new and advanced technologies in order to increase their SRI, rather than focusing on improving performance as measured by DRGs'.

Furthermore, most countries that have introduced DRG-based hospital payment systems have phased in the systems over several years, with the size of total hospital revenues related to DRG-based payment slowly increasing over time. Consequently, the incentives of such hospital payment were minimal at first, giving hospitals time to slowly adjust to the changing financial environment.

6.6 Conclusions: Maximizing the intended and avoiding unintended consequences

This chapter illustrates that DRG-based hospital payment systems in the 12 countries analysed for this volume do not conform to the basic model presented in section 6.4. All countries' hospital payment systems include other payment components: the cumulative effect of structural adjustments of weights or monetary conversion factors, of outlier payments, and additional payments can be assumed to moderate the incentives associated with the basic model of DRG-based hospital payment. The resulting intricately blended hospital payment systems are more likely to contribute to achieving the societal objectives of securing high-quality hospital care at affordable costs than any other hospital payment mechanism alone (Ellis & Mcguire, 1986).

One advantage of determining hospital payment on the basis of DRGs is that hospitals will be incentivized to increase their efforts in terms of coding of diagnoses and procedures, which will contribute to generating better hospital activity data. Yet, it is important to be aware that DRG-based hospital payment systems should always be accompanied by thorough monitoring systems that enable payers to reduce the information asymmetries, which would give rise to unintended consequences of the incentives that are inherent to DRG-based hospital payment systems. Furthermore, continuous refinement of DRG systems (see Chapter 4), and high-quality cost-accounting data (see Chapter 5) are essential for optimizing DRG-based hospital payment systems, and for assuring that payment rates are sufficiently related to the costs of care.

However, the country experiences presented in this book also suggest that governments do not need to be afraid of introducing DRG-based payment systems – as long as they do so carefully and over extended time periods, slowly increasing the share of DRG-based payments within the overall hospital payment system. The large number of alternative models – ranging from DRG-based case payment systems (operating within DRG-based negotiated budgets or not) to DRG-based budget allocation systems – illustrate that countries can tailor DRG-based hospital payment systems to the specific structure of their existing hospital payment system. If the effects of DRG-based hospital payment systems are carefully re-evaluated at regular intervals, ideally in close collaboration with all actors concerned, the incentives of DRG-based payment systems have the potential to contribute to achieving the intended consequences, as long as the unintended ones can be adequately controlled through the mechanisms described.

6.7 Notes

1 Even though some DRG-like PCSs do not define DRGs in the strict sense of the word (that is, groups are not diagnosis-related), this chapter uses the term DRGs to summarize all groups of patients defined by DRG systems or DRG-like PCSs (for further details see Chapter 4 or the relevant country-specific case study chapters in Part Two).

2 In fact, the extraordinarily high share of hospital revenues appearing to be determined by the DRG-based payment system in Austria is somewhat misleading, for example, as the state-specific monetary conversion factors in several of the federal states adjust – to a significant extent – for the structural characteristics of hospitals.

6.8 References

Berki, S.E. (1985). DRGs, incentives, hospitals, and physicians. *Health Affairs (Millwood)*, 4:70–6.

Böcking, W., Ahrens, U., Kirch, W., Milakovic, M. (2005). First results of the introduction of DRGs in Germany and overview of experience from other DRG countries. *Journal of Public Health*, 13:128–37.

Cots, F., Elvira, D., Castells, X., Sáez, M. (2003). Relevance of outlier cases in casemix systems and evaluation of trimming methods. *Health Care Management Science*, 6:27–35.

Ellis, R.P. (1998). Creaming, skimping and dumping: provider competition on the intensive and extensive margins. *Journal of Health Economics*, 17:537–55.

Ellis, R.P., McGuire, T.G. (1986). Provider behavior under prospective reimbursement – cost-sharing and supply. *Journal of Health Economics*, 5:129–51.

Farrar, S., Yi, D., Sutton, M. et al. (2009). Has payment by results affected the way that English hospitals provide care? Difference-in-differences analysis. *British Medical Journal*, 339:1–8.

Fetter, R.B. (1991). Diagnosis-related groups – understanding hospital performance. *Interfaces*, 21:6–26.

Frant, H. (1996). High-powered and low-powered incentives in the public sector. *Journal of Public Administration Research and Theory*, 6(3):365–81.

Hafsteinsdottir, E.J.G., Siciliani, L. (2009). DRG prospective payment systems: refine or not refine? *Health Economics*, 19(10):1226–39.

Kahn, K.L., Rogers, W.H., Rubenstein, L.V. et al. (1990). Measuring quality of care with explicit process criteria before and after implementation of the DRG-based prospective payment system. *Journal of the American Medical Association*, 264:1969–73.

Kimberly, J.R., de Pouvourville, G., D'Aunno, T., eds (2008). *The Globalization of Managerial Innovation in Health Care*. Cambridge: Cambridge University Press.

Lave, J.R. (1989). The effect of the Medicare prospective payment system. *Annual Review of Public Health*, 10:141–61.

Lave, J.R. (2003). Developing a Medicare prospective payment system for inpatient psychiatric care. *Health Affairs (Millwood)*, 22:97–109.

Levaggi, R., Montefiori, M. (2003). *Horizontal and Vertical Cream-Skimming in the Health Care Market*. DISEFIN Working Paper, 11/2003. Rochester, NY: Social Science Research Network (http://ssrn.com/abstract=545583, accessed 10 July 2011).

Martinussen, P.E., Hagen, T.P. (2009). Reimbursement systems, organizational forms and patient selection: evidence from day surgery in Norway. *Health Economics, Policy and Law*, 4:139–58.

MDS (2011). *Abrechnungsprüfungen der MDK in Krankenhäusern sind angemessen, wirtschaftlich und zielführend. Zahlen und Fakten der MDK-Gemeinschaft*. Essen: Medizinischer Dienst des Spitzenverbandes Bund der Krankenkassen e.V.

Miraldo, M., Goddard, M., Smith, P. (2006). *The Incentive Effects of Payment by Results*. York: University of York Centre for Health Economics (CHE Research Paper 19).

Newhouse, J.P., Byrne, D.J. (1988). Did Medicare's prospective payment system cause length of stay to fall? *Journal of Health Economics*, 7:413–16.

Schreyögg, J., Stargardt, T., Tiemann, O., Busse, R. (2006). Methods to determine reimbursement rates for diagnosis-related groups (DRG): a comparison of nine European countries. *Health Care Management Science*, 9:215–23.

Silverman, E., Skinner, J. (2004). Medicare up-coding and hospital ownership. *Journal of Health Economics*, 23:369–89.

Simborg, D.W. (1981). DRG creep: a new hospital-acquired disease. *New England Journal of Medicine*, 304:1602–4.

Steinbusch, P.J., Oostenbrink, J.B., Zuurbier, J.J., Schaepkens, F.J. (2007). The risk of up-coding in casemix systems: a comparative study. *Health Policy*, 81:289–99.

chapter seven

DRG-based hospital payment and efficiency: Theory, evidence, and challenges

Andrew Street, Jacqueline O'Reilly, Padraic Ward and Anne Mason

7.1 Introduction

Diagnosis-related groups (DRGs) were first used to pay hospitals in 1983 under the Medicare Program in the United States. This development was born out of a need to move away from an approach to hospital financing based on fee-for-service payments, which was seen as inherently inefficient and increasingly expensive. Since then, DRG-based hospital payment has been widely adopted internationally with the explicit objective of improving efficiency, principally because of its three overarching strengths, summarized here (see Chapter 2 for further details).

1. By relating provider revenue directly to their workload, DRG-based hospital payment offers greater transparency in the financing of health care.
2. Payments are based on patient characteristics (predominantly demographic and clinical). Fundamental to effective DRG-based hospital payment is an accurate description of the type of patients treated (casemix).
3. DRG-based hospital payment is a form of 'yard stick competition', designed to encourage greater efficiency in the absence of market competition.

Concentrating on the third strength, this chapter considers the relationship between DRG-based hospital payment and efficiency from theoretical and empirical perspectives. It thus first discusses the concepts 'efficiency' and 'yard stick competition'. Different hospital payment models are then compared in section 7.2, with the intention of indicating in each case the incentives for hospitals to pursue efficient behaviour, particularly in terms of maximizing output and minimizing cost. The empirical evidence regarding the impact of DRG-based hospital payment on efficiency is reviewed in section 7.3 by looking at studies that consider efficiency as defined by economists and those that focus on indicators of efficient practice. Finally, the chapter outlines in section 7.4 some key challenges associated with the use of DRG-based hospital payment. While economic theory suggests that this hospital payment system may provide incentives to encourage efficiency, there could be barriers (such as the system's particular design and operation) to realizing these incentives in practice.

'Efficiency' is a widely used term that can have various meanings. Economists make distinctions between technical, cost- and allocative efficiency. Technical efficiency is defined as maximizing output for given input levels or, in this context, treating as many patients as possible given the resources available. Hospitals are cost-efficient when they minimize costs for any given output level (closely related to, but distinct from, technical efficiency). Allocative efficiency can be defined for both outputs and inputs. The optimal output mix depends on the value of each output, which requires judgements to be made on the relative values of an appendectomy operation, a heart bypass and all other health care interventions. The optimal mix of inputs depends on the relative price of each input type, such as the salaries of doctors and nurses. Alongside these economic terms, reference is often made to things thought to be indicative of efficient behaviour, which – in the hospital sector – might include the number and type of patients treated, unit costs and length of stay, for example. The extent to which DRGs contribute to achieving these forms of efficiency depends on how they are used for payment purposes, which helps to determine the incentives hospitals face to pursue efficient behaviour.

Yard stick competition is designed to encourage providers to reduce their costs in contexts in which they face limited competitive pressure (Shleifer, 1985). If providers outperform others they benefit directly by retaining the generated financial surplus; if they underperform they generate deficits and, ultimately, risk bankruptcy. All providers, including the most efficient, are incentivized to continually reduce costs. Yard stick competition is effective when regulated prices are virtually independent of an individual provider's costs. Ideally, prices should reflect the supply costs of efficient providers, determined across all providers within the same industry.

However, it is not straightforward to identify efficient providers, especially if the regulator is poorly informed about the provider's costs, the exogenous influences on these costs and the level of effort expended by the provider (that is, their efficiency). This asymmetry of information is particularly problematic in the health care sector. In practice, price is often determined on the basis of the average cost of all or a sample of providers (see Chapter 5), although it may remain preferable to base it on 'best practice', set at the level of efficient high-quality providers that deliver care at costs below the average costs in other hospitals. In England, such 'best practice tariffs' have recently been introduced for certain high-volume areas (such as cholecystectomy, hip fractures, cataracts, and stroke), with significant unexplained variation in quality of clinical practice and clear evidence of what constitutes best practice (see Chapter 12).

7.2 Hospital payment models

To understand the role of DRG-based hospital payment in enhancing efficiency, we compare (simplified versions of) the three main forms of provider payment models used in hospital financing: cost-based reimbursement (also known as fee-for-service payment), the global budget model, and DRG-based payment.

7.2.1 Cost-based or fee-for-service reimbursement

With cost-based reimbursement, payments to hospitals are based on the cost incurred by each individual patient (plus potentially a profit margin). The main method of cost control is to specify a price list that details the unit payment for each 'item of service' (for example, medication, X-ray, procedure). Hospitals must therefore provide itemized bills for every patient treated, but there is no incentive to limit what treatments they provide per insured patient – the more diagnostic tests they perform, the more they get paid.

Stated formally, with cost-based reimbursement, hospital revenue (R^C) amounts to the number of patients treated (Q_i) multiplied by the unit cost of treatment (c_i), where i indicates a particular patient:

$$R^C = \sum_{i=1}^{I} [Q_i \times c_i] + Z^C \tag{1}$$

Z^C captures all other forms of revenue that hospitals receive, such as funds for teaching and research. In the hospital sector, cost-based reimbursement was primarily used in the United States during the 1960s and 1970s. This fuelled escalation in health care costs as hospitals engaged in a 'medical arms race', spending ever more on technologies and facilities to attract patients. Hospitals knew that they could reclaim the costs from health insurance companies as well as Medicare and Medicaid, the public insurance programmes for older people and those with low incomes.

7.2.2 Global budgets

Cost control is one of the key advantages of global budget arrangements, which have been used in many European health care systems, at least if the budget constraint is credible and binding, and a separation exists between a payer (also known as 'purchaser') and hospitals as providers of care. This division has traditionally been present in social health insurance systems and, since the 1990s, increasingly also in tax-funded systems (Robinson et al., 2005). A fixed payment is agreed in advance for a target level of activity – often specified at specialty level. Figure 7.1 illustrates the case in which a hospital receives a fixed payment ($\bar{R}$) for carrying out a pre-specified volume of health service activity ($\bar{Q}$).

Difficulties arise if there are deviations from the pre-specified volume. Some form of penalty must be imposed if the volume is not achieved. If the pre-specified volume – usually defined as the number of hospital cases – is exceeded

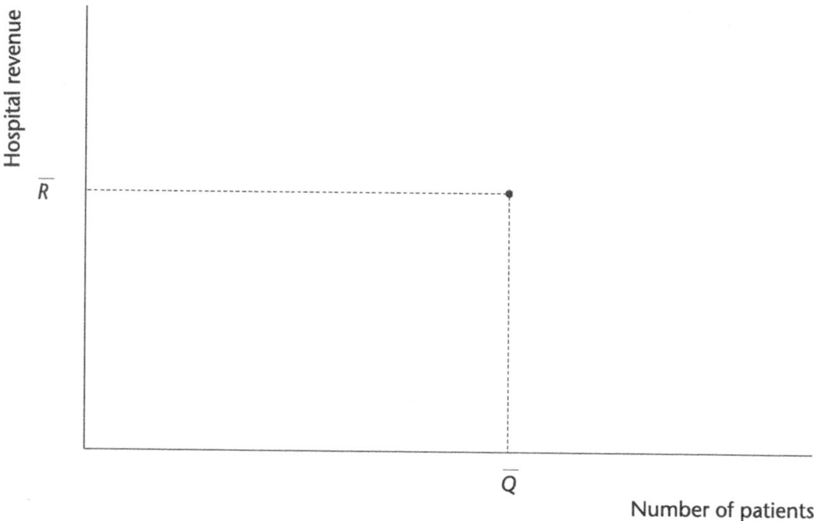

Figure 7.1 Hospital revenues under global budgets

Source: Street et al., 2007.

('overperformance'), the funder must either provide extra money or the hospital will refuse to do extra work, thereby creating waiting lists. 'Cost and volume' contracts were developed to deal with these problems, and we return to a DRG-based hospital payment form of these in the following subsection (7.2.3).

In more advanced global budget systems, activity is specified by specialty. Negotiations between the payer (whether this is a sickness fund or a health authority) and the hospital revolve around the monetary value of each specialty-level contract (B_s) and how much activity ($\overline{Q}_s$) – usually defined as cases per specialty – will be provided under this contract. The local specialty-level price (p_s) is the by-product of negotiations relating to total contract value and the volume of activity. In formal terms, with the approach to financing that uses global budgets, hospital revenue comprises the sum of its contracts across specialties (B_s):

$$R^G = \sum_{s=1}^{S} B_s + \mathbf{Z}^G = \sum_{s=1}^{S} [\overline{Q}_s \times p_s] + \mathbf{Z}^G \qquad (2)$$

where $\mathbf{Z}^G$ captures all other forms of revenue that hospitals receive within the framework of these payment arrangements.

7.2.3 DRG-based hospital payment

There are two key features of DRG-based hospital payment. (1) Activity is described using DRGs rather than by specialty. For instance, payment is made for a patient receiving a hip replacement rather than a patient treated in trauma and orthopaedics. (2) The reimbursement per DRG is to a large extent fixed in advance, as patient characteristics (especially the main diagnosis) determine the DRG category with its fixed 'price'. As this constituted a major shift from the 'retrospective' system of cost-based reimbursement, payment by DRGs was thus termed 'prospective' in the United States – a term which was inappropriate for systems with a global budget approach to financing (where instead 'activity-based' was used to describe the new payment system). As shown in Chapter 4, the 'prospective' nature of DRGs is also weaker if to a large extent procedures determine the DRG classification. However, whether driven by diagnosis or procedure, the 'price' of a DRG is wholly or at least partially independent of an individual provider's costs (see Chapter 5). In many jurisdictions, this fixed price is set nationally rather than locally (see Chapter 6).

The relationship between the unit price and amount of activity can take a number of forms. The main ones discussed here are:

1. linear payments, whereby the total payment equals price multiplied by quantity;
2. mixed payments, whereby hospitals receive additional payments (often in the form of lump sums) that are unrelated to activity levels;
3. marginal payments, whereby different prices are payable for the same type of activity, depending on the quantity provided;
4. mixed and marginal payments, which are a combination of (2) and (3).

To understand the differences between these payment arrangements, we consider how the total revenue received by a particular hospital is calculated.

Linear payments

With the most straightforward DRG-based hospital payment system, using linear payments, hospital revenue is determined simply by multiplying activity in each DRG (Q_j) by the fixed price per DRG ($\hat{p}_j$), where j indicates a DRG:

$$R^A = \sum_{j=1}^{J} [Q_j \times \hat{p}_j] \qquad (3)$$

Using this formulation, hospital revenue increases linearly with activity, as illustrated in Figure 7.2. If the hospital treats Q_0 patients it receives revenue amounting to only R_0; if Q_1 patients are treated, revenue increases to R_1. Clearly, then, the revenue consequences of changes in activity are much more transparent than within a system based on global budget arrangements.

Mixed payments

In almost all countries that have introduced DRG-based hospital payment, hospital revenue is not determined solely by the number of patients treated. Hospitals also receive revenue in other forms – for instance, to fund teaching and research, to compensate for different geographical costs, or to cover some element of the fixed costs of providing services. It has been formally demonstrated that such a 'mixed' hospital payment system creates better incentives than 'pure' systems (Ellis & McGuire, 1986; Barnum et al., 1995). The composition

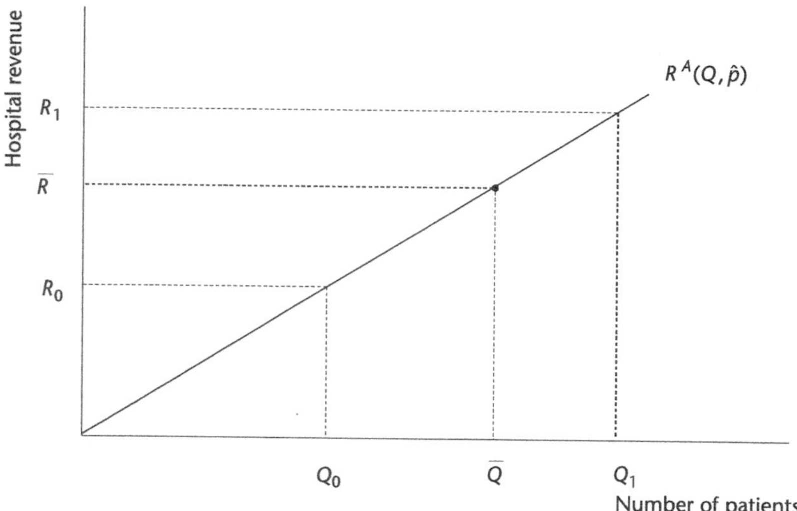

Figure 7.2 Hospital revenue under 'pure' DRG-based hospital payment

Source: Street et al., 2007.

of these other revenue forms is a matter of negotiation between the payer (or 'purchaser') and the hospital sector, and may vary between hospitals, between countries and over time. We define $\mathbf{Z}^A$ as capturing all these sources of revenue not related to health care activity within the category 'DRG-based hospital payment'. Then the revenue function becomes:

$$R^A = \sum_{j=1}^{J} [Q_j \times \hat{p}_j] + \mathbf{Z}^A \qquad (4)$$

Figure 7.3 shows how this arrangement changes the relationship between revenue and activity. Hospitals receive a fixed amount $\mathbf{Z}^A$ irrespective of the number of patients treated. On top of this, hospitals receive revenue in line with activity – but the unit price ($\hat{p}_j$) will be lower within the framework of this 'mixed' arrangement than within a 'pure' DRG-based system.

Marginal payments

DRG-based hospital payment can be modified to allow incentives to vary with supply. Quite often, DRG-based hospital payment is introduced to stimulate activity beyond existing levels. But unconstrained growth in activity may be undesirable. First, it undermines control over global expenditure – under the simple formulation (see equation (3)), expenditure may simply keep rising in line with activity. Second, hospitals may be able to expand activity at low marginal cost – perhaps because they have underutilized resources available – and, thus, this differential pricing may be used to exploit economies of scale. If so, there is an argument for reducing the unit price for additional activity.

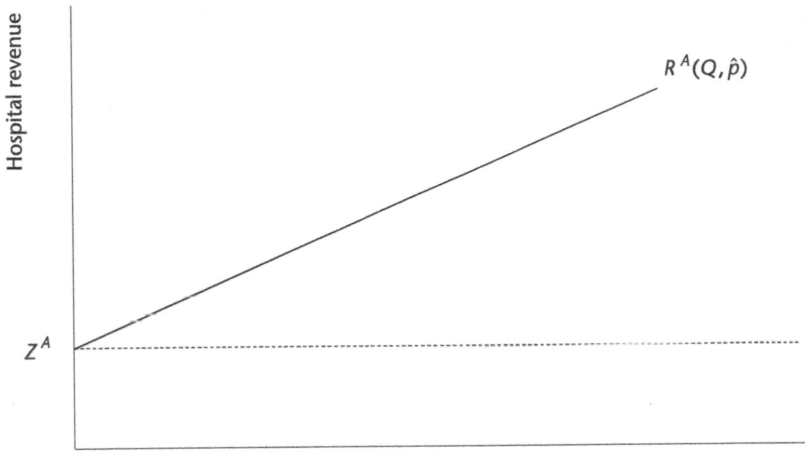

Figure 7.3 Hospital revenue under 'mixed' DRG-based hospital payment

Source: Street et al., 2007.

The resulting arrangements are akin to 'cost and volume' contracts. Two policy decisions are required.

1. A 'target' level of activity ($\overline{Q}_j$) should be defined for each hospital. In some countries, this is based on historical activity. Agreeing a target is more difficult where there is decentralized purchasing, such as in England, because the target has to be agreed between each purchaser and provider.
2. The price that should be paid for activity above the target level must be agreed – this is usually defined as some proportion (α) of the price up to the target level. Formally the revenue function can be expressed as:

$$R^A = \sum_{j=1}^{J} [\overline{Q}_j \times \hat{p}_j] + \sum_{j=1}^{J} [(Q_j - \overline{Q}_j) \times \alpha \hat{p}_j] + \mathbf{Z}^A \quad (5)$$

where $(Q_j - \overline{Q}_j)$ is non-negative and represents activity above the target and $\alpha\hat{p}_j$ is the price paid per unit of additional activity. If $\alpha = 0.5$, the price for additional activity is 50 per cent of that paid for activity up to the target; if $\alpha = 1$, the same price is paid (in which case equations (4) and (5) are equivalent); if $\alpha = 0$, the marginal price is zero, so there is no incentive for hospitals to undertake more activity; and if $\alpha > 1$, additional payments are higher than the base price, which creates very strong incentives to undertake additional work. This may be justified if marginal costs are high, as expansions in activity require additional investment.

Figure 7.4 shows how revenue changes under this arrangement, when the marginal price for additional activity is below the price for activity up to the target; that is, $0 < \alpha < 1$. This results in a 'kinked' revenue function.

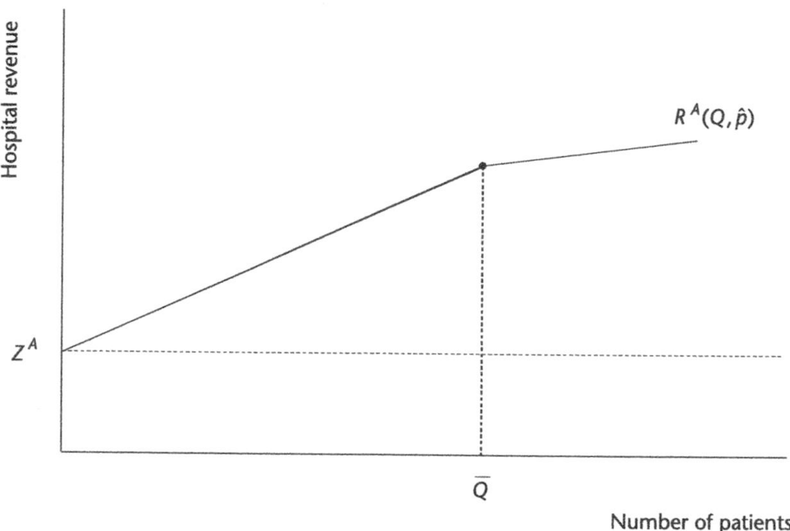

Figure 7.4 Hospital revenue under 'mixed' DRG-based hospital payment with marginal pricing

Source: Street et al., 2007.

7.2.4 Summary

Table 7.1 summarizes the main differences between the three hospital payment systems. Of course, it is important to be cognisant that the hospital payment systems implemented in practice are usually more complicated variants of the simplified models in the previous subsections.

The three models offer different incentives for achieving objectives relating to activity levels, expenditure control, quality of care and the three types of efficiency (Table 7.2). Incentives to increase activity exist in both cost-based and DRG-based hospital payment systems, with the relative strength of the incentives depending on how closely the link between reimbursement and activity levels is

Table 7.1 Main differences across hospital payment systems

System	*Description of patients*	*Amount of activity*	*Price per unit of activity*	*Basic formulation of revenue function*
Cost-based/fee-for-service	Individual	Unrestricted	Item of service	$R^C = \sum_{i=1}^{I} [Q_i \times c_i]$
Global budget	Per hospital/ specialty	Target/ historical	Locally agreed	$R^G = \sum_{s=1}^{S} B_s = \sum_{s=1}^{S} [\bar{Q}_s \times p_s]$
'Pure' DRG-based hospital payment	DRG	Unrestricted	Fixed prospectively	$R^A = \sum_{j=1}^{J} [Q_j \times \hat{p}_j]$

Source: Adapted from Street et al., 2007.

Table 7.2 Incentives offered by three hospital payment models

	Objective					
	Increase activity	*Expenditure control*	*Improve quality*	*Enhance efficiency*		
				Technical	*Cost*	*Allocative*
Cost-based/ fee-for-service	Strong	Weak	Strong*	Weak	Weak	Weak
Global budget	Weak	Strong	Moderate	Weak	Moderate	Moderate
'Pure' DRG-based hospital payment	Moderate	Moderate	Moderate	Strong	Strong	Moderate

*However, quality of care could be adversely affected, as the incentive to increase activity may lead to the provision of inappropriate and potentially harmful services (see Chapter 8 of this volume).

specified (WHO, 2000; Langenbrunner et al., 2005; Moreno-Serra & Wagstaff, 2010). DRG-based hospital payment performs better than cost-based reimbursement with regard to expenditure control, but not as well as global budgets (assuming that budgets are enforced). The potential for quality improvement under a DRG-based hospital payment system may be dependent on whether payments are adjusted for quality of care (see Chapter 8).

Where DRG-based hospital payment provides a fixed price per unit of activity, hospitals are incentivized to increase activity and minimize cost and, therefore, to improve technical efficiency. While cost-based reimbursement also encourages increased activity, there is no motivation to minimize inputs/costs (unless there is a fixed fee schedule). DRG-based hospital payment may offer incentives to improve allocative and cost-efficiency by encouraging providers to consider the prices and amount of inputs they use. It may also promote an efficient allocation of outputs if prices reflect their relative value but, in practice, most jurisdictions still base prices on costs. Nevertheless, overall, DRG-based hospital payment is likely to provide stronger incentives for efficiency compared to either of the alternatives.

7.3 Review of empirical evidence on DRG-based hospital payment and efficiency

The preceding discussion suggests that DRG-based hospital payment may enhance hospital efficiency, either by changing the focus of cost-based reimbursement from retrospective to prospective (as was the case in the United States), or by explicitly linking payment to activity in systems with global budgets (as in most European countries).

This section reviews recent empirical evidence from developed countries. Although improving hospital efficiency is generally a key motivation for introducing DRG-based hospital payment, relatively few studies have explicitly identified and quantified its impact. Rather, most research has concentrated on indicators of efficiency – such as activity and costs – which are more easily measured, but by definition provide only a partial picture. It is important to note, moreover, that the different starting points in the United States and Europe also imply different hypotheses about the impact of DRG-based payment; that is, moving from cost-based reimbursement to DRGs weakens the activity incentive and strengthens the expenditure control incentive – while the opposite is the case when moving from global budgets to DRG-based payment.

7.3.1 Impact on efficiency

Studies of the impact of DRG-based payment on hospital-level efficiency typically focus on technical efficiency and/or the broader concept of productivity (which incorporates scale, as well as technical, efficiency; see Coelli et al., 2005; Street & Häkkinen, 2010). Data envelopment analysis (DEA) – a well-established non-parametric method – is the most commonly applied approach, although some studies use regression-based (parametric) stochastic frontier analysis. Both methods have advantages and disadvantages (*inter alia*, Jacobs et al., 2006; Street & Häkkinen, 2010; Street et al., 2010) yet, reassuringly, studies that applied both techniques produce broadly consistent results (Gerdtham et al., 1999a, b; Dismuke & Sena, 1999).

Given the challenges inherent in undertaking cross-country efficiency comparisons, all but two of the studies summarized in Table 7.3 adopted a longitudinal perspective, comparing hospital efficiency before and after the introduction of a DRG system. However, the length of follow-up periods varies, complicating interpretation: where the time horizon is short, changes may not be sustained; conversely, a longer time frame may fail to establish a causal relationship, particularly if other reforms are implemented in the interim. Several studies explicitly highlight the difficulty in attributing changes in efficiency, or any of its indicators, to the introduction of DRG-based payment (Farrar et al., 2007; Audit Commission, 2008). Moreover, few studies assess the quality of care, despite the potential trade-off between quality and efficiency (see Chapter 8 of this volume).

Methodological caveats aside, findings relating to the impact of DRG-based payment on hospital efficiency are mixed. The reformed hospital payment system was associated with improved technical efficiency in Portugal (albeit narrowly assessed; Dismuke & Sena, 1999, 2001), Sweden (Gerdtham et al., 1999a, b) and Norway (Biørn et al., 2003; Hagen et al., 2006). By contrast, no positive impact was observed in the United States (Borden, 1988; Chern & Wan, 2000) and there were technological improvements but no technical efficiency gains in Austria (Sommersguter-Reichmann, 2000). The limited evidence on time-series changes to cost-efficiency – confined to Norwegian data – is also mixed (Biørn et al., 2003; Hagen et al., 2006). These divergent results may be explained by the country-specific starting points and contexts in which the hospital payment reforms were implemented, including different incumbent reimbursement mechanisms, the specification of DRG-based payment, and/or the simultaneous introduction of other health care reforms.

Table 7.3 Summary of recent studies examining the impact of DRG-based hospital payment on hospital efficiency

Country, Year of change to DRG-based hospital payment	*Study*	*Methodology*	*Variables*	*Results/Conclusions*
United States, 1983	Borden, 1988[a]	*Method:* DEA, ratio and regression analysis *Sample:*52 hospitals in New Jersey *Study period:* 1979–1984	*Outputs:* (1) Cases treated in each of the eight DRG categories with the highest volumes; (2) Cases treated in the remaining DRG categories *Inputs*: (1) Total FTEs; (2) Nursing FTEs; (3) Other non-payroll expenses; (4) Beds *Quality*: Not included	The hospital payment reform did not have a positive effect on technical efficiency
	Chern & Wan, 2000	*Method*: DEA *Sample*: 80 hospitals in Virginia *Study period*: 1984 & 1993	*Outputs*: (1) Casemix-adjusted inpatient discharges; (2) Visits to the ER and outpatient facilities *Inputs*: (1) Beds and service complexity; (2) Non-physician FTEs and weighted number of part-time personnel; (3) Operating expenses excluding payroll, capital and depreciation *Quality*: Not included	There was no statistically significant difference in technical efficiency between 1984 and 1993, but the percentage of efficient hospitals was higher in 1993
Portugal, 1990	Dismuke & Sena, 1999[b]	*Method*: Two stages: (1) DEA and maximum likelihood estimation of stochastic input requirement frontier; (2) Regression *Sample*: 2 DRGs: (1) Heart Failure and Shock; (2) Specific Cerebrovascular Disorders except Transient Ischaemic Attack *Study period*: 1992–1994	*Outputs*: (1) Number of live discharges within each DRG; (2) Number of dead discharges within each DRG *Inputs*: Utilization of: (1) CAT scanner; (2) Electrocardiogram; (3) Echocardiogram *Quality*: Distinguishes between desirable outputs (live discharges) and undesirable outputs (dead discharges)	Percentage paid through DRGs had a positive impact on productivity

Continued overleaf

Table 7.3 *Continued*

Country, Year of change to DRG-based hospital payment	*Study*	*Methodology*	*Variables*	*Results/Conclusions*
Portugal, 1990	Dismuke & Sena, 2001[b]	*Method*: Malmquist-Luenberger index *Sample*: 2 DRGs *Study period*: 1992–1994	*Outputs*: (1) Number of live discharges within each DRG; (2) Number of dead discharges within each DRG *Inputs*: Utilization of: (1) CAT scanner; (2) Electrocardiogram; (3) Echocardiogram *Quality*: As per Dismuke & Sena, 1999	DRG-based payment appears to have improved the productivity of the diagnostic technologies considered
Sweden, Early 1990s	Gerdtham et al., 1999b	*Method*: Two stages: (1) Modified DEA; (2) Regression *Sample*: 26 county councils *Study period*: 1993 & 1994	*Outputs*: (1) Surgical discharges; (2) Short-term internal medicine discharges; (3) Surgical operations in short-term care; (4) Physician visits in short-term surgical care; (5) Physician visits in internal medicine *Inputs*: (1) Total cost for short-term care; (2) Beds *Quality*: Not included	Hospital services were more efficient in county councils with internal markets and output-based reimbursement, compared to those with a budget-based approach. Potential cost-savings of approximately 13% by switching from budget- to output-based reimbursement
	Gerdtham et al., 1999a	*Method*: Multiple-output stochastic ray frontier model *Sample*: 26 county councils *Study period*: 1989–1995	*Dependent variables*: (1) Operations; (2) Discharges; (3) Physician visits *Independent variables*: (1) Cost; (2) Available beds; (3) Year; (4) Variables to capture the lead effects of reform; (5) Variables for the new reimbursement system; (6) Political majority; (7) Proportion of population aged over 70 years; (8) Proportion of private visits; (9) University hospital *Quality*: Not included	Move to output-based hospital payment increased technical efficiency by 9.7% on average

Austria, 1997	Sommersguter-Reichmann, 2000	*Method*: DEA/ Malmquist *Sample*: 22 hospitals *Study period*: 1994–1998	*Outputs*: (1) Patients treated in the outpatient care unit; (2) Credit points reported by each hospital, multiplied by a steering factor (to differentiate between hospital types) *Inputs*: (1) Labour FTEs; (2) Hospital beds; (3) Expenses for external medical services *Quality*: Not included	There was an improvement in technology between 1996 and 1998, but there was no improvement in technical efficiency
Norway, 1997	Biørn et al., 2003	*Method*: Two stages: (1) DEA; (2) Regression *Sample*: 48 hospitals *Study period*: 1992–2000	*Outputs*: (1) Casemix-adjusted discharges (including day care); (2) Outpatient visits weighted by the fee paid by the state for each visit *Inputs*: (1) Physician FTEs; (2) Other labour FTEs; (3) Medical expenses; (4) Total running expenses (for analysis of cost-efficiency) *Quality*: Not included	The introduction of DRG-based hospital payment improved technical efficiency, but results relating to the impact on cost-efficiency were varied
	Hagen et al., 2006	*Method*: Two stages: (1) DEA; (2) Regression *Sample*: 48 hospitals *Study period*: 1992–2003	*Outputs*: (1) Casemix-adjusted discharges; (2) Outpatient visits weighted by government reimbursement per visit *Inputs*: (1) Physician FTEs; (2) Other labour FTEs; (3) Medical expenses; (4) Total operating costs (for analysis of cost-efficiency) *Quality*: Not included	Technical efficiency increased after the reimbursement reform, but the effect on cost-efficiency was insignificant
Norway, 1997 and Finland	Linna et al., 2006	*Method*: DEA *Sample*: Finland – 47 hospitals and Norway – 51 hospitals *Study period*: 1999	*Outputs*: (1) DRG-weighted admissions; (2) Weighted outpatient visits; (3) Weighted day care; (4) Inpatient days *Inputs*: (1) Net operating costs *Quality*: Not included	The average level of cost-efficiency was lower in Norwegian hospitals

Source: Compiled by the authors based on the works listed in the 'Study' column.

Notes: ER: emergency room; FTE: full-time equivalent; [a]Studies hospitals in New Jersey, in which DRG-based payments were introduced for all payers in 1980; [b]Assesses the productivity and technical efficiency of diagnostic technologies only.

Taking the first of these, the potential for efficiency gains may depend on the pre-existing hospital payment system. Thus, where global budgets preceded DRG-based payment (as in Sweden, Portugal and Norway, detailed in Table 7.3), hospitals' technical efficiency apparently improved (although Linna and colleagues (2006) found lower cost-efficiency in Norwegian hospitals compared to their Finnish counterparts, despite the latter being understood to operate within a global budget framework). Conversely, DRG-based payment did not improve technical efficiency when it replaced retrospective, cost-based reimbursement (as in the United States) or per diem payments (as in Austria).

This apparent greater potential for efficiency gains when moving from global budgets cannot be regarded as definitive, because the operation of the national DRG-based payment system may itself act as a constraint. Hence, initial efficiency improvements in Sweden were subsequently negated when ceilings were imposed on hospital-activity levels (Gerdtham et al., 1999a, b; Anell, 2005; Kastberg & Siverbo, 2007), and analogous restrictions may also help to explain the lack of improvements in the United States and Austria (US Congress Office of Technology Assessment, 1985; Sommersguter-Reichmann, 2000; Böcking et al., 2005). Finally, it is difficult to isolate the impact of DRG-based payment when it is introduced as part of a wider health care reform programme, as was the case in Sweden when an internal market was also established (Gerdtham et al., 1999a, b).

7.3.2 Impact on indicators of efficiency: Activity, length of stay and costs

Table 7.4 summarizes studies that examined country-specific changes in indicators of efficiency. Following the introduction of DRG-based payment, hospital admissions increased in Australia (Ettelt et al., 2006; Street et al., 2007), Denmark (Street et al., 2007), England (Farrar et al., 2007; Audit Commission, 2008; Farrar et al., 2009), France (Or, 2009), Germany (Böcking et al., 2005; Hensen et al., 2008), Norway (Biørn et al., 2003; Kjerstad, 2003; Hagen et al., 2006; Magnussen et al., 2007), Spain (Cots, 2004, cited in Ellis & Vidal-Fernández, 2007) and, at least initially, in Sweden (Anell, 2005; Kastberg & Siverbo, 2007). However, in line with the hypotheses derived from the incentives indicated in Table 7.2, activity did not increase in the United States (US Congress Office of Technology Assessment, 1985; Davis & Rhodes, 1988; Guterman et al., 1988; Manton et al., 1993; Muller, 1993; Rosenberg & Browne, 2001). Results for Italy are mixed (Louis et al., 1999; Ettelt et al., 2006), while Moreoa-Serra & Wagstaff (2010) found no effect on activity countries in central and eastern Europe and central Asia that had introduced DRGs or other activity-based reimbursement systems. Of course, the aforementioned points regarding country-specific contexts and the difficulties in assigning causality also apply here.

The financial incentive to minimize costs under DRG-based hospital payment has often contributed to a shift from inpatient to day-case and/or outpatient settings (for example, in the United States and England, see Rosenberg & Browne, 2001 and Farrar et al., 2009, respectively) – this may also improve the quality of care, as well as efficiency, *ceteris paribus*. Indeed, DRG-based tariffs

Table 7.4 Summary of recent studies examining changes in indicators of hospital efficiency following the introduction of DRG-based hospital payment

Country, Year of change to DRG-based hospital payment	*Study*	*Study period*	*Methodology*	*Hospital activity*	*ALOS*	*Costs*	
						Unit/average	*Total*
United States, 1983	US Congress Office of Technology Assessment, 1985	1983–1984 and Review	Descriptive	–	–		
	Guterman et al., 1988	1983–1986	Descriptive (with some sub-group analysis)	–	–	+	+ (but at a slower rate)
	Davis & Rhodes, 1988	1984–1985	Descriptive	–	–		
	Kahn et al., 1990	1981/1982 & 1985/1986	Retrospective observational study (focusing on five diseases)		–		
	Manton et al., 1993	1982/1983 & 1984/1985	Descriptive (using life table models)	–	–		
	Muller, 1993	1970–1992	Autoregressive-integrated moving average models	–	–		
	Rosenberg & Browne, 2001	Review	Review	–	–		
Australia, 1993[a]	Ettelt et al., 2006	Review	Review	+		–	–
	Street et al., 2007	Review	Review	+			
Sweden, early 1990s	Anell, 2005	Review	Review	+	–		+
	Kastberg & Siverbo, 2007	Review	Review	+	–		+
Italy, 1995	Louis et al., 1999	1993–1996	Descriptive (with some sub-group analysis)	?	–		
	Ettelt et al., 2006	Review	Review	+	–		
Catalonia, Spain, 1997	Cots, 2004[b]	1993–2000	Descriptive	+		–	+ (but at a slower rate)

Continued overleaf

Table 7.4 *Continued*

Country, Year of change to DRG-based hospital payment	Study	Study period	Methodology	Hospital activity	ALOS	Costs	
						Unit/average	Total
Norway, 1997	Biørn et al., 2003	1992–2000	Descriptive	+			
	Kjerstad, 2003	1995–1998	Difference-in-difference model	+			
	Hagen et al., 2006	1992–2000	Descriptive	+			
	Magnussen et al., 2007	Review	Review	+			
Austria, 1997	Theurl & Winner, 2007	1989–2003	Econometric model with fixed effects		–		
Denmark, 2002	Street et al., 2007	Review	Review	+			
Germany, 2003	Böcking et al., 2005	Review	Review	+	–		
	Schreyögg et al., 2005	2003–2004 and Review	Descriptive		–		
	Hensen et al., 2008[c]	2003–2006	Descriptive	+	–		
England, 2003/2004	Farrar et al., 2007	2002/2003 & 2005/2006	Difference-in-difference framework	+	–	–	
	Audit Commission, 2008	2003/2004 & 2006/2007	Descriptive	+	–	?	
	Farrar et al., 2009	2003/2004 & 2005/2006	Difference-in-difference analysis	+	–	–	
France, 2004/2005	Or, 2009	2005 and Review	Descriptive	+			
OECD countries	Forgione & D'Annunzio, 1999	1984–1986 & 1994–1996	Descriptive		–		+
Various countries in central and eastern Europe as well as central Asia	Moreno-Serra &Wagstaff, 2010	1990–2004	Difference-in-difference model	=	–		+

Source: Compiled by the authors based on the works listed in the 'Study' column.

Notes: The changes following the introduction of DRG-based hospital payment are denoted by + for an increase, – for a decrease, = for no change, and ? for mixed effects; [a] DRG-based hospital payment was introduced in Victoria in 1993; [b] Not intended as a study of the effect of DRG-based hospital payment; [c] Relates to dermatology.

can be used to explicitly incentivize hospitals to increase day-case activity, as for example in England, where a common national tariff has been applied to most elective activity across inpatient and day-case settings (Epstein & Mason, 2006; Street et al., 2007). In the United States, the shift towards outpatient care may also be explained by the operation (until 2000) of a parallel retrospective cost-based reimbursement system for such treatment (Rosenberg & Browne, 2001).

Average length of stay generally declined following the move to DRG-based payment (for example, Kahn et al., 1990; Böcking et al., 2005; Moreno-Serra & Wagstaff, 2010), although some argue that this was merely consistent with a general trend (Rosenberg & Browne, 2001; Schreyögg et al., 2005). Discharge rates to post-acute institutions (typically less costly than acute facilities) usually increased. On average, the recorded severity of patients remaining in acute settings increased (Böcking et al., 2005), and assuming this was not simply changed coding practice, suggests limited potential for further reductions in length of stay *ceteris paribus* (Guterman et al., 1988; Rosenberg & Browne, 2001).

Finally, in the majority of cases, the introduction of DRG-based hospital payment was associated with higher total costs, partly due to higher activity levels (Forgione & D'Annunzio, 1999; Anell, 2005; Kastberg & Siverbo, 2007; Moreno-Serra & Wagstaff, 2010), whereas unit costs appear to have declined (Böcking et al., 2005; Farrar et al., 2009). In the United States the overall impact was reduced inflation in aggregate costs (Guterman et al., 1988). The initial experience with DRG-based payment in the Netherlands has been a lower rate of increase where prices are negotiated rather than set centrally and there is increased competition among hospitals and health insurers (see Chapter 23 of this volume).

In short, in some cases, hospital-level efficiency has improved following the introduction of DRG-based hospital payment, but establishing causation is difficult, due to confounding factors. Elsewhere its theoretically beneficial effects may have been somewhat offset by other features of the national health care system – such as limitations on activity and/or expenditure, or the pre-existing reimbursement system – leading to mixed results.

7.4 What are the key challenges?

7.4.1 Categorization problems may lead to unfair reimbursement or patient selection

Like any categorization system, DRGs cannot group patients perfectly on the basis of their expected resource requirements. Much health care is highly individualized, so defining a 'standardized package of care' is not straightforward. This would not create hospital payment problems if differences across providers were random, but if the differences across providers are systematic, then the reimbursement system becomes potentially unfair and may encourage hospitals to engage in up-coding or to 'dump' (that is, avoid) high-cost patients. These adverse consequences could be avoided, however, if the financial risks of such cases were shared between payer and hospital (see Part Two of this volume, along with chapters 5 and 6).

7.4.2 Independence in price-setting

In some countries, the number of hospitals may be insufficient to ensure that prices are independent of each hospital's costs. This has two implications. First, the regulator may be unable to determine whether costs are contaminated by inefficient behaviour, especially if provision is concentrated in only one or two hospitals. DRG-based hospital payment is then in danger of reducing to cost-based reimbursement – which embodies little incentive to improve efficiency. Second, this form of reimbursement may encourage collusion between providers in their reporting behaviour or in their efforts to reduce their costs. The likelihood of such behaviour increases if there are few providers that are well informed about each other's behaviour. Collusion will limit the scope for DRG-based hospital payment to deliver efficiency improvements. Where data are collected on a sampling basis, as in Germany, the sample must be representative of all hospitals; otherwise, unfair reimbursement may result (see chapters 5 and 14).

7.4.3 Control of expenditure

DRG-based hospital payment that adopts a simple price-per-unit-of-activity approach offers direct incentives to suppliers to increase activity levels. If marginal cost is lower than marginal revenue, the more providers 'do', the larger their financial surplus/profit. Increases in activity levels may therefore place severe pressure on funders' budgets. Consequently, a number of countries attempt to contain expenditure by a system of operating DRG-based hospital payment within a global budget framework (for example, Catalonia (Spain) and Sweden – see chapters 22 and 19, respectively). In France, local-level contracts were found to be more effective at controlling spending than macro-level mechanisms (see Chapter 13).

7.5 Conclusions

DRG-based hospital payment systems have the potential to enhance efficiency in the delivery of hospital services, more so than other hospital payment models. This is because there are clear incentives for hospitals to work harder, because they are paid according to the number of patients they treat, as well as to control their costs, because the prices they face are set independently of their own costs. These payment characteristics encourage providers to improve their technical and cost-efficiency and to seek allocative efficiency in their choice of input mix. In theory, DRG-based hospital payment can be used to support allocative efficiency in the overall mix of outputs produced by the hospital sector as a whole. This requires the price attached to each DRG to reflect its societal value. In practice, though, DRG prices are based on costs in almost all countries, so the pursuit of allocative efficiency in this sense has not been a feature of DRG-based hospital payment policy.

Empirical evidence is mixed in terms of the extent to which DRG-based hospital payment has improved efficiency. This is partly because of cross-country heterogeneity in how DRG-based hospital payment systems are operated (detailed in Part Two of this volume) and because attribution is complicated by the existence of confounding factors (such as changes being part of a wider reform package, or the country-specific design and operation of the reimbursement regime). It is generally agreed that DRG-based hospital payment affects indicators of efficiency, such as activity and length of stay, although the same caveats apply. Unintended consequences may include skimping (on quality), cost-shifting, patient selection or up-coding to higher priced DRGs (see Chapter 6).

While we have outlined simplified forms of DRG-based hospital payment, in practice the payment arrangements implemented in each country can be quite sophisticated (see the country-specific chapters in Part Two of this book). More complex formulations may reflect concerns over the ability of DRG classifications to describe casemix accurately, if the need to moderate incentives to undertake more activity in the pursuit of quality, or other regulatory objectives, such as an equitable geographical distribution of hospital provision. Such sophistication is not surprising: the provision of hospital care is a complex process, often requiring packages of care tailored to the individual patient and delivered under conditions of crisis and uncertainty, requiring co-ordination of health professionals both within and beyond the hospital. In the face of such complexity, the method by which payments are made must be sophisticated enough to provide clear incentives for what is desirable and to avoid creating perverse responses. Compared to cost-based reimbursement and global budgets, DRG-based hospital payment is able to embody such sophistication and, thereby, to provide clearer incentives for hospitals to improve their efficiency.

7.7 References

Anell, A. (2005). Swedish health care under pressure. *Health Economics*, 14:S237–54.

Audit Commission (2008). *The Right Result? Payment by Results 2003–2007*. London: Audit Commission (http://www.audit-commission.gov.uk/SiteCollectionDocuments/AuditCommissionReports/NationalStudies/The_right_result_PbR_2008.pdf, accessed 29 June 2011).

Barnum, H., Kutzin, J., Saxenian, H. (1995). Incentives and provider payment methods. *International Journal of Health Planning & Management*, 10:23–45.

Biørn, E., Hagen, T.P., Iversen, T., Magnussen, J. (2003). The effect of activity-based financing on hospital efficiency: a panel data analysis of DEA efficiency scores 1992–2000. *Health Care Management Science*, 6:271–83.

Böcking, W., Ahrens, U., Kirch, W., Milakovic, M. (2005). First results of the introduction of DRGs in Germany and overview of experience from other DRG countries. *Journal of Public Health*, 13:128–37.

Borden, J.P. (1988). An assessment of the impact of diagnosis-related group (DRG)-based reimbursement on the technical efficiency of New Jersey hospitals using data envelopment analysis. *Journal of Accounting and Public Policy*, 7:77–96.

Chern, J.Y., Wan, T.T. (2000). The impact of the prospective payment system on the technical efficiency of hospitals. *Journal of Medical Systems*, 24:159–72.

Coelli, T.J., Rao, D.S.P., O'Donnell, C.J. (2005). *An Introduction to Efficiency and Productivity Analysis*. New York, NY: Springer Science+Business Media.

Cots, F. (2004). La sostenibilidad del sistema hospitalario en Cataluña. El balance de una década [Viability of the hospital system in Catalonia. Balance after a decade]. *Gaceta Sanitaria*, 18:64–7.

Davis, C., Rhodes, D.J. (1988). The impact of DRGs on the cost and quality of health care in the United States. *Health Policy*, 9:117–31.

Dismuke, C., Sena, V. (1999). Has DRG payment influenced the technical efficiency and productivity of diagnostic technologies in Portuguese public hospitals? An empirical analysis using parametric and non-parametric methods. *Health Care Management Science*, 2:107–16.

Dismuke, C., Sena, V. (2001). Is there a trade-off between quality and productivity? The case of diagnostic technologies in Portugal. *Annals of Operations Research*, 107:101–16.

Ellis, R.P., McGuire, T.G. (1986). Provider behaviour under prospective reimbursement: cost sharing and supply. *Journal of Health Economics*, 5:129–51.

Ellis, R.P., Vidal-Fernández, M. (2007). Activity-based payments and reforms of the English hospital payment system. *Health Economics, Policy and Law*, 2:435–44.

Epstein, D., Mason, A. (2006). Costs and prices for inpatient care in England: mirror twins or distant cousins? *Health Care Management Science*, 9:233–42.

Ettelt, S., Thomson, S., Nolte, E., Mays, N. (2006). *Reimbursing Highly Specialised Hospital Services: The Experience of Activity-Based Funding in Eight Countries*. London: London School of Hygiene & Tropical Medicine.

Farrar, S., Sussex, J., Yi, D. et al. (2007). *National Evaluation of Payment by Results*. Aberdeen: University of Aberdeen Health Economics Research Unit.

Farrar, S., Yi, D., Sutton, M. et al. (2009). Has payment by results affected the way that English hospitals provide care? Difference-in-differences analysis. *British Medical Journal*, 339 b3047doi:10.1136/bmj.b3047.

Forgione, D.A., D'Annunzio, C.M. (1999). The use of DRGs in health care payment systems around the world. *Journal of Health Care Finance*, 26:66–78.

Gerdtham, U., Löthgren, M., Tambour, M., Rehnberg, C. (1999a). Internal markets and health care efficiency: a multiple-output stochastic frontier analysis. *Health Economics*, 8:151–64.

Gerdtham, U., Rehnberg, C., Tambour, M. (1999b). The impact of internal markets on health care efficiency: evidence from health care reforms in Sweden. *Applied Economics*, 31:935–45.

Guterman, S., Eggers, P.W., Riley, G., Greene, T.F., Terrell, S.A. (1988). The first 3 years of Medicare prospective payment: an overview. *Health Care Financing Review*, 9:67–77.

Hagen, T.P., Veenstra, M., Stavem, K. (2006). *Efficiency and Patient Satisfaction in Norwegian Hospitals*. Oslo: Health Organization Research Norway (HORN Working Paper 2006:1).

Hensen, P., Beissert, S., Bruckner-Tuderman, L. et al. (2008). Introduction of diagnosis-related groups in Germany: evaluation of impact on inpatient care in a dermatological setting. *European Journal of Public Health*, 18:85–91.

Jacobs, R., Smith, P.C., Street, A. (2006). *Measuring Efficiency in Health Care: Analytic Techniques and Health Policy*. Cambridge: Cambridge University Press.

Kahn, K.L., Keeler, E.B., Sherwood, M.J. et al. (1990). Comparing outcomes of care before and after implementation of the DRG-based prospective payment system. *Journal of the American Medical Association*, 264:1984–8.

Kastberg, G., Siverbo, S. (2007). Activity-based financing of health care – experiences from Sweden. *International Journal of Health Planning and Management*, 22:25–44.

Kjerstad, E. (2003). Prospective funding of general hospitals in Norway: incentives for higher production? *International Journal of Health Care Finance and Economics*, 3:231–51.

Langenbrunner, J.C., Orosz, E., Kutzin, J., Wiley, M.M. (2005). Purchasing and paying providers, in J. Figueras, R. Robinson, E. Jakubowski, eds. *Purchasing to Improve Health Systems Performance*. Maidenhead: Open University Press.

Linna, M., Häkkinen, U., Magnussen, J. (2006). Comparing hospital cost efficiency between Norway and Finland. *Health Policy*, 77:268–78.

Louis, D.Z., Yuen, E.J., Braga, M. et al. (1999). Impact of a DRG-based hospital financing system on quality and outcomes of care in Italy. *Health Services Research*, 34: 405–15.

Magnussen, J., Hagen, T.P., Kaarboe, O.M. (2007). Centralized or decentralized? A case study of Norwegian hospital reform. *Social Science & Medicine*, 64:2129–37.

Manton, K.G., Woodbury, M.A., Vertrees, J.C., Stallard, E. (1993). Use of Medicare services before and after introduction of the prospective payment system. *Health Services Research*, 28:269–92.

Moreno-Serra, R., Wagstaff, A. (2010). System-wide impacts of hospital payment reforms: evidence from central and eastern Europe and central Asia. *Journal of Health Economics*, 29:585–602.

Muller, A. (1993). Medicare prospective payment reforms and hospital utilization: temporary or lasting effects? *Medical Care*, 31:296–308.

Or, Z. (2009). Activity-based payment in France. *Euro Observer*, 11:5–6.

Robinson, R., Jakubowski, E., Figueras, J. (2005). Organization of purchasing in Europe, in J. Figueras, R. Robinson, E. Jakubowski, eds. *Purchasing to Improve Health Systems Performance*. Maidenhead: Open University Press.

Rosenberg. M.A., Browne, M.J. (2001). The impact of the inpatient prospective payment system and diagnosis-related groups: a survey of the literature. *North American Actuarial Journal*, 5:84–94.

Schreyögg, J., Tiemann, O., Busse, R. (2005). The DRG reimbursement system in Germany. *Euro Observer*, 7:4–6.

Shleifer, A. (1985). A theory of yard stick competition. *Rand Journal of Economics*, 16: 319–27.

Sommersguter-Reichmann, M. (2000). The impact of the Austrian hospital financing reform on hospital productivity: empirical evidence on efficiency and technology changes using a non-parametric input-based Malmquist approach. *Health Care Management Science*, 3:309–21.

Street, A., Häkkinen, U. (2010). Health system productivity and efficiency, in P.C. Smith, E. Mossialos, I. Papanicolas, S. Leatherman, eds. *Performance Measurement for Health System Improvement: Experiences, Challenges and Prospects*. Cambridge: Cambridge University Press.

Street, A., Scheller-Kreinsen, D., Geissler, A., Busse, R. (2010). *Determinants of Hospital Costs and Performance Variation: Methods, Models and Variables for the EuroDRG Project*. Berlin: Universitätsverlag der Technischen Universität Berlin (working Papers in Health Policy and Management Volume 3).

Street, A., Vitikainen, K., Bjorvatn, A., Hvenegaard, A. (2007). *Introducing Activity-Based Financing: A Review of Experience in Australia, Denmark, Norway and Sweden*. York: University of York Centre for Health Economics (CHE Research Paper 30).

Theurl, E., Winner, H. (2007). The impact of hospital financing on the length of stay: evidence from Austria. *Health Policy*, 82:375–89.

US Congress Office of Technology Assessment (1985). *Medicare's Prospective Payment System: Strategies for Evaluating Cost, Quality, and Medical Technology*. Washington, DC: United States Government Printing Office.

WHO (2000). *The World Health Report 2000 – Health Systems: Improving Performance*. Geneva: World Health Organization.

7.8 Summary of terms used in the equations

Symbol	*Description*
R^C, R^G, R^A	Hospital revenue under, respectively, cost-based reimbursement (*C*), global budgets (*G*) and DRG-based funding (*A*)
$\mathbf{Z}^C$, $\mathbf{Z}^G$, $\mathbf{Z}^A$	All sources of revenue not related to health to care activity under cost-based reimbursement, global budgets and DRG-based funding
Q	Activity
$\overline{Q}$	Target activity
I	Individual patient
S	Specialty
J	DRG
C	Unit cost
B_s	Specialty contract value
p_s	Locally agreed specialty-level price
$\hat{p}_j$	Prospectively fixed DRG price
α	Proportion of fixed DRG price paid for additional activity

chapter eight

DRGs and quality: For better or worse?

Zeynep Or and Unto Häkkinen

8.1 Introduction

Initially, in most European countries, diagnosis-related groups (DRGs) were introduced to better describe hospital services and to improve the measurement and management of hospital production (services). Increasing the transparency of care procedures and hence facilitating comparisons of hospitals' activity was seen as a way of improving quality of care in hospitals. Over time, DRGs have increasingly become the basis for hospital payment. However, the impact of DRG-based hospital payment systems on quality of care is not straightforward. These systems may present an inherent risk to quality of care because they directly incentivize hospitals to reduce the cost per stay, irrespective of outcomes. Hospitals are expected to reduce costs by cutting down unnecessary services and by improving efficiency through organizational changes. On the one hand, these changes may improve quality, if they improve clinical process and care management. On the other hand, providers may also 'skimp' on quality as a way of cost-saving, potentially placing the patient's health at risk.

There are many different ways through which DRG-based hospital payment systems may create perverse incentives (Ellis & McGuire, 1996; Miraldo et al., 2006), which could negatively affect care quality. In particular, hospitals may discharge patients earlier than clinically appropriate, omit medically indicated tests and therapies, or over-provide certain services, pushing the patient into a higher paying DRG in order to optimize the payments they receive. Despite greater awareness of the need for better monitoring of care quality and patient outcomes, basic information relating to the quality of services provided is lacking in most countries in which DRGs are used for hospital payment.

This chapter explores the possible impact of DRG-based hospital payment on quality of care. We first provide a theoretical discussion of how the quality of care might be affected in DRG-based payment systems. Quality is defined as any aspect of the service that benefits patients during the process of treatment, or improves health outcome after treatment (Chalkley & Malcomson, 1998). We do not focus here on issues related to patient selection and overspecialization (discussed further in Chapter 6 of this volume), but instead on care quality following hospital admission. We then review the available evidence concerning the impact of DRG-based payment on quality of care, including the experience of countries participating in the EuroDRG project. Finally, based on a review of the available literature on contracting and the results of a few experimental payment designs that explicitly take into account quality of care, we discuss how DRG-based payment systems can be adjusted for quality. We conclude with some recommendations for ensuring a DRG design which will not lead to deterioration in the quality of care.

8.2 What the theory suggests

In the health sector, the notion of quality is rather diffuse, since it is difficult to observe and quantify the quality of care provided. Quality of care is a multi-dimensional concept, covering effectiveness (appropriateness), safety, accessibility and responsiveness of care (Kelly & Hurst, 2006) but there is no agreement on how these should be measured. A useful and widely used approach is the one conceptualized by Donabedian (2003) that describes quality measures as being either structure-, process- or outcome-oriented in nature. Structural measures – such as qualification of medical staff or equipment levels – may represent conditions for the delivery of a given quality of health care, but they are not sufficient to ensure an appropriate care process. Process measures should be based on clinical evidence of the effectiveness of the process concerned and consistent with current professional knowledge (IOM, 2001). However, there is not always agreement on what is 'appropriate' in health care. Thus, process indicators may be more vulnerable to 'gaming' than outcome or structure measures. While outcome indicators are attractive, it is not always possible to assess the contribution of care to health outcomes which are influenced by other patient-level factors.

Information about quality – whether in terms of the care structure, process or medical outcomes – is particularly difficult to obtain. Moreover, in the hospital sector there are several sources of information asymmetries. Patients and purchasers may not be able to distinguish whether a bad medical outcome is attributable to the underlying disease or poor quality of care. Individual patients would have little experience with their specific problem to be able to compare different providers or care procedures. Finally, in some health systems, patients may not have a choice regarding which hospital to attend. The existence of information asymmetry implies that payers and patients will have to rely on the decisions made by the providers. In the 'agency theory' framework, the providers are 'experts' who act on behalf of their patients, but patients, providers and purchasers may have conflicting interests (Forgione et al., 2005). Providers are interested in recovering their costs, or maximizing profits, while achieving an acceptable level of quality in the market place. Public purchasers are interested in meeting the health care needs of the population, while controlling costs. They become economically concerned only when the marginal cost of lower quality exceeds the marginal benefits from cost-saving policies.

Therefore, the type and quality of treatment provided (clinical discretion) is a choice variable of the provider and is determined by multiple incentives. While some incentives are non-financial and can be induced by organizational culture, leadership, information systems, quality regulations, and so on, the economic incentives provided by the payment policy would also influence how providers behave in different situations.

As discussed in Chapter 7, under the most basic DRG-based hospital payment system, hospital revenue (R^A) increases linearly with the quantity of patients treated,[1] as follows:

$$R^A = \sum_{j=1}^{J} [Q_j \times \hat{p}_j] \tag{1}$$

where j refers to each DRG category, ($\hat{p}_j$) refers to the fixed payment for each patient treated in each DRG and (Q_j) to the volume of patients. Thus, under this formulation, hospitals will seek to increase the volume of their activity and are not incentivized financially to improve the quality of care provided (Street et al., 2007). In systems where there is an 'excess demand' (or undersupply), stimulating higher production by itself may help to improve quality by reducing long waiting times (accessibility).

However, in conditions in which it is possible to manipulate treatment thresholds or in which clinical discretion is high, quality of care may be at risk. For example, it is difficult to ascertain the right amount of diagnostic tests to be carried out, or in which circumstances a surgical procedure (such as a caesarean section) is justified.

In the literature on contracting, it is widely recognized that when some dimensions of the product/service are not visible (not specified in the contract) providers will be incentivized to withhold or 'economize' on the dimensions that are not verifiable (Chalkley & Malcomson, 1998; Levaggi, 2005). Given that the treatments provided in a DRG (content) are not always known (badly defined) the providers could decrease resources devoted to the services covered by the fixed (DRG) payment and seek to transfer the cost related to other aspects of care to other providers (cost-shifting). Moreover, Siciliani (2006) shows that when the information on average severity of the patient is known only by the provider, they (the hospital) are incentivized to over-provide high-intensity (surgical) treatment to low-severity patients.

In several countries in which DRG-based hospital payment has been introduced, there has been a significant reduction in the average length of stay (ALOS) (see Chapter 7). As reducing the length of stay in hospitals has been a policy objective in many countries (with or without DRG-based hospital payment), this could be seen as desirable. Shorter hospital stays reduce the risk of morbidity and may be preferred by patients. However, providers can also discharge patients prematurely, in an unstable condition. Unfortunately, it is difficult to assess to what extent reductions in length of stay are 'legitimate' and to what extent they are the result of premature discharges.

The way prices are set will have a significant impact on the cost-efficiency effort of providers (see Chapter 6) and, consequently, on quality. For example, moving from local prices to a national tariff would increase incentives to control costs. This may reduce incentives for improving quality if quality implies extra costs. Of course, quality would not be a concern in situations in which better quality induces costs savings. Moreover, if providers can increase their profits by treating more patients, they have an incentive to attract more patients – if multiple providers exist – by increasing quality (Farrar et al., 2007).

8.3 Evidence from the literature

The earliest and most comprehensive evidence on the impact of DRG-based hospital payment on quality comes from the Unites States, where a DRG-based hospital payment system known as the 'prospective payment system' was implemented in 1983, replacing a cost-based (or fee-for-service) reimbursement model. The following subsections first review evidence from the United States, before turning to experiences from Europe.

8.3.1 Evidence from United States studies

In one of the earliest and most significant studies, using a nationally representative sample of 14 012 patients hospitalized between 1981/1982 and 1985/1986, the RAND Corporation showed that a prospective payment system led to a 20 per cent rise in the likelihood that a patient was discharged from hospital in an unstable condition. However, mortality at 30 and 180 days following hospitalization was unaffected (Rogers et al., 1990). The study also looked at changes in a large number of variables defining the process of care, including cognitive skills of physicians and nurses, as well as technical diagnostic and therapeutic scales, and it suggested that while the process of care improved after the introduction of a prospective payment system (better nursing care, better physician cognitive performance), these improvements in hospital process began prior to the introduction of the prospective payment system and have continued after its implementation. Moreover, after the implementation of the prospective payment system, the ALOS decreased considerably, with no significant impact on readmission rates, and patients were diagnosed as having been more ill at the time of admission (Keeler et al., 1990: Kahn et al., 1991).

Other studies also suggested that since the introduction of the prospective payment system, hospitals have been treating a more severely ill inpatient population, since less severely ill patients were shifted to outpatient settings (Newhouse & Byrne, 1988), but it is not clear to what extent this reflects an improvement in care organization (better management of cases), and to what extent it is a selection effect or shift in coding practices. Some of the increase in severity of illness reflects hospitals' efforts to input more co-morbidity codes, leading to better financial rewards (Feinglass & Holloway, 1991).

In general, the introduction of DRG-based payment has significantly decreased both the ALOS and the rate of hospital admissions in the United States (Feinglass & Holloway, 1991). Despite the evidence of some adverse effects, some of the decline in the number of admissions and the ALOS appears to be related to improvements in organizational efficiency and quality (utilization of new technologies/procedures, development of home or ambulatory care, and so on).

For example, Schwartz & Tartter (1998) compared the experiences of patients who underwent colorectal cancer surgery before and after the implementation of DRG-based hospital payment, in order to identify changes in health care delivery. Studying a sample of 446 patients treated in a New York hospital they showed that the mean length of stay was 2.6 days shorter after the introduction of the DRG system, with a 1.1-day decrease in preoperative and 1.5-day decrease in postoperative length of stay. DRG patients had significantly less operative blood loss, fewer transfusions, shorter duration of surgery, and fewer post-operative complications than the patients treated before the DRG system was implemented. Measures of disease severity (admission hematocrit, tumour differentiation, and tumour size) and patient mix (age and gender) did not change. Schwartz and Tartter (1998) suggested that there have been improvements in operative techniques, but the surgeons may have modified certain aspects of treatment in order to reduce length of stay without adversely affecting the quality. The significant decrease in preoperative length of stay may be due to organizational changes, shifting preoperative assessment to out-patient settings.

Nevertheless, the prospective payment systems may have had contradictory effects for different patient groups, depending on the price incentives provided by the different DRGs. Gilman (2000) examined the effect of DRG refinement for HIV infection in 1994 in the United States, where the prices of non-procedural DRGs were generally lowered and those of procedural DRGs were raised. He demonstrated that in the New York State hospital length of stay for lower priced non-procedural DRGs declined by 3.3 days from 1992 to 1995, while length of stay for better paid procedural DRGs increased by 1.1 days on average over the same period.

However, the pressure for cost-containment created by the DRG-based payment system can also adversely affect care quality. Cutler (1995) demonstrated that the impact of prospective payment systems may depend on the hospitals' economic situation (efficiency) before the prospective payment system was implemented. Using a longitudinal dataset of about 40 000 hospital admissions (from 1981 to 1988) in New England, he showed that hospitals experiencing average price declines (historical costs higher than DRG prices) had a 'compression' of mortality rates, with more deaths occurring in hospital or within two months after discharge, while overall one-year death rates remained the same. Reductions in average prices (revenues) may force hospitals to cut back on treatment intensity and/or other inputs. Cutler also found that there was an increase in readmission rates caused by the introduction of the prospective payment system, without any apparent change in sickness levels.

In a similar (more recent) study, Shen (2003) showed that financial pressure from the prospective payment system adversely affected short-term health outcomes after treatment for acute myocardial infarction (AMI), but did not affect patient survival beyond one year after admission.

Some evidence from the United States suggests that the introduction of DRG-based payment in rehabilitation/nursing facilities had a similar impact on the quality of rehabilitative and post-acute care. After the implementation of the new payment approach, patients appeared to have shorter lengths of stay, with lower functional levels at discharge and higher institutional discharge rates (Gillen et al., 2007; Buntin et al., 2009). Moreover, both emergency readmissions and deaths within 60 days of discharge increased significantly for patients with chronic obstructive pulmonary disease (COPD), although some other outcomes of post-acute care were not affected (McCall et al., 2003).

8.3.2 Evidence from Europe

The evidence from Europe is scarce and less clear cut. In Sweden and Finland, where the incentives of DRG-based hospital payment are moderated by locally adjusted monetary conversion rates and additional payment components (see Chapter 6), it is believed that DRGs have helped with homogenizing care procedures and have improved inpatient care organization. However, in both countries there are no direct indicators of care quality, treatment and access associated with the DRG system. In Sweden, most hospitals contribute to quality registers, but quality monitoring appears to be independent of the DRG-based payment system. A longitudinal study of patient-reported quality of care in two Swedish hospitals suggested that the quality of care as perceived by patients – especially with respect to treatment by staff – decreased after the introduction of DRG-based payment (Ljunggren & Sjödén, 2001) but had no effect on quality of life after surgery (Ljunggren & Sjödén, 2003). The evidence from Sweden also confirmed that the introduction of DRG-based payments contributed to an increase in re-coding diagnoses and increased the number of secondary diagnoses recorded per case (Serdén et al., 2003). In Finland, comparison of outcomes across hospitals is based on specific diseases or procedures, and this information is used only for benchmarking.

An early study of four Norwegian hospitals suggests that the DRG-based payment system did not have any impact on hospital-acquired infections (Pettersen, 1995), although there was some evidence of cream-skimming in the immediate period after DRG-based hospital payment was introduced in Norway in 1997 (Martinussen & Hagen, 2009).

Using data from one region (Friuli) and 32 hospitals over the period 1993–1996, Louis and colleagues (1999) found for Italy – where a DRG-based payment system was introduced at national level in 1995 – that the total number of hospital admissions decreased by 17 per cent, while day-case hospital use increased sevenfold. They also found that the mean length of stay decreased (resulting in a 21 per cent decrease in hospital bed days) for most conditions, while severity of illness increased without any significant change in mortality or readmission rates.

A formal evaluation of DRG-based hospital payment in England, locally referred to as Payment by Results (PbR), also showed that while the ALOS has decreased significantly in settings in which PbR was implemented, little measurable change has occurred in the quality of care in terms of inpatient (in-hospital) mortality, 30-day post-surgical mortality and emergency readmissions after treatment for hip fracture (Farrar et al., 2009). The Audit Commission (2008) concluded that PbR has not had a measurable impact on quality of care in England.

No other formal evaluation of the impact of DRG-based payment on quality of care is available from other European countries. It appears that in most countries in which a DRG-based hospital payment system is introduced, the monitoring and reporting of care quality remains inadequate. For example, both in Germany and France, there is still no systematic information system to monitor readmission rates, postoperative mortality and complication rates.

In Germany, a survey of 30 hospitals in Lower Saxony suggested that the introduction of DRG-based payment did not create cream-skimming or early discharge problems in these hospitals (Sens et al., 2009). Based on interviews with hospital managers, health professionals and patients, the study suggested that service quality appeared to be steady over the period 2007–2008, and may even have improved due to better care organization, especially in large hospitals. Nevertheless, this study did not analyse any concrete measures of patient outcomes or care quality.

In France, there is evidence that up-coding might be a concern. External control efforts by the health insurance fund(s) revealed quickly that a significant proportion of the increase in day cases was due to incorrect coding of outpatient consultations (CNAM, 2006). While this problem has been partly resolved with stricter coding rules for day cases, introduced in 2007, further attention was required to address the pertinence of some day-case procedures, which have been increasingly significantly (see Chapter 13 of this volume).

8.4 Integrating quality into payment

Unintended adverse effects of DRG-based hospital payment systems on care quality could potentially be avoided by modifying the incentives of the payment system. If the payer/purchaser wants to improve quality of care, payments need to be adjusted in a way that rewards hospitals for the additional costs/effort involved in raising quality. Chalkley & Malcomson (1998) suggest, furthermore, that the form of the payment contract should take into account the type of provider (public, profit-making, non-profit-making) and should be adjusted carefully by the purchasers, depending on the objectives pursued (maintaining a certain level of quality while reducing costs, improving quality, and so on).

Different options exist for adjusting DRG-based hospital payment systems on the basis of quality of care. Simplified, there are three options: (1) the hospital level, (2) the level of a DRG-or all DRGs for one condition, and (3) the individual patient level.

Under the first option, total hospital income could be adjusted on the basis of hospital-level quality indicators:

$$R^A = \sum_{j=1}^{J} [Q_j \times \hat{p}_j] + p^h q^h \qquad (2)$$

where q^h is an index of quality measured at hospital level and p^h is payment (price) per unit change on this quality scale. Given the difficulties and cost of measuring treatment-specific outcomes at patient level, hospitals can be rewarded for quality improvements or progress in the care process, given a national framework. This is appropriate if quality is independent of the volume of activity. Otherwise, contracts using a price which varies by volume of patients treated could be more efficient (Chalkley & Malcomson, 1998).

One example of hospital-level quality adjustment is the approach adopted in England according to the Commissioning for Quality and Innovation (CQUIN) framework, which came into effect in April 2009. Within this framework, all acute trust hospitals collect patient-related outcome measures and report on quality in order to publish 'quality accounts' alongside their financial accounts. Subsequently, Primary Care Trusts (PCTs) can link a specific modest proportion of providers' income (agreed nationally) to the achievement of realistic locally agreed goals. In 2009/2010 the CQUIN payment framework covered 0.5 per cent of a provider's annual contract income (Department of Health, 2008), and this proportion increased to 1.5 per cent in 2010/2011 (Department of Health, 2010). Along a similar line, the Centers for Medicare and Medicaid Services (CMS) in the United States will lower DRG payments for all patients in hospitals – initially by up to 1 per cent – with above-average readmission rates for congestive heart failure, pneumonia and AMI from October 2012. Two years later, COPD, coronary artery bypass graft, percutaneous coronary intervention and other vascular procedures will be included in the calculation – and penalties will increase to 2 per cent in 2014 and 3 per cent in 2015.

Under the second option, when patient-level data are available on outcomes and/or treatment process(es), payments can be adjusted for certain DRGs based on the quality of all patients treated within that DRG. The aim is to encourage medical practice that is considered to be 'good quality' by moving away from pricing simply based on average observed costs per episode. However, this requires reliable indicators of patient-level data and agreement on what constitutes 'good quality'. In this case, both quality measurement and payments are DRG specific, as follows:

$$R^A = \sum_{j=1}^{J} [Q_j \times \hat{p}_j] + \sum_{j=1}^{J} [(q^i_j Q_j) \times p'_j] \quad (3)$$

where p'_j corresponds to the price for the 'good quality' care practice for patients of a given DRG (j), and quality is measured at individual DRG level. The price paid for good quality (p'_j) could be higher or lower than the average cost of an episode, depending on what is considered 'good' or 'best' compared to average/common practice. In England, 'best practice tariffs' have recently been introduced for four areas (cholecystectomy, hip fractures, cataracts and stroke), whereby significant unexplained variation in quality of clinical practice is observed and clear evidence of what constitutes best practice is available (Department of Health, 2011). Best practice tariffs are set to incentivize day-case activity for cholecystectomy, while for cataract treatment the price covers the entire care pathway, so that commissioners only pay for events in the best practice (streamlined elective cataract) pathway, in which patients are treated in a 'joined-up' and efficient manner. For hip fracture and stroke, prices are adjusted upwards if key clinical characteristics of best practice care are met (with corresponding lower payment for non-compliance).

In practice, outcome-based adjustment can also be carried out for specific diseases, such as AMI, stroke (Ash et al., 2003; Iezzoni, 2003) or for procedures deemed effective (Nashef et al., 1999) that are not related to specific DRGs. In Germany, one example of such a quality adjustment is the 'integrated care' contract between a large German sickness fund (*Techniker Krankenkasse*) and the Karlsruhe heart surgery hospital, which has been in place since 2005. Under the terms of the contract, the hospital receives higher payments for coronary bypass surgery patients if it scores above the national average on a set of heart surgery quality indicators, which are collected as part of the German external quality assurance system (see Busse et al., 2009). Similarly, in the Netherlands, the original purpose of introducing DBCs was to allow insurers to negotiate with hospitals regarding price, volume and quality of care (which purchasers are currently allowed to do for about 30 per cent of DBCs). However, it would appear that insurers and hospitals negotiate predominantly on price and volume, whereas quality plays only a minor role in the negotiation process.

However, it is challenging to integrate in the payment system an implicit set of clinical guidelines defining how to treat a homogeneous group of patients, approximating a contract that specifies what is 'good quality' for specific DRGs (Newhouse, 2003). Clearly, the condition for such contracts is a consensus on what constitutes 'good-quality' care in different clinical contingencies. The lack of clinical consensus on the guidelines to be used – even in cases of common problems, such as heart attacks – is well documented (Baker et al., 2008; Phelps, 2000) and remains a major obstacle to quality-based contracting. Whether or not best practice tariffs can contribute to improving quality remains to be seen.

The third option is to adjust payments for individual patients based on the quality of their treatment, independent of the DRG to which they are allocated. Hospital contracts could be simply modified to take into account the quality of care provided, as follows:

$$R^A = \sum_{j=1}^{J} [Q_j \times \hat{p}_j] + \sum_{j=1}^{J} [(q^i_j Q_j) \times p^i] \tag{4}$$

where q^i is the patient-level quality index (which could be simply 0, 1) and p^i is the price for individual-level quality (or non-quality). The revenue (R) of providers depends on the number of patients treated Q_j as well the quality of treatment and its price, irrespective of the DRG in which patients are placed. This requires reliable indicators of patient outcomes.

Developing such indicators is not always straightforward, as attributing a certain patient outcome to provider behaviour (rather than to patient health status) can be controversial. Indicators for bad (or good) quality, on which such penalties (or rewards) are based, will thus need to be very robust and subject to as little controversy as possible.

Patient-level quality adjustment policies so far have focused on disentangling complications (caused by the hospital) from co-morbidities (which the patient already has upon admission), as well as on readmissions.

The best-known example of this is the United States Medicare policy, whereby the CMS require hospitals to use 'present-on-admission' codes for both primary and secondary diagnoses when submitting claims for discharges. Since October 2008, diagnosis codes for ten selected conditions – such as pressure ulcers; 'dislocation of patella open' due to a fall; catheter-associated urinary tract infection – are excluded from consideration during the grouping process if they were not coded as being present on admission (that is, they were contracted during the hospital stay) (Department of Health and Human Services, 2008). Consequently, these codes cannot lead to the classification of patients into higher-paying DRGs, and Medicare no longer has to pay for the extra costs of these avoidable hospital-acquired conditions. It is estimated that about 15 per cent of the claims had a 'non-present on admission' diagnosis (Zhan et al., 2007). While this approach to reducing adverse events is considered attractive by some (McNair et al., 2009), others highlight the difficulty of determining what are avoidable adverse events (Provonost et al., 2008). Furthermore, ensuring accurate and thorough coding of hospital diagnoses is challenging. Penalizing or rewarding hospitals based on their diagnosis coding could heighten the risks of 'gaming' or coding manipulation (Iezzoni, 2009).

Another patient-based alternative for integrating quality into DRG-based hospital payment systems is to extend the treatment episode for which a DRG-based payment is granted; that is, by including outpatient visits, readmissions, and so on. In England and Germany, hospitals do not receive a second DRG payment if a patient is readmitted for the same condition within 30 days after discharge. Ideally, it is desirable to extend the payment for an integrated set of treatments, including outpatient visits, rehabilitation, and so on, but this is challenging and requires a sophisticated integrated information system. In the Netherlands, the DBC-based DRG system covers the whole spectrum of inpatient and outpatient care provided at hospitals, relating to a specific diagnosis from the first specialist visit to the end of the care process (treatment completed) and including inpatient days, outpatient visits, laboratory services, medical imaging services, medications, medical materials, (surgical) procedures, and so on. Consequently, as long as a patient is treated for the same condition, the hospital does not receive an extra payment. However, the Dutch system does not provide incentives to reduce postoperative infections or readmission rates, since these are coded as new DBCs.

Of course, it is also possible to have a system which combines different approaches, for example: quality adjustments at the patient level with a global payment/adjustment for quality at the hospital level. However, and essential prerequisite for any quality-based payment adjustments to the hospital payment system is the availability of information on quality of care. Therefore, several countries have increased their efforts to collect quality information (for example, BQS/AQUA[2] in Germany (Busse et al., 2009), COMPAQH in France) but routinely available information on patient outcomes is still scarce. The importance of having better information regarding the quality of care is evidenced by the existence of specific financial incentives to hospitals for reporting quality information. For example, Medicare in the United States encourages hospitals to participate in public reporting of quality information. Those hospitals that do not report on 10 measures of quality (defined by the Hospital Quality Alliance) receive a 0.4 per cent reduction in their DRG prices. In Germany, hospitals are financially penalized if they report quality information for less than 80 per cent of treated cases (Busse et al., 2009). The pertinence of using the act of reporting quality data as a proxy for quality of care delivery is questionable, but – when data are available – hospitals can also be offered positive incentives for their effort or extra payments can be made for stimulating innovative approaches to improving quality and patient safety. However, caution is called for before implementing any such schemes, as providers could be destabilized if their revenues fluctuate significantly from one year to another.

8.5 Conclusions

The effects of DRG-based hospital payment systems on patient outcomes and quality of care have long been debated. In many countries, health professionals have expressed concern that these systems may lead to a focus on cost-containment efforts at the expense of quality of care. Based on theoretical considerations and a review of the available literature, this chapter suggests that DRG-based payment systems may represent risks for quality of care, but may also provide opportunities for quality improvements. The introduction of DRGs has increased transparency and has facilitated comparison and standardization of care. The pressure for efficiency introduced by DRG-based payment systems might help to improve organization of care, accelerate the adoption of technology, and hence improve quality. Nevertheless, hospitals can also skimp on quality as a way of saving costs by manipulating the services/care provided to patients. Technology adoption rates may decelerate if new technologies do not induce cost-savings (see Chapter 9). At the same time, these potential adverse effects are not inevitable consequences of DRG-based hospital payment and can be addressed by carefully designing the payment scheme.

The evidence from the United States suggests that, on the one hand, the introduction of DRG-based payment has improved organizational efficiency and quality of care in some areas, in particular by stimulating better options for ambulatory and home care. On the other hand, there is evidence that the cost-containment pressure created by the introduction of DRG-based payment can have an adverse impact on patient outcomes in terms of readmission and mortality rates. Different patient groups can also experience various impacts, depending on the price incentives provided by different DRGs. Particular attention appears to be necessary to ensure that high-severity groups are adequately accounted for in the DRG system, in order to avoid quality of care being adversely affected for these patients.

In Europe, despite the widespread introduction of DRG-based hospital payment systems since the early 2000s, the available research evaluating the systems' impact on care quality and patient outcomes is too limited to draw any firm conclusions. The limited evidence so far does not suggest that the introduction of DRG-based hospital payment had a significant impact on patient outcomes (as measured by readmission and mortality rates). Thus, some of the adverse effects observed in the United States are not confirmed by evidence from Europe. Clearly, the impact of DRGs on quality would depend on the model adopted and the regulatory and health care context of each country. Because DRG-based hospital payment systems in Europe generally speaking did not replace fee-for-service systems, but rather replaced per diem-based payments or global budgets (see Chapter 2), the effect of DRG-based hospital payments on quality of care might also be different in Europe from that experienced in the United States. In addition, the pressure to contain costs is possibly weaker in many European countries than in the United States, because of the stronger presence of both public providers and public regulator in the hospital sector. If this is true, any adverse impact on quality would also be weaker.

In basic DRG-based hospital payment systems, health care providers are not explicitly rewarded for improving quality. Therefore, these schemes need to be refined in order to integrate direct incentives for improving quality. This chapter provides some examples of how this could be carried out. Nevertheless, caution is called for when implementing any such schemes. A balance needs to be struck between the positive motivational effects and the potentially destabilizing effect of penalties for providers (Maynard & Bloor, 2010). Also, providers may focus too much on those areas in which payments are linked to measured quality improvements, to the detriment of some other (non-measured) aspect(s) of care. Therefore, careful piloting and evaluation of such schemes is essential.

DRG-based hospital payment provides an opportunity to better measure quality of care in hospitals. Thus, it becomes possible to improve quality by providing explicit incentives for higher quality procedures/treatments, penalizing 'poor-quality care' or granting funds for improving patient outcomes. This requires continuous refinement of data and indicators for monitoring quality of care. In many countries, information on patient outcomes and process quality is not routinely collected. However, if financing arrangements become more sophisticated, the demand for and supply of information regarding quality of health care will surely increase.

8.6 Notes

1 In practice, in all countries, hospitals receive some fixed payments independent of their activity to cover the fixed costs of providing certain services, such as education and research. For the sake of simplicity, these are not discussed here.

2 Federal Office for Quality Assurance/AQUA-Institute for Applied Quality Improvement and Research in Health Care.

8.7 References

Ash, A.S., Posner, M.A., Speckman, J. et al. (2003). Using claim data to examine mortality trends following hospitalization for heart attack in Medicare. *Health Services Research*, 38:1253–62.

Audit Commission (2008). *The Right Result? Payment by Results 2003–2007*. London: Audit Commission (http://www.audit-commission.gov.uk/SiteCollectionDocuments/AuditCommissionReports/NationalStudies/The_right_result_PbR_2008.pdf, accessed 29 June 2011).

Baker, L., Fisher, E.S., Wennberg, J. (2008). Variations in hospital resource use for Medicare and privately insured populations in California. *Health Affairs*, 27(2):123–34.

Buntin, M., Colla, C., Escarce, J. (2009). Effects of payment changes on trends in post-acute care. *Health Services Research*, 44(4):1188–210.

Busse, R., Nimptsch, U., Mansky, T. (2009). Measuring, monitoring, and managing quality in Germany's hospitals. *Health Affairs (Millwood)*, 28:294–304.

Chalkley, M., Malcomson, J.M. (1998). Contracting for health services when patient demand does not reflect quality. *Journal of Health Economics*, 17:1–19.

CNAM (2006). *Contrôles et lutte contre les abus et les fraudes*. Paris: Caisse National d'Assurance Maladie (http://www.securite-sociale.fr/institutions/fraudes/fraude.htm, accessed 4 July 2011).

Cutler, D.M. (1995). The incidence of adverse medical outcomes under prospective payment. *Econometrica*, 63(1):29–50.

Department of Health (2008). *Using the Commissioning for Quality and Innovation (CQUIN) Payment Framework*. London: Department of Health.

Department of Health (2010). *Using the Commissioning for Quality and Innovation (CQUIN) Payment Framework – A Summary Guide*. London: Department of Health.

Department of Health (2011). *Best Practice Tariffs*. London: Department of Health (http://www.dh.gov.uk/en/Managingyourorganisation/NHSFinancialReforms/DH_105080, accessed 27 July 2011).

Department of Health and Human Services (2008). *Changes to the Hospital Inpatient Prospective Payment Systems and Fiscal Year 2009 Rates*. Washington, DC: Federal Register (Vol. 73, No. 84).

Donabedian, A. (2003). *An Introduction to Quality Assurance in Health Care*. Oxford: Oxford University Press.

Ellis, R.P., McGuire, T.G. (1996). Hospital response to prospective payment: Moral hazard, selection and practice style effects. *Journal of Health Economics*, 15:257–77.

Farrar, S., Sussex, J., Yi, D. et al. (2007). *National Evaluation of Payment by Results*. Aberdeen: University of Aberdeen Health Economics Research Unit.

Farrar, S., Yi, D., Sutton, M. et al. (2009). Has payment by results affected the way that English hospitals provide care? Difference-in-differences analysis. *British Medical Journal*, 339:1–8.

Feinglass, J., Holloway, J.J. (1991). The initial impact of the Medicare prospective payment system on United States health care: a review of the literature. *Medical Care Review*, 48(1):91–115.

Forgione, D.A., Vermeer, T.E., Surysekar, K., Wrieden, J.A., Plante, C.A. (2005). DRGs, costs and quality of care: an agency theory perspective. *Financial Accountability & Management*, 21(3):291–307.

Gillen, R., Tennen, H., McKee, T. (2007). The impact of the inpatient rehabilitation facility prospective payment system on stroke program outcomes. *American Journal of Physical Medicine & Rehabilitation*, 86(5):356–63.

Gilman, B.H. (1999). Measuring hospital cost-sharing incentives under refined prospective payment. *Journal of Economics and Management Strategy*, 8(3):433–52.

Gilman B.H. (2000). Hospital response to DRG refinements: the impact of multiple reimbursement incentives on inpatient length of stay. *Health Economics*, 9(4):277–94.

Iezzoni, L.I. (2003). *Risk Adjustment for Measuring Health Care Outcomes*. Chicago: Health Administration Press.

Iezzoni, L. (2009). Reinvigorating the quality improvement incentives of hospital prospective payment. *Medical Care*, 47(3):269–71.

IOM (2001). *Crossing the Quality Chasm: A New Health System for the 21st Century*. Washington DC: National Academy Press.

Kahn, K., Draper, D., Keeler, E. et al. (1991). *The Effects of the DRG-Based Prospective Payment System on Quality of Care for Hospitalized Medicare Patients*. Pittsburgh, PA: RAND Corporation.

Keeler, E.B. (1990). What proportion of hospital cost differences is justifiable? *Journal of Health Economics*, 9:359–65.

Kelly, E., Hurst, J. (2006). *Health Care Quality Indicators Project: Conceptual Framework Paper*. Paris, Organisation for Economic Co-operation and Development (OECD Health Working Papers, No. 23).

Levaggi, R. (2005). Hospital health care: pricing and quality control in a spatial model with asymmetry of information. *International Journal of Health Care Finance and Economics*, 5(4):327–49.

Ljunggren, B., Sjödén, P.O. (2001). Patient-reported quality of care before vs. after the implementation of a diagnosis-related groups (DRG) classification and payment system in one Swedish county. *Scandinavian Journal of Caring Sciences*, 15(4):283–94.

Ljunggren, B., Sjödén, P.O. (2003). Patient-reported quality of life before, compared with after a DRG intervention. *International Journal for Quality in Health Care*, 15(5): 433–40.

Louis, D., Yuen, E.J., Braga, M. et al. (1999). Impact of a DRG-based hospital financing system on quality and outcomes of care in Italy. *Health Services Research*, 34(1 Pt 2): 405–15.

Martinussen, P., Hagen, T. (2009). Reimbursement systems, organisational forms and patient selection: evidence from day surgery in Norway. *Health Economics, Policy and Law*, 4:139–58.

Maynard, A., Bloor, K. (2010). Will financial incentives and penalties improve hospital care? *British Medical Journal*, 340:c88.

McCall, N., Korb, J., Petersons, A., Moore, S. (2003). Reforming Medicare payment: early effects of the 1997 Balanced Budget Act on post-acute care. *The Milbank Quarterly*, 81(2):277–303.

McNair, P., Borovnicar, D., Jackson, T., Gillett, S. (2009). Prospective payment to encourage system-wide quality improvement. *Medical Care*, 47(3):272–8.

Miraldo, M., Goddard, M., Smith, P. (2006). *The Incentive Effects of Payment by Results*. York: University of York Centre for Health Economics (CHE Research Paper 19).

Nashef, S.A.M., Roques, F., Michel, E. et al. (1999). European system for cardiac operative risk evaluation (EuroSCORE). *European Journal of Cardio-thoracic Surgery*, 16:9–16.

Newhouse, J.P. (2003). Reimbursing for health care services. *Economie Publique*, 13:3–31.

Newhouse, J.P., Byrne, D.J. (1988). Did Medicare's prospective payment system cause length of stay to fall? *Journal of Health Economics*, 7:413–16.

Pettersen, K.I. (1995). Hospital infections as quality indicators. DRG-based financing, did it change therapeutic quality? [in Norwegian] *Journal of the Norwegian Medical Association*, 115(23):2923–7.

Phelps, C.E. (2000). Information diffusion and best practice adoption, in J.P. Newhouse, A. Culyer, eds. *Handbook of Health Economics*. Amsterdam: North Holland Press.

Pronovost, P., Goeschel, C., Wachter, R. (2008). The wisdom and justice of not paying for 'preventable complications'. *Journal of the American Medical Association*, 299(18): 2197–9.

Rogers, W.H., Draper, D., Kahn, K.L. et al. (1990). Quality of care before and after implementation of the DRG-based prospective payment system. A summary of effects. *Journal of the American Medical Association*, 264:1989–94.

Schwartz, M.H., Tartter, P.I. (1998). Decreased length of stay for patients with colorectal cancer: implications of DRG use. *Journal for Healthcare Quality*, 20(4):22–5.

Sens, B., Wenzlaff, P., Pommer, G., von der Hardt, H. (2009). *DRG-induzierte Veränderungen und ihre Auswirkungen auf die Organisationen, Professionals, Patienten und Qualität*. Hanover: Zentrum für Qualität und Management im Gesundheitswesen, Einrichtung der Ärztekammer Niedersachsen.

Serdén, L., Lindqvist, R., Rosen, M. (2003). Have DRG-based prospective payment systems influenced the number of secondary diagnoses in health care administrative data? *Health Policy*, 65(2):101–7.

Shen, Y.C. (2003). The effect of financial pressure on the quality of care in hospitals. *Journal of Health Economics*, 22(2):243–69.

Siciliani, L. (2006). Selection of treatment under prospective payment systems in the hospital sector. *Journal of Health Economics*, 25(3):479–99.

Street, A., Vitikainen, K., Bjorvatn, A., Hvenegaard, A. (2007). *Introducing Activity-Based Financing: A Review of Experience in Australia, Denmark, Norway and Sweden*. York: University of York Centre for Health Economics (CHE Research Paper 30).

Zhan, C., Elixhauser, A., Friedman, B., Houchens, R., Chiang, Y. (2007). Modifying DRG-PPS to include only diagnosis present at admission. *Medical Care*, 45(4):288–91.

chapter nine

Technological innovation in DRG-based hospital payment systems across Europe

Wilm Quentin, David Scheller-Kreinsen and Reinhard Busse

9.1 Introduction

Technological innovation in health care is highly valued by patients, clinicians and politicians (Rettig, 1994), as advances in medical technology have greatly improved the ability to prevent, diagnose and treat a large number of diseases and conditions, leading to reduced mortality and better quality of life in many countries (Atella & The TECH Investigators, 2003; Cutler & McClellan, 2001; Cutler, 2007; Tunstall-Pedoe et al. 2000). At the same time, technological innovation is a major driver of increasing health care costs (Weisbrod, 1991; Cutler et al., 1998a; Congressional Budget Office 2008), and policies have been devised with the aim of balancing technological innovation and affordability (Schreyögg et al., 2009).

The hospital payment system is one important factor influencing the implementation of technological innovation in health care (Greenhalgh et al., 2004; Banta, 1983; Torbica & Cappellaro, 2010; Atella & the Tech Investigators, 2003; Cappellaro et al., 2011), especially as many new technologies are first used in the inpatient sector. Ever since the introduction of diagnosis-related group (DRG)-based hospital payment systems, there have been concerns that these systems may not provide the right set of incentives to encourage the desired adoption and use of technological innovations in health care (OTA, 1983; Garrison & Wilensky, 1986; MedPAC, 2001; Shih & Berliner, 2008). Consequently, mechanisms have been developed by most countries using DRG-based hospital payment systems to account for technological innovation in health care (MedPAC, 2003; Clyde et al., 2008; Schreyögg et al., 2009; Henschke et al., 2010).

This chapter aims to (1) clarify the relationship between DRG-based hospital payment systems and technological innovation; and (2) to describe how the 12 countries included in this book attempt to overcome the potential problems for technological innovation associated with DRG-based hospital payment systems. The following section (9.2) provides a theoretical overview of the relationship between technological innovation, hospital costs and quality, in order to explain how DRG-based hospital payment systems can potentially affect the adoption and diffusion of technological innovations. Subsequently, section 9.3 presents a comparative analysis of the analysed countries' policy responses to the problems of encouraging technological innovations and incorporating them formally into DRG-based hospital payment systems. Section 9.4 summarizes the findings and draws some conclusions for European countries regarding how best to deal with technological innovations in the context of DRG-based hospital payment systems.

9.2 Technological innovation and DRG-based hospital payment in theory: Costs, quality and the adequacy of payment

9.2.1 Technological innovation: Costs and quality

Technological innovation is often defined as the practical application and diffusion of ideas or knowledge (Goodman, 2004). In health care, innovations can potentially refer to all categories of medical technology, such as drugs, devices, equipment and supplies, medical and surgical procedures, support systems and organizational and managerial systems (Banta et al., 1978). Technological innovation may be incremental, consisting of small improvements of existing services; or it may comprise radical changes, such as replacing surgical therapy with new medical therapy. Finally, technological innovation may occur as a transfer or adaptation of existing technology from one setting to another, for example the shift of certain procedures from inpatient settings to day care.

When analysing the implications of DRG-based hospital payment systems for the adoption and diffusion of technological innovation in health care, it is essential to consider the effects of technological innovations on hospital costs and quality. Table 9.1 illustrates possible effects of technological innovations on hospital costs: such innovations may increase or decrease capital costs, operating costs or both (OTA, 1983). Yet, the overall effect on hospital costs depends on the interplay of various factors. For example, in large or highly specialized hospitals, an increase in capital costs might be compensated by reductions in operating costs, if capital costs can be distributed among a sufficiently large number of patients. In small or less-specialized hospitals, the effect of the same technological innovation on costs may be different. Furthermore, it is important to bear in mind that technological innovations may be related to costs of all hospital services (for example, the introduction of electronic medical records) or may only affect the costs of treating a small and very specific group of patients (for example, the introduction of drug-eluting stents).

Table 9.1 Possible effects of technological innovation on hospital costs

Technological innovation	*Effect on costs*		
	capital	*operating*	*total*
Cost-increasing technology	+	+	+
Cost-decreasing technology	–	–	–
Capital cost-increasing technology	+	–	+/–
Operating cost(s)-increasing technology	–	+	+/–

Source: OTA, 1983, with modifications.

Quality in health care can be defined as any aspect of health services that benefits patients during the process of treatment or improves health outcome after treatment (see Chapter 8). In theory, the effect of technological innovation on 'quality' can be positive, neutral or negative. Figure 9.1 illustrates different theoretical combinations of costs and quality that can result from the introduction of technological innovations, using a graphical illustration similar to that of the cost–effectiveness plane (Black, 1990). Technological innovations can increase both costs and quality (A), increase quality while decreasing costs (B), decrease both costs and quality (C), or increase costs while decreasing quality (D).

Whether or not the incentives of DRG-based hospital payment systems produce socially desirable effects depends on the specific combination of costs and quality; that is, it depends on the quadrant (A to D) into which the new technology would be classified. Technologies falling into quadrant B would be always desirable, whereas technologies falling into quadrant D should never be

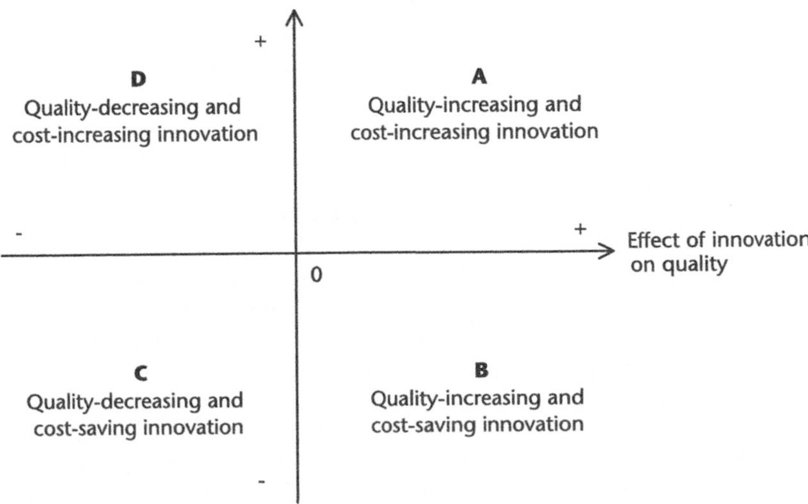

Figure 9.1 Effects of innovation on cost and quality

Source: Adapted from Black, 1990.

adopted. For technologies falling into quadrants A and C, things are more complicated (Cutler & McClellan, 2001). For quadrant A, the country-specific willingness to pay for a given increase in quality determines whether these technological innovations should be used in hospitals. Conversely, for technologies falling into quadrant C, it depends on the extent to which countries are willing to forego quality in exchange for a decrease in costs.

However, the effects (especially long-term effects) of technological innovation on quality (and on costs) are often difficult to identify at the time, when innovations are first introduced into hospital practice (Mowatt et al., 1997). In fact, a variety of technologies have been found to be ineffective or even harmful after having been widely adopted and used (Goodman, 2004). Consequently, policy-makers face considerable uncertainty when making decisions about technological innovations.

9.2.2 DRG-based hospital payment systems: Incentives against technological innovation?

Under DRG-based hospital payment systems, clinicians are free to decide on the exact set of technologies that they want to employ when treating a given patient. However, as outlined in Chapter 6, DRG-based hospital payment systems provide a specific set of incentives to hospitals that are likely to have an effect on shaping the clinicians' decisions. This subsection investigates how these incentives may influence the use of technological innovations in hospitals. Under the most basic DRG-based hospital payment system, introduced in Chapter 6, hospitals are paid a predetermined fixed payment rate per case. Consequently, hospitals are encouraged to keep their average costs below the payment rate in order to avoid making a loss. Thus, the two dominant incentives of a basic DRG-based hospital payment system encourage hospitals to (1) reduce costs per admission, and (2) increase the number of admissions (OTA, 1983).

The effects of these incentives on the hospitals' willingness to adopt and to use technological innovations are summarized in Table 9.2. Hospitals are likely to invest in technological innovations that reduce total costs per admission. They may purchase new diagnostic equipment or electronic drug interaction monitoring systems if these can be shown to reduce costs per stay – for example, by reducing length of stay. In cases in which technological innovations are cost neutral, or in which increases in one area can be compensated by decreasing costs in another area, DRG-based hospital payment systems should have no effect on the introduction of technological innovations. Furthermore, as technological innovation often increases capital costs, DRG-based hospital payment systems might encourage the specialization of hospitals (if separate funding for capital costs is unavailable), concentrating the adoption of technological innovations in centres with sufficiently large numbers of patients. In addition, as hospitals bear the financial risk of average costs rising above the payment rate, hospitals are likely to make use of economic evaluations before introducing certain technological innovations.

As far as many cost-decreasing, cost-neutral or cost-increasing but quality-decreasing technological innovations are concerned (quadrants B to D in

Table 9.2 Incentives of DRG-based hospital payment systems and effects related to technological innovation

Main incentives	*Effects related to technological innovation*
1. Reduce costs per admission	• Promoting the use of cost-decreasing technological innovations • Encouraging the concentration of capital cost-increasing innovations in fewer institutions, leading to specialization of hospitals for certain technologies • No effect on technological innovations that are cost neutral • Discouraging the introduction of cost-increasing technologies • Encouraging HTAs before introduction of new technologies
2. Increase number of admissions	• Encouraging the use of technologies promoting hospital reputation • Promoting the use of technological innovations valued by patients/admitting physicians

Source: Based on OTA, 1983.

Figure 9.1), DRG-based hospital payment provides incentives that are likely to be in line with societal objectives: they encourage adoption of technological innovations in quadrant B and C, and inhibit technological innovation in quadrant D. However, economic evaluations and country-specific value-judgements are required in cases in which cost-decreasing technological innovations are accompanied by decreases in quality (quadrant C), as it should be determined whether the decrease in quality outweighs the reduction in costs (Drummond et al., 2005).

Problems with DRG-based hospital payment occur when technological innovations improve quality but are associated with increased costs per admission (quadrant A in Figure 9.1). In most countries, DRG-based payment rates are at least remotely related to the average costs of treating cases in other hospitals in the past (see Chapter 5). When technological innovations are introduced, hospitals are paid according to historical cost patterns that do not reflect the (potentially) higher costs of using technological innovations. Consequently, disincentives exist for hospitals to adopt and use cost-increasing technological innovations until the payment system is updated to account for their extra costs. Patient access to quality-increasing technological innovations that also increase costs could be delayed because, in general, it takes some time for enough information regarding the costs of using a technological innovation in routine practice to be generated.

In some cases, the disincentive for using technological innovations under DRG-based hospital payment systems might be counterbalanced by the second kind of incentive (Table 9.2), which is to increase the number of admissions. In competitive environments, and if certain technological innovations are thought to improve hospital reputation or to stimulate admissions by physicians, hospitals are likely to react by offering these services (OTA, 1983). Of course, particular design features of each country's DRG system and its DRG-based hospital payment system (see Chapter 6 of this volume) are likely to modify the strength of the basic incentives of these systems. For example, several countries (such as France, Germany, Ireland, Poland, and Spain (Catalonia)) provide additional funding for capital costs, thus exempting a significant proportion of hospital costs (particularly relevant in the context of innovations that increase capital costs) from the incentives of DRG-based hospital payment. Similarly, the availability of funding from sources other than the DRG-based hospital payment system may modify the incentives of DRG-based hospital payment systems. For example, hospitals receiving extra funding for teaching or research are more likely to be in a better position to adopt technological innovations.

Yet, as evidenced by the existence of specific payment instruments for technological innovations in most countries across Europe (see section 9.3), DRG-based hospital payment systems alone seem to be perceived as providing insufficient incentives for the desired introduction of technological innovations that increase quality but also increase cost.

9.3 Technological innovation and DRG-based hospital payment in practice: 12 European countries in comparison

As illustrated in the country-specific studies in the Part Two of this volume, and as shown by Scheller-Kreinsen et al. (2011) DRG-based hospital payment systems in most countries are updated at regular intervals. These long-term mechanisms ensure that technological innovations are eventually formally incorporated into the DRG-based hospital payment system, either through updates of the DRG system (see Chapter 4), or through updates of the payment rate (see Chapter 6). In addition, almost all countries have developed certain short-term payment instruments that encourage the use of quality-increasing technological innovations that also increase costs, within the time period during which the DRG-based hospital payment system does not yet account for the technological innovation.

Figure 9.2 illustrates the short-term payment instruments and long-term updating mechanisms used to encourage and incorporate technological innovation in the DRG-based hospital payment system. On the left, the figure shows the short-term payment instruments used to encourage the use of quality-increasing technological innovations that also increase costs. These can be completely outside the system (extreme left) or can be associated to the DRG-based hospital payment system (in the middle). On the right, the figure presents mechanisms to incorporate technological change into the systems, either by updating the DRG system – that is, the patient classification system (PCS) – or by adjusting the payment rate. When updating the PCS, several options exist: (1) cases can be reassigned to different DRGs, (2) existing DRGs can be split, and (3) new DRGs can be created when necessary.

A common challenge for policy-makers when devising payment policies is to find the right balance between two conflicting goals (Schreyögg et al., 2009). On the one hand, they need to provide sufficient incentives for hospitals to make use of quality-increasing technological innovations that also increase

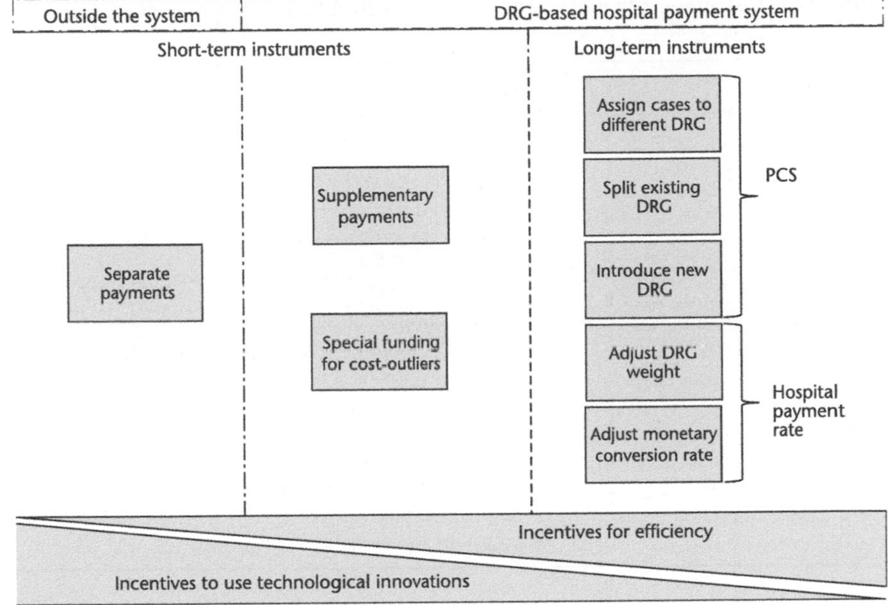

Figure 9.2 Short-term payment instruments and long-term updating mechanisms

costs, in order to assure patient access. On the other hand, they need to keep expenditure for technological innovations under control. If short-term instruments provide additional payments for selected technological innovations, these payments introduce incentives that may distort clinical decision-making and can lead to inefficiencies related to over-provision of these services and escalating health care costs (MedPAC, 2001). These conflicting incentives are illustrated by the bars at the bottom of Figure 9.2. Specific incentives to use technological innovations should decrease as technologies become more formally incorporated into the system (although exceptions are conceivable, as discussed later). Conversely, incentives for providers to make efficient use of resources increase once the use of technological innovations is no longer encouraged through specific payment incentives.

9.3.1 Short-term instruments across Europe to encourage the use of technological innovation

In the countries analysed in this book, three different short-term instruments are employed to encourage the use of quality-increasing technological innovations that also increase costs: (1) separate payments, (2) supplementary payments and (3) special funding for cost-outliers. Table 9.3 shows that these three types of short-term instruments can be represented in different forms.

Separate payments can take two forms: (1) fee-for-service payment, negotiated nationally or locally, as is used in Germany (see Box 9.1); or (2) retrospective reimbursement of hospital-reported total costs, as is used by some county

Table 9.3 Instruments to encourage the use of technological innovation and types of associated payments

Instrument	*Type of payment*
Outside DRG system	
Separate payments	• fee-for-service (based on weighted costs or negotiated payment) • retrospective reimbursement of reported costs per case
Inside DRG system	
Supplementary payments	• fee-for-service • retrospective reimbursement of costs above standard rate • payment of weighted costs
Special funding for cost-outliers	• retrospective reimbursement of costs above a statistically determined threshold • fixed payments (based on weighted costs or negotiated payment) • payment of weighted costs

councils in Sweden. Both payment instruments are designed to encourage the use of technological innovations when information regarding associated costs and effects is still relatively scarce. Separate payments do not necessarily require procedure codes to have been assigned to procedures, or drugs to be entered in specific lists. The associated flexibility allows some countries, such as France, to make decisions at the level of the individual patient; for example, whether or not to pay for experimental cancer drugs (see Chapter 13). Consequently, access to new therapies in France (particularly in terms of cancer treatment) remains one of the most generous in Europe (de Pouvourville, 2009). However, the disadvantages of extensively using a system of separate payments have also been experienced in France, where expenditure on new drugs has rocketed (Cour de Comptes, 2009).

Box 9.1 Separate payment to German hospitals under NUB regulations

In Germany, the New Diagnostic and Treatment Methods Regulation (NUB) was introduced as part of the 2005 Hospital Remuneration Act (KHEntgG). It provides extrabudgetary funding in the form of negotiated fee-for-service payments to selected hospitals using technological innovations. Hospitals wishing to be reimbursed via NUBs for their use of technological innovations must take several steps before being reimbursed. First, hospitals must apply – with a description of the new technology and of associated costs – to the Institute for the Hospital Remuneration System (InEK), which is responsible for managing the German diagnosis-related groups (G-DRG) system. If the application is accepted, individual providers must successfully negotiate with the sickness funds concerning the size of the payments to be made. Finally, each hospital must conclude a contractual agreement with the sickness funds to receive NUB reimbursement for its use of the technology. Negotiated NUB payments are valid for only one year and hospitals need to reapply to the InEK if they want to continue to use a technology in subsequent years. Since the introduction of this approach in 2005, it has been shown that acceptance for NUB reimbursement often represents the first step in the process of incorporating new technologies into the DRG system (Henschke et al., 2010).

Source: Henschke et al., 2010.

In contrast to separate payments, supplementary payments and cost-outlier funding are relevant for technological innovations, but are also used to improve the general coherence of the DRG system by excluding certain high-cost technologies or high-cost patients and reimbursing them separately (see Chapter 4 and Chapter 6). Both instruments take a specific DRG payment rate as a starting point and justify additional payments in terms of substantial differences between incurred costs and standard payment rates.

Supplementary payments are made on top of the 'standard' DRG payment rate if specific technologies (including new and innovative ones) are applied. The amount to be paid on top of the standard rate can be negotiated or can take the form of retrospective reimbursement of reported costs (per case) above the standard rate of individual providers. In some countries costs are weighted across providers before being paid; that is, average costs per patient category are calculated and reimbursed ('payment of weighted costs'). The necessary administrative processes for establishing a relationship between a procedure (a technological innovation) and a DRG require some time, which may contribute to slowing down the adoption of technological innovations by hospitals. In some cases, a procedure code needs to be assigned to a technological innovation before supplementary payments can be made, thus prolonging the process of providing reimbursement for technological innovations.

In countries in which special funding for cost-outliers is available, the way technologies (including new and innovative ones) influence homogeneity of resource use of patients within DRGs determines whether special funding is made available on top of standard payment rates. Cost-outlier funding builds on detailed retrospective statistical analysis of cost data. Different variants of this instrument exist (see Table 9.3). In addition, many countries provide extra payments for length-of-stay outliers (see Chapter 6) but these instruments are not particularly relevant to technological innovation, as technological innovation may contribute to a reduction in the length of stay, for example, when new, minimally invasive surgical procedures lead to faster patient recovery and discharge (Simpson et al., 2005).

Table 9.4 presents the distribution of the outlined short-term payment instruments across the 12 countries. Separate payments are the most frequently used payment instrument. Surprisingly, cost-outlier funding for cost-increasing technological innovation is used only in Estonia, Finland and some Swedish county councils. Some countries with DRG-based budget-allocation systems (such as Austria and Portugal) do not make use of any short-term payment instruments.

Table 9.4 The application of short-term reimbursement instruments in 11 European countries (plus Catalonia)

	Instruments used to provide extra payments for technological innovations		
	Separate payments	*Supplementary payments*	*Cost-outlier funding*
Austria	No	No	No
Catalonia (Spain)*	Yes (for certain high-cost procedures)	No	No
England/ United Kingdom	Yes (for up to three years)	Yes (for certain high-cost services)	No
Estonia	Yes (for certain high-cost services)	No	Yes
Finland	Depending on hospital district, both instruments are used		No
France	Yes	Yes	No
Germany	Yes	Yes (for certain high-cost services)	No
Ireland	Yes	No	No
Netherlands	Yes (for certain high-cost drugs)	Yes (envisaged to start in 2011)	No
Poland	No	Yes (for certain high-cost services)	No
Portugal	No	No	No
Sweden	Depending on the county council, all instruments are used		

Source: Compiled by the authors on the basis of information presented in the country-specific chapters in Part Two of this volume.

*In Spain hospital financing is decentralized. The information presented here refers to Catalonia, where a DRG system is used that determines 35 per cent of hospital reimbursement.

All extra payments provide strong incentives to hospitals to apply technological innovations, as they exempt the selected technologies from the incentives of DRG-based hospital payment. However, as already mentioned, they may favour the use of certain procedures, drugs or technological equipment over existing technologies included within the DRG-based system, which may reduce efficiency of hospital care (MedPAC, 2001). Furthermore, extra funding may produce 'winners' and 'losers' in the hospital market, as it is likely to lead to higher payments for hospitals that play a strong role in technology dissemination (for example, at university hospitals, at the expense of other hospitals) (MedPac, 2001).

9.3.2 Long-term updating mechanisms in European DRG-based hospital payment systems: Incorporating technological innovations

In terms of incorporating technological innovations into DRG-based hospital payment systems, the processes of updating the PCS and the payment rate are essential. Table 9.5 presents the frequency of updates and the time-lag to data used for updates in 12 countries across Europe, as these two factors determine how fast a DRG-based hospital payment system is able to respond to technological innovations. Neither of the updating mechanisms are specifically targeted at incorporating technological innovations, but they are intended to

Table 9.5 Frequency of updates and time-lag to data used for updates across 12 European countries

	DRG-based hospital payment system			
	PCS		*Payment rate*	
	Frequency of updates	*Time-lag to data*	*Frequency of updates*	*Time-lag to data*
Austria	Annual	2–4 years	4–5 years (updated when necessary)	2–4 years
England/United Kingdom	Annual	Minor revisions annually; irregular overhauls about every 5–6 years	Annual	3 years (but adjusted for inflation)
Estonia	Irregular (first update after 7 years)	1–2 years	Annual or following update of fee-for-service fees	1–2 years
Finland	Annual	1 year	Annual	0–1 year
France	Annual	1 year	Annual	2 years
Germany	Annual	2 years	Annual	2 years
Ireland	Every 4 years, linked to Australian updates of AR-DRGs	Not applicable (imported AR-DRGs)	Annual (linked to Australian relative-weight updates)	1–2 years
Netherlands	Irregular	Not standardized	Annual or when considered necessary	2 years, or based on negotiations
Poland	Irregular (planned twice per year)	1 year	Annual update only of base rate	1 year
Portugal	Irregular	Not applicable (imported AP-DRGs)	Irregular	2–3 years
Spain (Catalonia)	Biennial	Not applicable (imported 3-year-old CMS-DRGs)	Annual	2–3 years
Sweden	Annual	1–2 years	Annual	2 years

Source: Compiled by the authors on the basis of information presented in the country-specific chapters in Part Two of this volume.

ensure that the DRG-based payment systems are always adapted to current practice patterns and treatment costs.

Both the PCS and the payment rate are updated annually in the majority of countries, but there are remarkable exceptions. In 2010, Estonia updated its DRG system for the first time since the introduction of the Nordic PCS (NordDRGs) to the country in 2003. Ireland currently uses Australian Refined (AR-)DRGs, which are updated every four years (see Chapter 15 of this volume). Austria is an interesting outlier with regard to the adjustment of payment rates, as DRG weights are not updated regularly, but are adjusted only for specific DRGs when deemed necessary by policy-makers. The data used for updates vary considerably between countries. In Finland, data are used from the current year to update the DRG system for the next year, and DRG weights are recalculated as soon as data become available (during the same year). In most countries, however, data both for updating the PCS and for adjusting DRG weights or prices are at least two years old.

In addition, the mechanisms to introduce new codes for new procedures, drugs and medical devices affect the way in which DRG systems can incorporate technological innovations. Frequent updates of codes facilitate more rapid adoption and incorporation of technological innovations into DRG systems. Rare updates increase the length of time before technological innovations can be systematically incorporated.

As already mentioned, technological innovations can alter treatment costs in different ways. Countries collecting detailed bottom-up hospital cost-accounting information (see Chapter 5) are clearly in a better position to precisely identify the effect of technological innovations on hospital costs using routinely available information. When technological innovations increase (or decrease) costs for a well-defined subset of patients, adjusting the PCS is the best method of incorporating technological innovations into the DRG-based hospital payment system. However, the incentives to modify the PCS should be closely monitored: if a new DRG is introduced – for example, for using a specific innovative medical device in a broadly defined group of patients – providers could be incentivized to over-provide the technological innovation to patients that would not benefit from the innovative technology.

When technological innovations increase the costs of all services bundled in one DRG or the costs of all hospital services, updates to the payment rate are the best approach to incorporating them into the DRG-based hospital payment system. In order to increase payment for a specific DRG, DRG weights can be recalculated. In order to increase funding for all hospital services, countries not operating a relative-weight approach can inflate raw tariffs by the appropriate amount. Countries using a relative-weight approach have different options. They can either adjust the base rate to account for proportionate increases in costs (for example, a 5 per cent increase of all hospital costs), or they can adjust the base rate and recalculate relative weights if technological innovations increase costs for all cases by a fixed amount.

9.4 Conclusions: Encouraging and incorporating technological innovations in European DRG-based hospital payment systems: Scope for improvement

In many European countries, there are concerns that DRG-based hospital payment systems do not provide the right set of incentives to ensure that patients have timely access to technological innovations. Our discussion of the theoretical incentives of DRG-based hospital payment systems to adopt and use technological innovations in hospitals has revealed that these concerns should be important only for the specific case of those technological innovations that increase quality and are accompanied by a significant increase in total costs per case.

The second part of the chapter illustrates that most (but not all) countries analysed in this book have complemented their DRG-based payment systems with specific short-term payment instruments targeted at encouraging the adoption and use of technological innovations. However, additional payments for technological innovations exempt these technologies from the inherent efficiency incentives of DRG-based hospital payment systems. In fact, generous separate payment methods (such as fee-for-service payments) may lead to a distortion of clinical decision-making and a significant increase in spending on those technological innovations for which separate payments are available (as evidenced in France). Furthermore, as short-term payment incentives are often introduced for technological innovations at a time when rigorous analyses of their (long-term) effects are not yet available, there is a risk that the additional payments inadvertently incentivize the use of cost-increasing technological innovations that are quality neutral or even result in a decrease in the quality of health care.

Therefore, short-term payment instruments should be employed very carefully, and incorporated only after careful assessments have been made concerning the likely effects of the concerned technology on quality of care. In the United States, short-term payment instruments are intended to be limited to technological innovations offering either considerable quality improvements over existing technologies, or offering options for diagnosis or treatment of previously untreatable conditions (Clyde et al., 2008). Unfortunately, in several European countries (such as Germany and France), the introduction of short-term payment instruments for technological innovations seems to be more directly linked to the criteria of higher costs than to the criteria of demonstrating considerable quality improvements.

If countries should want to provide short-term payment incentives for technological innovations with expected significant quality improvements but for which the evidence remains uncertain, one possible approach is the so-called Coverage with Evidence Development (CED) (Hutton et al., 2007). Under CED approaches, payments for technological innovations are provided only for a limited period of time and on the condition that continuing evaluation is carried out (see Box 9.2 for an example from the Netherlands).

Box 9.2 Coverage with evidence development in the Netherlands

In 2006, new regulations were introduced in the Netherlands regarding expensive (and orphan) inpatient drugs. The regulations specify that an innovative drug can be provisionally included on the expensive (or orphan) drug list(s) for up to four years, which allows hospitals to receive separate payments for these drugs even before their cost–effectiveness has been formally established. The conditions for a drug to be included on a list are that (1) added therapeutic value is demonstrated; (2) a plan for the assessment of cost–effectiveness in daily clinical practice is approved by the pharmaceutical advisory committee; and (3) the drug expenses account for over 0.5 per cent (for the expensive drugs category) or 5 per cent (for orphan drugs) of the annual hospital drug budget. If all three conditions are met, hospitals can receive separate payments amounting to 80 per cent (for expensive drugs) (and 100 per cent for orphan drugs) of the purchase price of drugs placed on the expensive (and orphan) drug list(s). After three years, the data generated in the context of the assessment plan are used to inform decisions about providing further funding for the innovative or (orphan) drug(s).

Source: Delwel, 2008.

Given that most DRG-based hospital payment systems are updated at regular intervals, the change of treatment patterns and costs resulting from the introduction of technological innovations should ultimately be reflected by the DRG-based hospital payment system. Countries with frequent updates of their DRG system and of the payment rate – and with a short time-lag between data collection and using the information collected for DRG-based hospital payment – are clearly in a better position to incorporate technological innovations into their systems. However, if updates of the system lead to the introduction of specific new DRGs for technological innovations (such as for drug-eluting stents), the effect may be similar to that of introducing separate payments for technological innovations; namely, introducing strong incentives to make use of the specific technology. More generally, therefore, the issue of incorporating technological innovations into DRG systems highlights the trade-off that exists between providing adequate funding for specific procedures and the intention to promote efficiency by leaving to clinicians the decisions regarding which procedures to use.

Furthermore, in the context of an emerging common European hospital market, there is scope for increasing cooperation across countries in terms of technological innovations. Cooperation appears to be particularly beneficial in the field of assessing the effect of technological innovations on quality. As envisaged by article 15 of the recently adopted European Union (EU) *Directive on the Application of Patients' Rights in Cross-Border Healthcare* (European Parliament and Council, 2011), a European network of health technology assessment (HTA) agencies could assess technological innovations using a common set of criteria in order to avoid duplication of work and individual analyses in each Member State (Kristensen, 2008). If sufficient evidence is available to demonstrate considerable improvements in quality, decentralized decisions regarding whether or not to introduce short-term payment instruments for these technologies could then be made by governments, self-governing bodies or local payers within Member States, in a manner similar to the decentralized approaches used in Finland, Germany (see Box 9.1) or Sweden. The advantage would be that the available evidence could be assessed more efficiently, while payment decisions would still be made according to national or local value-judgements, which is necessary because differences are likely to exist in the willingness to pay for a given increase in quality.

Empirical research on the effects of DRG-based hospital payment systems in terms of the adoption and diffusion of technological innovations is difficult to design and is relatively scarce. Research relating to the effects of DRG-based payment systems on the adoption, implementation and use of technological innovations has rarely taken into account the different approaches to encouraging and incorporating technological innovations within the family of DRG-based payment systems (Torbica & Cappellaro, 2010; Packer et al., 2006; Bech et al., 2009). Short-term payment instruments and long-term updating mechanisms differ greatly across countries. Future empirical cross-country investigations – for example of the determinants of the implementation and use of technological innovation – should take these differences into account and test empirically whether and how the different identified approaches affect the implementation and use of technological innovation.

9.5 References

Atella, V., the TECH Investigators (2003). The relationship between health policies, medical technology trends, and outcomes: a perspective from the TECH global research network, in OECD. *A Disease-Based Comparison of Health Systems. What is Best and at What Cost?* Paris: Organisation for Economic Co-operation and Development.

Banta, H.D. (1983). Social science research on medical technology: utility and limitations. *Social Science & Medicine*, 17(18):1363–1369.

Banta, H.D., Behney, C.J., Andrulid, D.P. (1978). *Assessing the Efficacy and Safety of Medical Technologies*. Washington, DC: Office of Technology Assessment.

Bech, M., Christiansen, T., Dunham, K., et al. (2009). The influence of economic incentives and regulatory factors on the adoptions of treatment technologies: a case study of technologies used to treat heart attacks. *Health Economics*, 18(10):1114–1132.

Black, W.C. (1990). The CE plane: a graphic representation of cost–effectiveness. *Medical decision-making: an international journal of the Society for Medical Decision-Making*, 10(3):212–214.

Cappellaro, G., Ghislandi, S., Anessi-Pessina, E. (2011). Diffusion of medical technology: the role of financing. *Health Policy*, 100(1):51–59.

Clyde, A.T., Bockstedt, L., Farkas, J.A., Jackson, C. (2008). Experience with Medicare's new technology add-on payment program. *Health Affairs*, 27(6):1632–1641.

Congressional Budget Office (2008). *Technological Change and the Growth of Health Care Spending*. Washington, DC : Congressional Budget Office.

Cour de Comptes (2009). *La Securité Sociale, chapitre 7, La mise en place de la T2A: Bilan à mi-parcours*. Paris: Cour de Comptes.

Cutler, D.M. (2007). The lifetime costs and benefits of medical technology. *Journal of health Economics*, 26(6):1081–1100.

Cutler, D.M., McClellan, M. (2001). Is technological change in medicine worth it? *Health Affairs*, 20(5):11–29.

Cutler, D.M., McClellan, M., Newhouse, J.P. (1998a). What has increased medical care spending bought? *The American Economic Review*, 88(2):132–136.

Cutler, D.M., McClellan, M., Newhouse, J.P., Remler, D. (1998b). Are medical prices declining? Evidence for heart attack treatment. *The Quarterly Journal of Economics*; 113(4):991–1024.

Delwel, G.O. (2008). *Leidraad voor Uitkomstenonderzoek ten behoeve van de beoordeling doelmatigheid intramurale geneesmiddelen [Guideline for Outcomes Research in Support of Assessing Efficiency of Intramural Drugs]*. Diemen: College voor Zorgverzekeringen.

Drummond, M.F., Sculpher, M.J., Torrance, G.W., O'Brien, B.J., Stoddart, G.L. (2005). *Methods for the Economic Evaluation of Health Care Programmes*. Oxford: Oxford University Press.

European Parliament and Council (2011). *Directive 2011/24/EU of 9 March 2011 on the Application of Patients' Rights in Cross-Border Healthcare*. Brussels: Official Journal of the European Union (L88/45-L88/65).

Garrison, L.P., Wilensky, G.R. (1986). Cost-containment and incentives for technology. *Health Affairs*, 5(2):46–58.

Goodman, C.S. (2004). *HTA 101. Introduction to Health Technology Assessment*. Falls Church, VA: The Lewin Group.

Greenhalgh, T., Robert, G., MacFarlane, F., Bate, P., Kyriakidou, O. (2004). Diffusion of innovations in service organizations: systematic review and recommendations. *Milbank Quarterly*, 82(4):581-629.

Henschke, C., Bäumler, M., Weid, S., Gaskins, M., Busse, R. (2010). Extrabudgetary ('NUB') payments – a gateway for introducing new medical devices into the German inpatient reimbursement system? *Journal of Management and Marketing in Healthcare*, 3(2): 119–33.

Hutton, J., Trueman, P., Henshall, C. (2007). Coverage with evidence development: an examination of conceptual and policy issues. *International Journal of Technology Assessment in Health Care*, 23:425–32.

Kristensen, F.B. (2008). Transnational collaboration on health technology assessment – a political priority in Europe, in M.V. Garrido, F.B. Kristensen, C.P. Nielsen, R. Busse, eds. *Health Technology Assessment and Health Policy-Making in Europe: Current Status, Challenges and Potential*. Copenhagen: WHO Regional Office for Europe on behalf of the European Observatory on Health Systems and Policies.

MedPAC (2001). Accounting for new technology in hospital prospective payment systems, in MedPAC *Report to the Congress. Medicare Payment Policy*. Washington, DC: Medicare Payment Advisory Commission.

MedPAC (2003). Payment for new technologies in Medicare's prospective payment system, in MedPAC *Report to the Congress: Medicare Payment Policy*. Washington, DC: Medicare Payment Advisory Commission.

Mowatt, G., Bower, D.J., Brebner, J.A. et al. (1997). When and how to assess fast-changing technologies: a comparative study of medical applications of four generic technologies. *Health Technology Assessment*, 1:1–149.

OTA (1983). *Diagnosis-Related Groups (DRGs) and the Medicare Program: Implications for Medical Technology – A Technical Memorandum*. Washington, DC: Office of Technology Assessment.

Packer, C., Simpson, S., Stevens, A. (2006). International diffusion of new health technologies: a ten-country analysis of six health technologies. *International Journal of Technology Assessment in Health Care*, 22(4):419–28.

de Pouvourville, G. (2009). Les hôpitaux français face au paiement prospectif au cas: la mise en ouvre de la tarification à l'activité. *Revue Economique*, 60(2):457–70.

Rettig, R.A. (1994). Medical innovation duels cost-containment. *Health Affairs*, 13(3): 7–27.

Scheller-Kreinsen, D., Quentin, W., Busse, R. (2011). DRG-based hospital payment systems and technological innovation in 12 European countries. *Value in Health*, 14(8).

Schreyögg, J., Bäumler, M., Busse, R. (2009). Balancing adoption and affordability of medical devices in Europe. *Health Policy*, 92(2–3):218–24.

Shih, C., Berliner, E. (2008). Diffusion of new technology and payment policies: coronary stents. *Health Affairs*, 27(6):1566–76.

Simpson, S., Packer, C., Stevens, A., Raftery, J. (2005). Predicting the impact of new health technologies on average length of stay: development of a prediction framework. *International Journal of Technology Assessment in Health Care*, 21(4):487–91.

Torbica, A., Cappellaro, G. (2010). Uptake and diffusion of medical technology innovation in Europe: what role for funding and procurement policies? *Journal of Medical Marketing*, 10(1):61–9.

Tunstall-Pedoe, H., Vanuzzo, D., Hobbs, M. et al. (2000). Estimation of contribution of changes in coronary care to improving survival, event rates, and coronary heart disease mortality across the WHO MONICA Project populations. *Lancet*, 355(9205):688–700.

Weisbrod, B.A. (1991). The health care quadrilemma: an essay on technological change, insurance, quality of care, and cost-containment. *Journal of Economic Literature*, 29(2):523–52.

chapter ten

Moving towards transparency, efficiency and quality in hospitals: Conclusions and recommendations

Reinhard Busse and Wilm Quentin

10.1 Introduction

Part One of this book has provided comparative information from 12 European countries about the specific characteristics of their diagnosis-related group (DRG) systems, about how these systems are used for hospital payment and about the progress that has been made in moving towards transparency, efficiency and quality in hospitals. Part Two provides more detailed information from the 12 European countries and facilitates insights into the strengths and problems of DRG systems and DRG-based hospital payment systems in each of these countries. Together, the two parts of the book demonstrate a great degree of diversity in the specific design features of DRG systems and DRG-based hospital payment systems across countries, but at the same time they reveal that most countries are struggling with similar issues in their pursuit of common goals.

This chapter draws together the findings from Part One and Part Two in order to address the question raised in the title of this book; namely, whether we are moving towards transparency, efficiency and quality in European hospitals. In addition, the chapter makes specific recommendations for policy-makers regarding how best to design DRG-based hospital payment systems given country-specific aims and objectives, and it explores the potential for cooperation across European countries in designing and developing DRG systems and DRG-based hospital payment systems – a process, which could ultimately lead to the emergence of European DRGs as the answer to common problems in this field in European countries.

The next section (10.2) summarizes the country experiences and draws on findings of the available literature presented, especially in Chapters 7 and 8, in order to provide an overview of the status quo. That is: where are we now, in terms of transparency, efficiency, and quality in hospitals? Subsequently, section 10.3 makes recommendations for both types of countries – those preparing the introduction of DRG systems, and those optimizing existing systems. This section is structured according to the three building blocks introduced in Chapter 3; namely, the DRG system itself, hospital cost information, and actual DRG-based hospital payment. Finally, section 10.4 draws conclusions from the vast experience summarized in this book and aims to look into the future of DRGs in Europe, including the potential for coordinating, and eventually harmonizing DRG systems and DRG-based hospital payment in Europe.

10.2 Where are we now?

In almost all European countries in which DRGs have been introduced since the mid-1980s, the most important aims related to their introduction included increasing transparency, improving efficiency and assuring quality of hospital care (see Chapter 2). Today, after more than a decade of experience with using DRGs in most European countries, it is time to consider whether the extensive use of DRGs in the 12 countries included in this book has contributed towards achieving these aims. The country chapters in Part Two and the extensive literature searches carried out for chapters 7 and 8 on the effects of DRG-based hospital payment systems on efficiency and quality of care provide a solid foundation for approaching this question. The following subsections discuss how far European countries have moved towards achieving each of these aims.

10.2.1 Moving towards transparency?

Following the introduction of DRGs and DRG-based hospital payment systems, transparency of hospital services and costs has substantially improved in all countries, essentially for four interrelated reasons: (1) DRGs provide a concise measure for reporting hospital activity; (2) DRGs facilitate performance comparisons of costs, efficiency and quality; (3) hospitals are incentivized to increase their efforts in coding diagnoses and procedures; and (4) hospitals are encouraged to improve their cost-accounting systems (see Chapter 5).

First, because DRGs aggregate the confusingly large number of patients treated by hospitals into a small number of groups of patients with similar clinical characteristics and similar resource-consumption patterns, they provide a concise and meaningful measure of hospital outputs (Fetter et al., 1976; Goldfield, 2010). Prior to the introduction of DRGs, hospital activity was reported either on the basis of highly aggregated measures, such as the number of provided bed days and the number of discharged patients, or on the basis of very detailed measures, such as the main diagnoses or procedures of all patients. However, because none of these measures summarized patients with similar clinical characteristics and similar resource-need patterns, they could not meaningfully reflect hospital activity. Today, the vast majority of hospitals in all countries – often including hospitals with different ownership (profit-making versus non-profit-making) and different levels of specialization (for example, teaching hospitals versus general hospitals) – are required to prepare detailed activity reports that specify the number and type of DRGs provided. These are usually made available to the public and help to overcome agency problems that existed prior to the introduction of DRGs, because purchasers did not have a meaningful measure for hospital activity.

Second, regulators, payers and hospital managers in most countries (for example, Finland, France, Ireland and Spain) are starting to use DRGs for hospital performance comparisons. They compare resource use of hospitals by assessing whether patients in one DRG are staying significantly longer in one hospital than in another, for example, or whether one hospital is significantly more costly than another when treating patients within the same DRG. Similarly, quality is compared by determining whether patients assigned to a particular DRG have a higher rate of complications in one hospital than in another, and efficiency is assessed by using DRGs as a measure of hospital output.

Third, because hospitals receive higher DRG-based payments if they 'code' (input) all relevant diagnoses and procedures, they have strong incentives to improve their coding practices. In many countries, clinicians, nurses or documentation assistants are specifically trained in order to improve their coding skills. Consequently, almost all countries find that information about diagnoses and procedures in hospitals has improved considerably since the introduction of DRGs. In addition, payers have introduced auditing systems to assure that the provided information is correct, which further increases the reliability of the available information. However, at the same time, the coding-related administrative workload has been of concern for clinicians in many countries.

Fourth, as discussed in Chapter 5, the introduction of DRG-based hospital payment has influenced cost-accounting practices in hospitals. On the one hand, regulators have mandated improved and standardized cost-accounting systems in hospitals, while on the other hand, hospitals have been incentivized to improve their cost-accounting systems for management purposes. Consequently, the quality of cost information has improved in most countries.

However, if patients within a DRG do not adequately account for differences between patients – that is, if DRGs are not sufficiently homogeneous – they are an inadequate measure of hospital activity and, consequently, hospital performance comparisons on the basis of DRGs will be unfair. Therefore, the methods used for ensuring that DRG systems are an adequate measure of hospital activity are highly important, particularly because innovations are continuously changing the way hospital services are provided. In addition, performance comparisons on the basis of DRGs need to take into account that certain factors may be beyond the control of hospitals (for example, treating a larger share of socially disadvantaged patients or having higher labour costs), which are not accounted for in the DRG system. Furthermore, while DRGs have contributed to increased transparency of hospital services within countries, transparency of hospital services across countries remains limited because different DRG systems are used in different countries, thus preventing – or at least severely complicating – comparisons of hospital activity and performance across borders except where the same systems are in use.

10.2.2 Moving towards efficiency?

As discussed in Chapter 7, although improving hospital efficiency is generally a key motivation for introducing DRG-based hospital payment systems, there are relatively few studies that have explicitly identified and quantified the impact of these systems on efficiency using established data-driven methods such as data envelopment analysis (DEA) or stochastic frontier analyses. Rather, most research has concentrated on indicators of efficiency – such as activity and length of stay – which are more easily measured, but by definition provide only a partial picture of efficiency.

Existing studies using DEA or stochastic frontier analyses – both with their own particular limitations (Street et al., 2010) – have produced mixed evidence on the extent to which DRG-based hospital payment has contributed to higher efficiency levels in hospitals. The studies reviewed in Chapter 7 reported that the introduction of DRG-based hospital payment was associated with improved technical efficiency in Portugal, Sweden and Norway, but that no positive impact was observed in the United States and in an Austrian study. On the one hand, this mixed evidence could be related to the considerable differences in the design and operation of DRG-based hospital payment systems in different countries and to heterogeneity in the hospital payment systems that existed prior to the introduction of DRG-based hospital payment. On the other hand, studies may have underestimated (or overestimated) the effect of DRG-based hospital payment on efficiency because attribution of efficiency changes to a hospital payment reform in longitudinal studies is complicated by the existence of confounding factors, such as changes being part of wider reform packages, and because detected changes could merely represent changes in documentation practice. In addition, because of an almost complete absence of data, it remains unknown whether the effect of the potential unintended consequences of DRG-based hospital payment systems (such as overtreatment of admitted patients ('gaming') or increased admissions of patients for unnecessary services (see Chapter 6)) could have led to reduced allocative (output) efficiency.

There is generally agreement in the literature that the introduction of DRG-based hospital payment systems has led to increased activity and reduced length of stay, and it is consequently often assumed that hospital efficiency has improved. For example, studies have found that hospital admissions increased following the introduction of DRG-based hospital payment in Australia, Denmark, England, France, Germany, Norway and, at least initially, in Sweden, while results for Italy are mixed (see Table 7.4 in Chapter 7). Hospital activity did not increase in the United States, but this is in line with the expected effects of DRG-based hospital payment when replacing a fee-for-service system. Yet, of course, the aforementioned points regarding country-specific contexts and the difficulties in attributing causality also apply here.

Mostly based on the evidence of these studies, the authors of the country-specific chapters in Part Two come to similar conclusions. In Austria and England, for example, DRG-based hospital payment is thought to have contributed to increased efficiency. In the chapters on Estonia, Germany, Ireland, Poland, Portugal, Sweden and the Netherlands, the authors do not directly comment on the effect of DRG-based hospital payment on efficiency but they highlight rather positive trends in costs, length of stay or productivity. For Finland and Spain (see chapters 18 and 22), DRG-based hospital payment is thought to have had only minimal effects on efficiency because country-specific design features imply that hospitals are not exposed to strong incentives for efficiency improvement (see Chapter 6). By contrast, in Chapter 13, Or and Bellanger come to a rather negative conclusion about the effect of the French GHM system on efficiency, which seems to be strongly influenced by the results of an evaluation by the Auditor's Office (Cour des Comptes, 2009).

In summary, while the evidence remains limited because of the above-mentioned difficulties in measuring and detecting efficiency changes (and in attributing them to the introduction of a specific payment system), the bulk of the literature and most of the authors in this book assume that DRG-based hospital payment systems have had a somewhat positive effect on efficiency. However, it is also clear that DRG-based hospital payment systems can have unintended consequences, such as 'cream-skimming', 'up-coding', overtreatment/'gaming', supplier-induced demand, and so on (see Chapter 6). If these unintended consequences are not accounted for by the specific design features of the payment system or by the regulatory and institutional context, they might threaten to outweigh any efficiency improvements that could be expected as a result of the introduction of DRG-based hospital payment systems.

10.2.3 Moving towards quality?

The effect of DRGs on quality of care has always been highly controversial: there have been major concerns on the part of health professionals in many countries that DRG-based hospital payment systems might compromise quality of care because hospitals are incentivized to reduce costs. However, at the same time, proponents of the use of DRGs have argued that quality of care could in fact be improved, because DRGs contribute to increased transparency in the quality of care and because hospitals are incentivized to invest in quality improvements that lead to reduced costs (for example, infection control measures or improved surgical techniques).

As discussed in Chapter 8, the effect of DRGs on quality of care has been assessed in numerous studies from the United States and – more recently – also in studies from Europe. The reviewed evidence from the United States has produced a multifaceted picture: some studies found that processes of care (for example, as measured by physician and nurse cognitive performance) improved following the introduction of DRG-based hospital payment (Kahn et al., 1990b), even though these changes could not be directly attributed to the hospital payment reform (Rogers et al., 1990). At the same time, a larger proportion of patients were found to have been discharged in unstable conditions after the implementation of DRG-based payment (Kosecoff et al., 1990), but mortality at 30 and 180 days following hospitalization was unaffected (Kahn et al., 1990a). It appeared that quality of care improved in certain hospitals and certain areas of care, such as colorectal cancer surgery (Schwartz & Tartter, 1998), but was worse in other areas of care (Gilman, 2000), in particular in hospitals for which the introduction of DRG-based payment implied high levels of financial pressure (Cutler, 1995). In summary, studies from the United States suggest that quality of care was, in general, not significantly affected by the introduction of DRG-based hospital payment, as it did not compromise the long-term trend towards improved quality of care in hospitals (Rogers et al., 1990). However, the effect on quality needs to be closely monitored because there could be adverse effects for certain patient groups in certain hospitals and because a trend towards more unstable discharges emerged after the implementation of DRGs.

In Europe, the available research evaluating the impact on care quality and patient outcomes is too limited to draw any firm conclusions, in particular because evidence is available only from a limited number of countries. In England, little measurable change was found in the quality of care following the introduction of DRG-based payment, in terms of in-hospital mortality, 30-day post-surgical mortality, and emergency readmissions after treatment for hip fracture (Farrar et al., 2009). In Germany, 30-day post-discharge mortality significantly decreased during the introduction period of DRG-based hospital payment, and a large number of quality indicators were found to have improved over the same period of time (Fürstenberg et al., 2011). In Norway and Italy, studies did not find that quality decreased following the introduction of DRG-based payment (see Chapter 8), while one study from Sweden showed that patient-perceived quality of care decreased after the introduction of DRG-based hospital payment (Ljunggren & Sjödén, 2003).

In general, it seems that quality was not adversely affected by the introduction of DRG-based hospital payment in most European countries. However, of course, the impact of DRG-based hospital payment on quality of care always depends on the country-specific design features of the systems and the regulatory and health care context(s) in question. The effect of DRG-based hospital payments on quality of care might be different in Europe from that in the United States because (1) DRG-based hospital payment systems in most countries did not replace fee-for-service systems (as was the case in the United States) but rather global budgets, which were already partly adjusted for activity measured in cases or bed days (see Chapters 2 and 7); and because (2) there is a much stronger public sector presence in the provision of health care in Europe than in the United States.

Surprisingly, only very few countries explicitly adjust DRG-based hospital payments on the basis of information regarding quality in hospitals. One notable exception is England, where the Commissioning for Quality and Innovation (CQUIN) framework allows purchasers to link a moderate proportion of hospitals' income (that is, 1.5 per cent in 2010/2011) to the achievement of locally negotiated quality goals. In the Netherlands, insurers can negotiate with hospitals regarding price, volume and quality of care for about 30 per cent of Dutch DRGs (Diagnose Behandeling Combinaties, DBCs – see Chapter 23). However, apparently insurers and hospitals negotiate predominantly on price and volume, while quality plays only a minor role in the negotiation process. Instead of adjusting DRG-based hospital payment for quality, most countries reward quality improvements through specific budgets that are independent from DRG-based hospital payment (see Chapter 8).

One problem relating to quality adjustments of DRG-based hospital payments is that in many European countries, information on quality in hospitals is still insufficient. However, data quality (at least in terms of diagnoses and procedures) has been found to have improved considerably following the introduction of DRGs in many countries. In addition, the authors of the country-specific chapters in Part Two of this book (see, for example, Chapter 13 on France or Chapter 14 on Germany) highlight that national quality measurement programmes have been introduced in recent years. If these data are found to provide valid and reliable indicators for the quality of care, it is likely that there will be increased efforts to use such data also for payment purposes, called pay-for-performance (P4P).

10.3 Improving transparency, efficiency and quality in hospitals: Recommendations for DRG systems and DRG-based hospital payment systems

As highlighted in the previous section (10.2), the specific design features of DRG systems and of DRG-based hospital payment systems are of utmost importance because they determine whether countries will be able to reap the potential benefits of these systems in terms of transparency, efficiency and quality in hospitals. This section takes up again the three main building blocks of DRG-based hospital payment systems introduced in Chapter 3; namely, the DRG system for patient classification purposes, hospital cost information, and the actual DRG-based hospital payment (see section 3.2 and Figure 3.1 in Chapter 3), and makes recommendations concerning the most important issues that need to be considered when introducing, revising, extending or harmonizing DRG systems and DRG-based hospital payment systems. The section does not provide detailed instructions in the sense of a 'how to' manual, as readers interested in this kind of information can find it in existing publications (see Langenbrunner et al., 2009; Cashin et al., 2005).

However, before turning to the building blocks of DRG-based hospital payment systems, three questions should be explored, which must represent the starting point for introducing DRGs.

First, is the political situation favourable to the introduction of a DRG system or of a DRG-based hospital payment system?

While this may seem to be an obvious point, the politics of health policy-making are too often overlooked (Eggleston et al., 2008). The introduction of DRG systems has been influenced by political agendas, along with the structure of political and health care systems, by the presence or absence of supporters and by the general economic and political context (D'Aunno et al., 2008). If these factors are not conducive to the introduction of a DRG system, the adoption of DRGs could be delayed or the application of DRGs could be limited to only certain regions or to a subset of hospitals. Furthermore, as noted in the chapter on Poland (Chapter 20), in a generally positive economic environment, the availability of additional financial resources may be able to assure support from various actors that would otherwise be opposed to the reform.

Second, is the institutional and legal context adequate for the introduction of DRGs and DRG-based hospital payment?

One prerequisite for DRG-based hospital payment to work is that purchasers and providers are separate entities. Public hospitals need to have a certain degree of autonomy for managing health care resources, for example, as autonomized organizations with decision rights regarding how to manage hospital resources (Busse et al., 2002; Langenbrunner et al., 2009). Purchasers need to have the capacity for managing the DRG system, for monitoring potential unintended consequences, and for negotiating contracts with private (profit-making or non-profit-making) hospitals. Furthermore, the legal and institutional context should not prevent the (intended) reorganization of care; for example, moving the provision of certain services from acute inpatient hospital care to outpatient care or long-term care settings.

Third, what is the intended purpose of using DRGs?

As illustrated in the country-specific chapters in Part Two and as summarized in Chapter 2, the purpose of using DRGs can change over time. Often countries begin using DRGs with the aim of improving transparency of hospital activity. While this can already be ambitious – in terms of DRG system development/ adjustment, management capacities and hospital data requirements – the (intended and unintended) effects of using DRGs merely as a measure of hospital activity are likely to be rather limited. Once countries have gathered experience with a DRG system and have gained confidence in the ability of the system to reflect adequately hospital activity, countries have always started moving towards using DRGs for determining a progressively increasing proportion of hospital revenues. Other countries have introduced DRGs directly with the purpose of using them for hospital payment. The purpose – namely, hospital activity measurement or hospital payment (in DRG-based case payment or DRG-based budget allocation systems) – implies different requirements for the capacity of purchasers and providers, and for the building blocks of the systems.

10.3.1 DRG systems

Countries planning to introduce DRG systems have two options: (1) they can develop a new DRG system from scratch (as described by Cashin and colleagues (2005)), or (2) they can import one of the already-existing DRG systems from abroad. Chapter 4 shows that most countries included in this book have adopted DRG systems that were originally developed abroad. Those first experimenting with DRGs in England, Portugal, France and Ireland used different versions of DRG systems developed in the United States as the starting point. Subsequently, several countries adopted DRG systems from the United States, either Health Care Financing Administration (HCFA-)DRGs or All Patient (AP-) DRGs (as in Ireland, Spain and Portugal). More recently, Australian Refined (AR-)DRGs have been adopted by a large number of countries in Europe, also going beyond those included in this book (for example, Ireland as well as Slovenia (Don, 2003), Croatia (Voncina et al., 2007) and Romania (Radu et al., 2010)). AR-DRGs served as the origin for developing the German DRG (G-DRG) system, which have in turn become the starting point for the development of DRGs in Switzerland. Finally, Poland has developed its own DRG system on the basis of the English system. Given that developing a new DRG system is a highly complex process, requiring several years of work (and which will not necessarily lead to a superior system compared to the existing ones), adopting a DRG system from abroad – at least as a starting point for country-specific modifications – appears to be the preferable solution.

When deciding which DRG system to adopt, countries need to consider a wide range of issues, such as the adequacy of the system for the national hospital context (in terms of clinical acceptability, cost homogeneity, and existing coding systems for diagnoses and procedures), the availability of training material and technical support systems (for example, software applications), and the costs related to obtaining copyright for using the system, in particular if the DRG system is produced by private enterprises (Don, 2003). Ideally, alternative DRG systems are evaluated using available data from hospital discharge summaries in order to reveal differences in the adequacy of alternative systems for the country-specific context (Aisbett et al., 2007). The additional administrative costs of coding diagnoses and procedures, installing necessary information technology (IT) systems, and enabling data transfer between providers and purchasers should also be considered when introducing DRGs. In particular, start-up costs may be higher if a DRG system is chosen that is based on coding systems for diagnoses and procedures that are not yet used in the country – but this does not need to be prohibitive, as shown by the case of Ireland, which adopted the Australian coding system when changing from HCFA-DRGs to AR-DRGs in 2003 (see Chapter 15).

Historically, most countries that introduced DRG systems initially did so for the classification of acute hospital inpatients. The reason for excluding outpatients, day cases, rehabilitation and psychiatric care from DRGs was that diagnoses were found to be a bad predictor of resource consumption and that dominant procedures were absent in psychiatric and rehabilitation facilities (Lave, 2003; Cotterill & Thomas, 2004). However, in recent years many countries have extended their DRG systems to account for day cases and sometimes have even included outpatient activity (see Figure 10.1 and Chapter 4). Furthermore, similar to the situation in the United States, where DRG-like systems were introduced for rehabilitation facilities in 2002 and for psychiatric facilities in 2005 (MedPAC, 2008, 2010), a number of European countries (such as England, France and Germany) are extending the concept of DRGs to other types of hospital care (namely, rehabilitation or psychiatric facilities) or have plans to do so in the near future (see Chapter 4 and the relevant country-specific chapters in Part Two).

Because hospital activity in most European countries is progressively expanding into day-case and/or outpatient settings, it is important for countries to explicitly consider these areas of care when designing or updating their DRG systems. Some DRG systems – such as NordDRGs, AR-DRGs, and the French system of patient classification (GHMs) – have been explicitly designed to take into account day-case and/or outpatient activity, which is important because otherwise an increasingly important share of hospital activity would be left out of the systems.

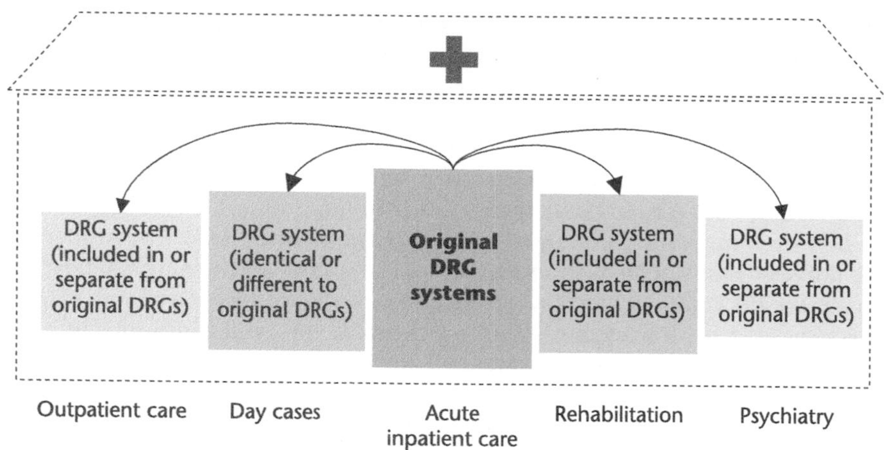

Figure 10.1 Extension of DRG systems from acute inpatient care to other sectors

The purposes of using DRG systems – that is, contributing to transparency in the hospital sector and paying hospitals fairly for provided services – can only be achieved if the defined groups of patients are sufficiently homogeneous in terms of treatment costs. Otherwise, performance comparisons on the basis of DRGs do not adequately control for differences in patients within the same groups; and hospital payment for a large number of patients is not appropriate – it can be either too high or too low. In order to ensure homogeneous groups of patients, DRG systems need to consider the most important determinants of resource consumption as classification variables. This can be achieved only if detailed information relating to treatment costs in hospitals (see subsection 10.3.2 and Chapter 5) is available for designing and updating the system. In addition, consultation mechanisms must be established, which can ensure that input from medical professionals is considered by the responsible DRG institutions during the process of updating and designing the system. This is also important because the selection of classification variables must carefully consider the incentives of using certain variables (such as specific procedures) for defining DRGs. If the DRG system is used for hospital payment, that system should ideally produce neutral incentives for alternative treatment options, in order to ensure that patients are treated according to their medical needs – and not according to profit considerations. Under such circumstances, decisions regarding which treatment options to choose can be left to clinicians.

As part of the attempt to increase resource homogeneity of DRGs, almost all systems have seen an expansion in the number of groups over the past few years (see Chapter 4). Today, the German G-DRG system defines 1200 DRGs, the English HRG system consists of about 1400 HRGs, and the French GHM system comprises almost 2300 groups. However, an increasingly large number of groups also brings about problems. First, with an increasingly large number of groups, it becomes more difficult to reliably calculate relevant and significant differences in the average treatment costs of patients within different DRGs. Therefore, it does not seem to be a coincidence that larger European countries are operating systems with a larger number of groups because larger countries should be better able to reliably calculate average costs of patients within relatively poorly populated DRGs.[1] Second, a more complex system is likely to define groups which are less clearly distinguishable from each other. The problem is not so much that hospitals would have difficulties grouping patients into the appropriate DRGs, because all countries use software tools for the classification of patients, but rather that, if the criteria used for grouping of patients into different DRGs are less distinguishable, it becomes increasingly difficult for purchasers or regulators to audit hospital activity and to detect whether hospitals are engaging in up-coding or gaming (see Chapter 6).

In addition, regular updates of DRG systems are important in order to account for changes in medical practice and hospital resource consumption, as well as to incorporate technological innovation. Chapter 9 has shown that most countries regularly update their DRG systems, albeit at different frequencies and with a different time-lag between data collection and using those data for updating the DRG system. Obviously, countries with frequent updates of their DRG system and with a short time-lag between data collection and use of the information for DRG-based hospital payment are in a better position to (1) correct the DRG system if unintended consequences of using a particular classification variable are detected (for example, unexplained increases in certain procedures); and (2) incorporate technological innovations into their systems. In fact, while it is important to have a good DRG system, it is at least as important to have a well-designed system for monitoring the effects of DRGs and to update and optimize the system over time.

Finally, DRG systems can be designed to facilitate attempts to incorporate quality into DRG-based hospital payment systems (for details see subsection 10.3.3). For example, Medicare in the Unites States demands that hospitals code into the system whether primary and secondary diagnoses were present on admission (Department of Health and Human Services, 2008). If certain diagnoses were not present on admission, they are excluded from consideration during the grouping process. Additionally, for certain high-volume DRGs in disease areas in which clear consensus exists regarding what constitutes best practice (for example, cholecystectomy, hip fracture, and stroke), it would be worth expanding on the concept introduced in the United Kingdom (Department of Health, 2011), to explicitly use such best practice care processes instead of the average across all hospitals. This would ideally lead to more clearly specified groups of patients with more homogeneous care processes, aligned with best practice guidelines. Obviously, if used for payment, such a process needs to be accompanied by appropriate measures to ensure that hospitals do not cut costs by under-providing services.

10.3.2 Hospital cost information

Chapters 2 and 5 have highlighted the importance of accurate cost-accounting information for the development of DRG systems and for the calculation of DRG payment rates. However, the availability of high-quality cost-accounting information is not a prerequisite for the introduction of DRG systems. Many countries originally introduced DRG systems and cost weights from abroad also because they did not have the necessary information for developing their own systems (as was the case in Ireland, Poland, Portugal and Spain). These countries adjusted imported DRG weights to the local cost context, using highly aggregated cost-accounting data and a set of internal DRG cost weights (see for example Chapter 22) or used data from a previously existing fee-for-service system for the calculation of weights (see for example Chapter 20). Nevertheless, even though it is possible to start using DRGs without having high-quality cost-accounting information, countries usually realize with the passing of time that better data are required in order to verify that the system and payment rates are adequate for the local cost context.

Therefore, standardized (sometimes mandatory) cost-accounting systems have been introduced in at least a sample of hospitals in most of the countries included in this book. Most frequently, data for the refinement of DRG systems and for the calculation of DRG weights are collected from a selected number of hospitals that use comparable cost-accounting systems meeting predefined quality standards (for example, in Finland, France, Germany and Sweden). However, the size of the hospital sample varies considerably, between 6 per cent in Germany and 62 per cent in Sweden. Other countries require all hospitals to report their activity and unit costs annually to their regulatory authority, but have fewer demands in terms of the quality and level of detail of this information (for example, England). In addition, the time-lag varies between data collection and the use of these data to readjust the DRG system and the DRG payment rates (see Chapter 9).

In countries in which cost-accounting data are collected from hospitals, this information is generally used to set DRG weights (the basis of DRG payment rates) at the average costs of cases within a DRG. However, average costs are usually calculated only after having excluded outliers through trimming (Schreyögg et al., 2006). This is because a relatively small number of high-cost outliers usually accounts for a relatively large proportion of total costs of all cases within a DRG. Consequently, calculating DRG weights on the basis of average costs of all cases (including outliers) would lead to an overvaluation of DRG weights for most cases. Recently, England has moved away from the concept of using average costs for determining DRG weights for a small number of high-volume DRGs (for example, hip fracture, cholecystectomy, stroke). For these DRGs, weights are set to reflect costs of efficient high-quality providers instead of average costs. However, this does not mean that cost-accounting data become less important. Quite the contrary; very reliable and comparable cost-accounting data are needed to be able to identify efficient providers, and to be sure that lower costs in certain hospitals are not the result of inaccuracies in the cost-accounting methodology.

When cost-accounting information is used to determine DRG weights, it is important that only those cost categories are included in the calculation of average costs that are paid for through the DRG-based hospital payment system. This is important because many countries use specific budgets or other payment systems for certain cost categories or certain activities (see subsection 10.3.3). For example, capital costs are not included in DRG weights in some countries (such as Germany, Ireland and Spain), whereas other countries include capital costs in the calculation. Whether to include capital costs when setting DRG weights depends on the objectives that countries want to achieve. Including capital costs in DRG weights will imply stronger incentives of the DRG-based hospital payment system for the reorganization of care, possibly leading to the concentration of large-scale equipment or certain specialties in fewer hospitals. While the reorganization of care can be an intended objective, it must be borne in mind that this could also compromise accessibility of services in poorly populated rural areas.

There has been some debate about which cost-accounting methodology is preferable (Tan, 2009). At a theoretical level, there is consensus that bottom-up micro-costing generates the highest quality of data for developing DRG systems and for calculating DRG weights (but also for hospital managers in terms of planning and controlling) because it allows differences in resource consumption and costs for individual patients to be identified. However, bottom-up micro-costing is also very demanding in terms of its impact on hospital information systems, data requirements and analytical complexity. Top-down micro-costing is more feasible because consumed resources are not valued for individual patients but for the average patient (see Chapter 5). In addition, top-down micro-costing has been found to be a fairly accurate alternative to bottom-up micro-costing, and it is possible to combine both methods and to restrict bottom-up micro-costing only to the most important cost components (Tan et al., 2009). By contrast, gross-costing produces relatively inaccurate estimates because it is unable to trace consumed resources to individual patients.

When deciding on the size of the data sample of cost-collecting hospitals, there seems to be a trade-off between collecting high-quality cost-accounting information and the goal of ensuring that a large and representative sample of hospitals contributes to a national cost database. More complex cost-accounting systems – collecting more detailed patient-level information using a bottom-up micro-costing approach – are also more costly to operate, which may make the data-collection exercise prohibitively costly if it is extended to a large number of hospitals. Concerning this trade-off, the Netherlands seem to have struck an interesting balance between representativeness and data quality, by collecting resource-use data from all hospitals (assuring representativeness of the data) and unit costs using bottom-up micro-costing from a small sample of hospitals.

Because collecting detailed cost-accounting information requires additional work from hospitals, regulatory authorities in some countries have started to provide monetary incentives to hospitals if they comply with predefined cost-accounting standards. For example, in France, the Regional Health Agencies (ARSs) pay the equivalent of the yearly salary for a financial controller for hospitals contributing to the national cost database (ENCC). In Germany, the national DRG institute (the InEK) pays hospitals a lump sum for participating in the data-collection exercise, and a variable amount of money related to the number of delivered cases and their data quality. In addition, because cost-accounting information is of such high importance, almost all countries that collect cost-accounting data have also implemented monitoring systems to verify the accuracy of the delivered data. However, if better cost-accounting information is collected in hospitals, this does not only contribute to more accurate data for regulators; in addition, hospital managers find this information useful because it enables the identification of the most important cost components and facilitates comparisons of resource consumption for similar patients across different hospitals.

10.3.3 DRG-based hospital payment

The countries included in this book have, in general, implemented one of two main models of DRG-based hospital payment systems: (1) DRG-based case payment systems (in Estonia, England, Finland, France, Germany, Poland, the Netherlands and Sweden) and (2) DRG-based budget allocation systems (in Austria, Ireland, Portugal and Spain; see Chapter 6). In DRG-based case payment systems, each discharged patient is grouped into the applicable DRG, and hospitals receive a payment per case that is determined by the weight of that DRG (after monetary conversion and relevant adjustments). In DRG-based budget allocation systems, the available regional or national hospital budget is distributed to individual hospitals on the basis of the number and type of DRGs that those hospitals produced (namely, the casemix of the hospitals) during one of the previous years, or that they are expected to produce in the current year. The existence of these alternative models facilitates the adjustment of the DRG-based hospital payment system to the country-specific context and to the pre-existing hospital payment system.

Adjusting DRG-based hospital payment to the country-specific context and to take account of the pre-existing payment system is important because new hospital payment systems should be introduced carefully over extended periods of time, in order to allow purchasers to monitor the potential unintended consequences and to give hospitals the necessary time to adjust to the changing context. Almost all countries included in this book have introduced DRG-based hospital payment systems over many years, usually operating the new DRG-based hospital payment system simultaneously with the pre-existing system and slowly increasing the share of total hospital revenues related to DRGs. For example, in Ireland, the share of hospital budgets that is determined on the basis of DRG-based budget allocation has increased progressively from 15 per cent in 2001 to 80 per cent in 2010. In Estonia, DRG-based case payment initially accounted for only 10 per cent of hospital payment in 2004, with the rest being determined on the basis of fee-for-service charges. Later, the proportion of DRG-based case payments as a percentage of total hospital payments per discharge was progressively increased to 70 per cent in 2007.

As explained in Chapter 6, there are three main incentives for hospitals resulting from DRG-based hospital payment systems:

(1) to reduce costs per treated patient,
(2) to increase revenues per patient, and
(3) to increase the number of patients.

These incentives can have both intended and unintended consequences. Therefore, it is important for countries to take into account the unintended consequences when designing their DRG-based hospital payment systems as part of the overall hospital payment system.

Concerning the first incentive, it is important that hospitals are adequately paid for the costs of provided services because, otherwise, they may reduce costs beyond acceptable levels and, in particular, may try to avoid high-cost patients. Therefore, a whole set of different mechanisms is used by European countries in order to avoid these unintended consequences: first, in order to adequately account for high-cost cases, all countries except for the Netherlands and Spain provide per diem-based additional payments to hospitals for outlier cases that stay in hospitals for longer than a specified length-of-stay threshold (for example, Austria, Germany, France, England, Ireland and Portugal) or additional fee-for-service payments for cases that exceed a specified cost threshold (for example, Estonia, Finland and Sweden). Second, additional payments are provided for certain high-cost services that are not adequately financed through the normal DRG-based payment system (for example, for certain high-cost drugs or devices), and some countries have defined specific DRGs for intensive care treatment according to the length of stay in these departments (such as in Germany), or finance treatment in intensive care units (ICUs) on the basis of per diem-based surcharges (such as Austria). Third, procedures have come to play a much more important role in most European DRG systems (see Chapter 4) compared to the DRG systems originally developed in the United States. Fourth, several countries have introduced adjustment factors to take into account structural differences between hospitals and to provide adequate payments to different kinds of hospitals (see Chapter 6).

In order to avoid hospitals being able to increase revenues per treated patient through up-coding or gaming, several countries have installed systems for regular auditing. For example, in Germany, the regional medical review boards of the sickness funds send teams to randomly selected hospitals to audit patients' medical records in order to evaluate whether they are correctly coding and treating patients (MDS, 2011). In 2009, 12 per cent of all hospital cases were audited by the sickness funds, resulting in average claw-back sums of around €800 per audited case. In France, a total of 1 per cent of hospital discharges were audited by the Regional Hospitalization Agencies (ARHs) in 2006, which found that 60 per cent of evaluated records had some kind of coding error. It is important for regulators to monitor both the adequacy of hospital treatment and whether it was really necessary for patients to be treated as inpatients.

Countering the third incentive of DRG-based hospital payment systems – that is, to increase the number of patients – several countries have introduced global expenditure control measures. For example, some countries are operating their DRG-based case payment systems within predefined volume limits. In Germany, DRGs are used to negotiate 'revenue budgets', which limit (to a certain degree) the total amount of money that hospitals can earn from DRG-based case payments. If hospitals provide more DRGs than agreed, they have to pay back at the beginning of the next year a certain percentage of the DRG-based case payments that they earned in excess of the negotiated revenue budgets (and they are rewarded with increased payments per case if they remained below the budget). By contrast, in the Netherlands, hospitals do not receive any payments for those cases treated in excess of the budget set prospectively which cannot be negotiated between insurers and hospitals.

Similarly, aiming to achieve expenditure control, France and Poland adjust national DRG-based case-payment rates in order to stay within global expenditure targets. However, in France, this approach is criticized for not being transparent enough, because payment rates are progressively set independently of average costs. Instead, Or and Bellanger (see Chapter 13 of this volume) argue in favour of clear volume targets for hospitals.

As chapters 6 and 8 have shown, all three DRG-inherent incentives may both improve or compromise quality of care. Although quality has been of continuous concern for policy-makers across Europe, it is still relatively rarely explicitly taken into account in existing DRG-based hospital payment systems. However, as evidenced by the examples presented in Chapter 8, it is possible to refine these systems to integrate direct incentives for improving quality. For example, DRG-based payments can be adjusted at the hospital level by increasing payments for all patients treated by one hospital, if one hospital provides above-average quality as measured through hospital-level quality indicators. Similarly, it is possible to increase payments to a hospital for all patients falling into one DRG if the hospital scores above average on DRG-specific quality indicators, or to adjust payments for individual patients if quality can be more robust monitored at the individual patient level (see Table 10.1). Yet, an essential prerequisite is that reliable quality indicators are developed and that more robust data about quality of care are collected in hospitals. Consequently, most countries have started collecting more detailed information regarding quality in hospitals in order to ensure that care quality is not compromised by the cost-reduction incentives of DRG-based hospital payment systems.

In addition, as discussed in Chapter 9, it is important that countries take into account the effect that DRG-based hospital payment may have on the adoption and use of technological innovations. Chapter 9 showed that most (but not all) countries included in this book have complemented their DRG-based payment systems with specific short-term payment instruments targeted at encouraging the adoption and use of technological innovations. However, short-term payment instruments should be employed very carefully, and granted only after careful assessment of the likely effects of the technology in question on costs, as well as quality of care. They should be limited to technological innovations that offer either considerable quality improvements over existing technologies, or options for diagnosis and treatment of previously untreatable conditions. Otherwise, if countries should want to provide short-term payment incentives for technological innovations with expected significant quality improvements but for which the evidence remains uncertain, one possible approach is that of so-called Coverage with Evidence Development (CED) (see Chapter 9, and Hutton and colleagues (2007)).

The payment of hospitals in all countries therefore consists of a highly sophisticated mix of different payment mechanisms that aim to modify the type and strength of the incentives of DRG-based hospital payment. The resulting intricately blended payment systems – incorporating elements of fee-for-service payment, per diem payment and global budgets – are more likely to contribute to achieving the societal objectives of securing high-quality hospital care at affordable costs than any other hospital payment mechanism alone (Ellis & McGuire, 1986).

Table 10.1 Options for integrating quality into DRG-based hospital payment systems and examples from selected countries in Europe and the United States

Type of payment adjustment/ calculation	*Mechanism*	*Examples*
Hospital based	• Payment for entire hospital activity is adjusted upwards or downwards by a certain percentage • Hospital receives specific budgetary allocation unrelated to activity	• Predefined quality results are met/not met (for example, in England) • Overall readmission rate is below/above average or below/above agreed target (for example, in the United States) • Hospitals install new quality improvement measures (for example, in France)
DRG/disease based	• Payment for all patients with a certain DRG (or a disease entity) is adjusted upwards or downwards by a certain percentage • DRG payment is not based on average costs but only on costs of those hospitals delivering 'good quality'	• Insurers negotiate with hospitals that DRG payment is higher/lower if certain quality standards are met/not met (for example, in Germany and the Netherlands) • DRG payment for all hospitals is based on 'best practice'; that is, costs incurred by efficient, high-quality hospitals (for example, in England)
Patient based	• No payment is made for a case • Payment for an individual patient is adjusted upwards or downwards by a certain amount	• Readmissions within 30 days are not paid separately but as part of the original admission (for example, in England and Germany) • Complications (that is, certain conditions that were not present upon admission) cannot be used to classify patients into DRGs that are weighted more heavily (for example, in the United States)

Figure 10.2 illustrates that DRG-based hospital payments generally account for only part of total hospital revenues. In the figure, the DRG-based payments – which are often operated partially and/or during the implementation phase simultaneously with a pre-existing hospital payment system (such as global budgets or fee-for-service payments) – constitute the basis of hospital revenues. These DRG-based hospital payments are often already adjusted for high-cost cases through outlier payments, as well as for quality and/or for structural differences between hospitals through structural adjustment factors.

On top of this, hospitals may receive additional payments for specific activities for DRG-classified patients, for example for certain expensive drugs, for certain services that are not adequately accounted for in the DRG system, and for certain cost-increasing technological innovations. Such payments may be integrated to different degrees into the DRG-based hospital payment systems, for example in the form of 'unbundled HRGs' in England or supplementary payments in Germany.

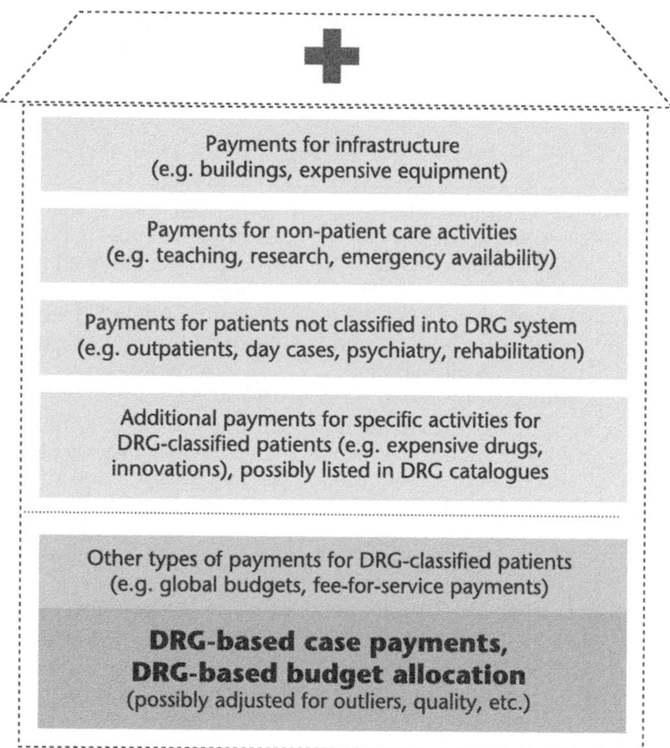

Figure 10.2 DRG-based hospital payment within the mix of total hospital revenues

A further element of hospital revenue originates from payments for patients not classified into the DRG system. The extent of these payments depends on both the types of activities hospitals are undertaking (for example, whether outpatients constitute a large part of their activity) and whether these have been incorporated into the DRG system (see Figure 10.1).

Furthermore, certain hospitals usually receive additional payments or budgets for non-patient care activities, such as teaching and research (although some countries may account for the extra costs of teaching and research within their DRG-based budget allocation model by operating separate systems for teaching hospitals and non-teaching hospitals – see, for example, Chapter 15) or emergency availability. Finally, several countries pay separately for capital investments (buildings and expensive equipment) or for certain structural quality measures, such as infection control programmes.

10.4 Conclusions: Future of DRG systems in Europe

Based on the experiences of the 12 countries included in Part Two of this book, the previous section has made recommendations regarding how best to design DRG systems, how to improve hospital cost information and how to maximize the intended consequences of DRG-based hospital payment systems, while avoiding the unintended ones. These recommendations may contribute towards improved national DRG systems and better DRG-based hospital payment systems in different countries. However, because the goals of European countries and the problems they face are highly similar, it is at least worth considering the benefits of increased cooperation, coordination and harmonization of DRG systems in Europe.

Currently, six of the twelve countries included in this book develop, update and operate their own national DRG systems. The other six countries use either imported DRG systems from abroad (for example, from Australia and the United States) or a national version of the common Nordic system of patient classification (NordDRGs). Each country with a national DRG system analyses its own national database to improve resource homogeneity of DRGs; develops and updates its own cost-accounting guidelines; has developed its own national consultation mechanisms with medical professionals; develops national software applications; evaluates technological innovations; updates national procedure coding systems, and so on. This raises two important questions: (1) Do all countries have the finances and skills to do this? And (2) is it worth it?

In regard to the first question, the answer – at least for smaller countries – is a clear 'no'. For practical reasons, without pan-European cooperation, these countries will always need to import certain important elements of their DRG systems. Further, if they have to do so anyway, it is not evident why imported DRG systems from outside Europe – which are used in several European countries – should be better able to define homogeneous groups of patients in these countries than a common European DRG system. In regard to the second question, one might argue that these efforts were worthwhile if the resulting national DRG systems were really tailor-made to achieve national objectives and better adjusted to the country-specific context than a multi-country solution. Before the EuroDRG project (which inspired this book), we did not know whether this was the case, because the ability of different DRG systems to define homogeneous groups of patients (in terms of clinical meaningfulness and costs) had not been assessed across European countries.

If the factors to explain cost differences (in terms of the patient characteristics and diagnoses as well as procedures performed and services provided) were sufficiently similar across European hospitals (and the parallel work of the EuroDRG project – to be published in 2012 – shows that this is the case), there would be a case for cooperation in terms of the development of DRG systems in Europe. The benefits would include: (1) avoiding duplication of work, (2) improving knowledge exchange in the refinement of DRG systems, (3) increasing transparency of hospital services across countries, and (4) facilitating cross-border movements of patients and payments. However, similar to the historical emergence of DRG systems as a result of political decisions, a coordination of European DRG systems – and, ultimately, possibly a harmonized DRG system – is likely to emerge only if there is sufficiently strong political will to support the emergence of a common European hospital market, as well as an increasing level of mobility of European patients. While this may be an unrealistic scenario in the short term, the recent *Directive on the Application of Patients' Rights in Cross-Border Healthcare* (European Parliament and Council, 2011) demonstrates that now is the time to start such a discussion.

The NordDRG system (see Chapter 16) provides an example of the feasibility of developing a common DRG system for a group of countries. NordDRGs emerged from existing cooperation between Nordic countries in the development of a common procedure classification system, and the presence of a common problem across Nordic countries during the mid-1990s; namely, how to convert the national or imported DRG systems from using the International Classification of Diseases (ICD) 9th revision for the coding of diagnoses to the ICD-10 codes. Consequently, countries amalgamated their efforts to develop a common DRG system that would replace existing national systems and imported DRG systems from abroad. The example of NordDRGs shows that a common DRG system does not prevent the adaptation of the common system to meet country-specific needs. Since the very beginning of NordDRGs, several countries have developed national versions of the system, and DRG weights are always calculated separately for each country. In addition, country-specific modifications of the underlying classifications of diagnoses and procedures exist, adding further detail where necessary but conforming to the general logic of the systems. Every year, NordDRGs are jointly updated by the Nordic Casemix Centre and country-specific modifications are then added to the updated version of the common NordDRG system.

The example of NordDRGs suggests that a first requirement for a common European DRG system (which could be called the 'EuroDRG' system) would be to harmonize the coding of diagnoses and procedures, or – as a second-best option – to develop a mapping system that would allow translation of codes from different coding systems into a common European coding system. The Hospital Data Project as part of the European Union (EU)'s Health Monitoring Programme has suggested a common – albeit for patient classification purposes, too rudimentary – format for hospital activity data, to improve comparability (Kiwa Prismant, 2008). For the coding of diagnoses, an agreement on a coding system should be relatively unproblematic, since the ICD-10 is already used for cause-of-death statistics in all countries. For procedures, an agreement could be more difficult to reach. This is testified by four decades of work, but the as yet unfinished attempt to develop such an international classification system, initially termed the International Classification of Procedures in Medicine (ICPM), and later the International Classification of Health Interventions (ICHI). European countries may consider not waiting for this development to be finished but to coordinate their efforts based on their own coding and patient classification systems.

As a starting point, the EuroDRG project has not only compared the DRG systems and their effects on transparency, efficiency and quality (in this volume), but has also compared in depth the classification of patients into DRGs across the DRG systems for 10 episodes of care. A common EuroDRG system could draw on the best features of national DRG systems, such as the most relevant classification variables, concepts for the definition of severity groups (for example, the patient clinical complexity levels (PCCLs), as used in AR-DRGs and G-DRGs; see Chapter 4) or the definition of short-stay groups, as in NordDRGs. However, detailed cost information collected on the basis of a standardized cost-accounting system from a sufficiently large and representative sample of hospitals from all participating countries would be necessary in order to test the ability of such a EuroDRG system to define homogeneous groups of patients across different countries.

A common EuroDRG system would not need to be employed in all countries and all hospitals from the beginning. It could initially be used only for the purpose of increasing transparency, possibly even coexisting simultaneously with national DRG systems, which could continue to be used for payment purposes for a limited time period – similar to the current situation in Spain (see Chapter 22). Furthermore, country examples included in this book show that it is possible to use DRG systems only for a subset of voluntarily participating hospitals (for example, as is the case in Ireland; see Chapter 15) or for certain regions (as in Spain; see Chapter 22). Similarly, EuroDRGs could initially be used only in certain countries, in certain hospitals interested in international performance comparisons, or for those patients treated in countries in which they are not permanent residents.

The starting point of this book (see Chapter 1) was the problem formulated by Dr. Eugene Codman in 1913: 'Really the whole hospital problem rests on one question: What happens to the cases? [...] We must formulate some method of hospital report showing as nearly as possible what are the results of the treatment obtained at different institutions.' While this book has demonstrated that DRGs have contributed to improved transparency *within* hospitals, the concept of DRGs has one important drawback: they are almost always restricted to one hospital stay, and providers are not encouraged to take into account the long-term effects of their treatment(s) in terms of continuity of care, patient outcomes and, ultimately, population health. While certain modifications of DRG-based hospital payment systems – such as not-paying for readmissions in England and Germany – aim to overcome (parts of) these problems, measuring the wider performance of hospitals in terms of the named outcomes remains a major obstacle. In this respect, only the Dutch DBCs have the advantage of defining groups on the basis of the treatment that is necessary for a specific condition, independent of the number of outpatient visits, diagnostic tests and inpatient admissions. Therefore, future developments of DRGs should be linked to efforts that aim to measure and ultimately increase the performance of health systems as a whole.

10.5 Note

1 The Netherlands may be considered an exception to this rule but they are currently in the process of reducing the complexity of their system; see Chapter 23.

10.6 References

Aisbett, C., Wiley, M.M., McCarthy, B., Mulligan, A. (2007). *Measuring Hospital Casemix: Evaluation of Alternative Approaches for the Irish Hospital System*. Dublin: Economic and Social Research Institute (ESRI Working Paper No. 192).

Busse, R., van der Grinten, T., Svensson, P. (2002). Regulating entrepreneurial behaviour in hospitals: theory and practice, in R.B. Saltman, R. Busse, E. Mossialos, eds. *Regulating Entrepreneurial Behaviour in European Health Care Systems*. Buckingham: Open University Press.

Cashin, C., O'Dougherty, S., Yevgeniy, S. et al. (2005). *Case-Based Hospital Payment Systems: A Step-By-Step Guide for Design and Implementation in Low- and Middle-Income Countries*. Bethesda, MD: United States Agency for International Development (USAID) ZdravPlus Project.

Cotterill, P.G., Thomas, F.G. (2004). Prospective payment for Medicare inpatient psychiatric care: assessing the alternatives. *Health Care Financing Review*, 26(1):85–101.

Cour des comptes (2009). *La Securité Sociale, chapitre 7, La mise en place de la T2A: Bilan à mi-parcours*. Paris, Cour des comptes (February).

Cutler, D. (1995). The incidence of adverse medical outcomes under prospective payment. *Econometrica*, 63(1):29–50.

D'Aunno, T., Kimberly, J.R., de Pouvourville, G. (2008). Conclusions: the global diffusion of casemix, in J.R. Kimberly, G. de Pouvourville, T. D'Aunno, eds. *The Globalization of Managerial Innovation in Health Care*. Cambridge: Cambridge University Press.

Department of Health (2011). *Best Practice Tariffs*. London: Department of Health (http://www.dh.gov.uk/en/Managingyourorganisation/NHSFinancialReforms/DH_105080, accessed 27 July 2011).

Department of Health and Human Services (2008). *Changes to the Hospital Inpatient Prospective Payment Systems and Fiscal Year 2009 Rates*. Washington, DC: United States Department of Health and Human Services.

Don, H. (2003). Implementing DRGs in Slovenia: why the Australian variant was selected. *Australian Health Review*, 26:50–60.

Eggleston, K., Shen, Y.C., Lau, J., Schmid, C.H., Chan, J. (2008). Hospital ownership and quality of care: what explains the different results in the literature? *Health Economics*, 17(12):1345–62.

Ellis, R.P., McGuire, T.G. (1986). Provider behavior under prospective reimbursement – cost-sharing and supply. *Journal of Health Economics*, 5(2):129–51.

European Parliament and Council (2011). *Directive 2011/24/EU of 9 March 2011 on the Application of Patients' Rights in Cross-Border Healthcare*. Brussels: Official Journal of the European Union (L88/45-L88/65).

Farrar, S., Yi, D., Sutton, M. et al. (2009). Has payment by results affected the way that English hospitals provide care? Difference-in-differences analysis. *British Medical Journal*, 339:b3047.

Fetter, R.B., Thompson, J.D., Mills, R.E. (1976). A system for cost and reimbursement control in hospitals. *Yale Journal of Biology and Medicine*, 49:123–36.

Fürstenberg, T., Laschat, M., Zich, K. et al. (2011). *G-DRG Begleitforschung gemäß §17b Abs. 8 KHG: Endbericht des zweiten Forschungszyklus*. Siegburg: Institut für das Entgeldsystem in Krankenhaus (InEK).

Gilman, B.H. (2000). Hospital response to DRG refinements: the impact of multiple reimbursement incentives on inpatient length of stay. *Health Economics*, 9(4):277–94.

Goldfield, N. (2010). The evolution of diagnosis-related groups (DRGs): from its beginnings in casemix and resource use theory, to its implementation for payment and now for its current utilization for quality within and outside the hospital. *Quality Management in Health Care*, 19(1):3–16.

Hutton, J., Trueman, P., Henshall, C. (2007). Coverage with evidence development: an examination of conceptual and policy issues. *International Journal of Technology Assessment in Health Care*, 23:425–32.

Kahn, K.L., Keeler, E.B., Sherwood, M.J. (1990a). Comparing outcomes of care before and after implementation of the DRG-based prospective payment system. *Journal of the American Medical Association*, 264(15):1984–8.

Kahn, K.L., Rogers, W.H., Rubenstein, L.V. et al. (1990b). Measuring quality of care with explicit process criteria before and after implementation of the DRG-based prospective payment system. *Journal of the American Medical Association*, 264(15):1969–73.

Kiwa Prismant (2008). *Hospital Data Project Phase 2: Final Report. The Need for Metadata and Data*. Utrecht: Kiwa Prismant.

Kiwa Prismant (2010). *Kengetallen Nederlandse Ziekenhuizen 2009 [Key Numbers Dutch Hospitals 2009]*. Utrecht: Dutch Hospital Data.

Kosecoff, J., Kahn, K.L., Rogers, W.H. et al. (1990). Prospective payment system and impairment at discharge. The 'quicker-and-sicker' story revisited. *Journal of the American Medical Association*, 264(15):1980–3.

Langenbrunner, J., Cashin, C., O'Dougherty, S. (2009). *Designing and Implementing Health Care Provider Payment Systems. How-To Manuals*. Washington, DC: World Bank (http://siteresources.worldbank.org/HEALTHNUTRITIONANDPOPULATION/Resources/Peer-Reviewed-Publications/ProviderPaymentHowTo.pdf , accessed 5 September 2011).

Lave, J.R. (2003). Developing a Medicare prospective payment system for inpatient psychiatric care. *Health Affairs*, 22(5):97–109.

Ljunggren, B., Sjödén, P. (2003). Patient-reported quality of life before, compared with after a DRG intervention. *International Journal for Quality in Health Care*, 15(5): 433–40.

MDS (2011). *Abrechnungsprüfungen der MDK in Krankenhäusern sind angemessen, wirtschaftlich und zielführend. Zahlen und Fakten der MDK-Gemeinschaft*. Essen: Medizinischer Dienst des Spitzenverbandes Bund der Krankenkassen e.V.

MedPAC (2008). *Rehabilitation Facilities (Inpatient) Payment System*. Washington, DC: Medicare Payment Advisory Commission.

MedPAC (2010). *Psychiatric Hospital Services Payment System*. Washington, DC: Medicare Payment Advisory Commission.

Radu, C., Chiriac, D.N., Vladescu, C. (2010). Changing patient classification system for hospital reimbursement in Romania. *Croatian Medical Journal*, 51(3):250–8.

Rogers, W.H., Draper, D., Kahn, K.L. et al. (1990). Quality of care before and after implementation of the DRG-based prospective payment system. A summary of effects. *Journal of the American Medical Association*, 264(15):1989–94.

Schreyögg, J., Stargardt, T., Tiemann, O., Busse, R. (2006). Methods to determine reimbursement rates for diagnosis related groups (DRG): a comparison of nine European countries. *Health Care Management Science*, 9(3):215–23.

Schwartz, M.H., Tartter, P.I. (1998). Decreased length of stay for patients with colorectal cancer: implications of DRG use. *Journal for Healthcare Quality*, 20(4):22–5.

Street, A., Scheller-Kreinsen, D., Geissler, A., Busse, R. (2010). Determinants of hospital costs and performance variation: methods, models and variables for the EuroDRG project. *Working Papers in Health Policy and Management*, 3:1–44.

Tan, S.S. (2009). *Micro-costing in Economic Evaluations: Issues of Accuracy, Feasibility, Consistency and Generalizability*. Rotterdam: Erasmus Universiteit Rotterdam.

Tan, S.S., Rutten, F.F., van Ineveld, B.M., Redekop, W.K., Hakkaart-van Roijen, R.L. (2009). Comparing methodologies for the cost estimation of hospital services. *European Journal of Health Economics*, 10:39–45.

Voncina, L., Strizrep, T., Dzakula, A. (2007). The introduction of DRGs in Croatia. *Eurohealth*, 13(1):4–5.

Part Two

chapter eleven

Austria: Inpatient care and the LKF framework

Conrad Kobel and Karl-Peter Pfeiffer

11.1 Hospital services and the role of DRGs in Austria

11.1.1 The Austrian health system

In Austria responsibility for coordination and planning of health care provision and financing has been traditionally shared between the federal Government, the nine states, called *Länder* in German, and their municipalities. In addition, several self-governing bodies representing physicians and pharmacists play an important role. Although the Ministry of Health delegates many tasks to the states or to the self-governing bodies, it remains by far the most influential actor in health policy-making and nationwide planning. It is responsible for supervision of the health insurance funds, enforcement of bills, and regulation of the training of health care professionals (Hofmarcher & Rack, 2006).

In general the Ministry of Health is responsible for enacting legislation, while the implementation of health care-related legislation is the responsibility of the states. However, states can also pass legislation concerning the inpatient sector. In practice, the Federal Health Commission and the Health Platforms at state level – composed of the state governments, the social health insurance institutions and the federal Government – are the most influential actors in terms of the actual implementation. In addition, the physicians' chambers, municipalities, patients and hospital owners are represented in the Health Platforms (Hofmarcher & Rack, 2006).

An agreement according to the Federal Constitution (B-VG) Article 15a between the states and the federal Government is signed and adjusted every four years to establish and coordinate the constitutional duties. As part of this agreement the Austrian Structural Plan for Health is elaborated (ÖBIG, 2008), which guarantees nationwide standards in health care. Regarding inpatient care, the plan specifies standards for bed capacities and the availability of infrastructure (such as major technological equipment) in hospitals. The states are obliged to ensure that these standards are met, which is achieved through regional health plans that specify regional standards for health care providers and their structural characteristics.

Since the early 1990s, expenditures on health have increased rapidly, both in absolute terms and as a share of gross domestic product (GDP). Total health expenditures (not including long-term care) grew from about €10 billion (7.4 per cent of GDP) in 1990 to almost €26 billion (9.2 per cent of GDP) in 2008 (Statistics Austria, 2010). In the same period, the share of public expenditure for health slightly increased from 73.4 per cent in 1990 to 76.9 per cent in 2008 (Statistics Austria, 2010).

In the statutory health insurance (SHI) system, membership is mandatory for almost 99 per cent of the population and depends either on profession or region of residence. SHI funds therefore do not compete. Income-related contributions to SHI are shared equally between employers and employees. Together this amounts to about 46 per cent of health care expenditure. Another 30 per cent of expenditure is paid from taxes. A total of 24 per cent is paid as co-payments either by additional private health insurance or out-of-pocket payments by patients (Thomson et al., 2009).

All SHI funds are organized in the Federation of Austrian Social Insurance Institutions, which administers delegated tasks from the federal Government and the states, such as contracting with the Austrian Physicians' Chamber or the Austrian Pharmacists' Association on prices for outpatient services and reimbursement of medications. Outpatient care is mainly provided by three types of providers: individual self-employed physicians, outpatient clinics and hospital outpatient departments.

Inpatient care is to a great extent provided by public or non-profit-making hospitals (see subsection 11.1.2) and is financed through State Health Funds (*Landesgesundheitsfonds* in German; SHF), which are supervised and managed by the respective State Health Platforms (BMGFJ, 2008e). Since 1997, resources from the SHFs have been allocated to hospitals on the basis of the Austrian performance-oriented hospital financing framework (*Leistungsorientierte Krankenanstaltenfinanzierung* in German; LKF). The introduction of the LKF framework shifted hospital budget allocation for most inpatient services in most hospitals away from a per diem-based system to one that allocates a significant proportion of hospital budgets on the basis of a diagnosis-related group (DRG)-like patient classification system.

To distinguish between the general hospital financing framework, that is, the LKF framework and the patient classification system (PCS), we will refer to the latter as the LKF-PCS, although the term is not used in Austria. The LKF framework applies to all inpatient services covered by SHI, including rehabilitation and psychiatric care. The LKF-PCS applies only to (most) areas of acute inpatient hospital care. All public and non-profit-making hospitals are primarily financed through the LKF framework.

Private profit-making hospitals, on the other hand, obtain their funds primarily through out-of-pocket payments by patients and from private health insurance companies. In addition, the nationwide Private Hospitals Financing Fund (PRIKRAF), which is exclusively funded by SHIs, pays private profit-making hospitals for health services covered by private health insurance. PRIKRAF allocates financial resources to hospitals exclusively on the basis of the same system of DRG-type hospital budget allocation that is used in public and private non-profit-making hospitals (Hofmarcher & Rack, 2006).

A more detailed description of the Austrian health care system can be found in Hofmarcher and Rack (2006).

11.1.2 Hospital services in Austria

Austrian hospitals provide a broad range of services. Amongst others, the Federal Hospitals Act (KAKuG) defines as hospitals (BMGFJ, 2008b) the following types of institutions:

- general hospitals for all patients without distinction according to gender, age or type of medical care provided;
- special hospitals for the examination and treatment of patients with particular illnesses or patients in particular age groups, or for other special purposes;
- convalescent homes for patients in need of medical care and special nursing care while they convalesce;
- homes for chronically ill patients in need of medical care and special nursing care;
- maternity clinics and maternity homes;
- sanatoria – hospitals specially equipped to provide higher standards of board and accommodation;
- independent outpatient health care centres (X-ray clinics, dental care centres and similar facilities) – organizationally independent facilities for the examination or treatment of patients who do not require inpatient care.

Table 11.1 provides an overview of the hospital infrastructure in Austria. In 2006 there were 264 registered hospitals equipped with 63 354 beds, which corresponds to 7.66 beds per 1000 residents and a utilization level of 32.5 admissions per 100 residents. All Austrian hospitals together provided more than 18 million bed days (BMGFJ, 2008b) in 2006.

There were 183 acute care hospitals in 2006, providing 52 894 beds. Of those, 133 were public or private non-profit-making hospitals funded by the SHFs. They provided 92 per cent of beds in acute care hospitals. A total of 43 hospitals were private profit-making hospitals. The remaining 7 were prison or military hospitals. Hospitals funded by the SHF had an average length of stay (ALOS) of 5.71 days (without day cases and long-term care) (BMGFJ, 2008b). For the remainder of this chapter we focus on acute care hospitals.

The sources of financing for inpatient care in Austria are regulated nationwide by the Article 15a B-VG treaties. The federal Government, states, local authorities and health insurance funds contribute to a global national budget, which is then allocated to the SHFs based on state quotas. While health insurance funds pay a flat fee, the federal Government, the states and local authorities pay based on fixed percentages of value-added taxes. In addition, in most states, payments to balance structural deficits by local authorities and the state are also included

Table 11.1 Hospital infrastructure in Austria

	Hospitals	*Beds*	*Hospitals*	*Beds*
	Absolute no.		*% of total*	
Non-acute care hospitals	81	10 460	30.7	16.5
Acute care hospitals	183	52 894	69.3	83.5
hospitals funded by SHF	133	48 870	50.4	77.1
hospitals funded by PRIKRAF[a]	43	4031	16.3	6.4
Total	264	63 354	100.0	100.0

Source: BMGFJ, 2008b.

[a] Applies to certain cases/services.

in the budgets (Hofmarcher & Rack, 2006). The sum of all financial contributions to SHFs determines the global budget of resources available for the financing of hospital services provided in that state for a given year (Table 11.2).

Financing of acute care hospitals is regulated by the national LKF framework, which provides the basis for resource allocation from SHFs to hospitals. The LKF framework consists of two areas: (1) the core area (*Kernbereich* in German) that is made up of the nationwide DRG-like patient classification system (the LKF-PCS); and (2) a state-specific steering area (*Steuerungsbereich* in German). When the LKF framework was introduced, the idea of the steering area was to enable quality-related payments and to allow for a transitional period before hospital resource allocation would be exclusively based on the LKF-PCS. Yet, states continue to use the steering area for different purposes, such as assuring higher payments to university hospitals, providing additional resources to hospitals in alpine areas or compensating for deficits of hospitals (see subsection 11.5.3).

Table 11.2 Payments to the SHFs in 2005

	%			
	Federal Government[a]	*States*	*Local authorities*	*Health insurance institutions*
Burgenland	11.3	45.3	3.6	39.8
Carinthia	11.7	33.2	8.0	47.2
Lower Austria	10.7	31.0	20.9	37.5
Salzburg	12.4	32.1	10.7	44.8
Styria	18.7	34.6	1.3	45.4
Tyrol	22.8	17.9	15.5	43.8
Upper Austria	13.0	22.5	16.8	47.7
Vienna	15.6	39.1	1.7	43.5
Vorarlberg	12.5	25.6	14.3	47.6
Austria	**14.7**	**31.6**	**9.9**	**43.8**

Source: Based on Grossmann & Hauth, 2007.

[a] Including payments for university teaching hospitals.

11.1.3 Purpose of the Austrian LKF-PCS

During the 1980s and 1990s, cost inflation in the Austrian health care system and in particular in the inpatient sector exceeded annual growth of GDP. Austria was spending more on inpatient care than the average of the EU15 countries (belonging to the European Union before May 2004) and had one of the longest ALOS (OECD, 2010). The old per diem-based hospital financing system did not provide incentives for cost–effectiveness or for a reduction in lengths of stay. In addition, transparency in terms of hospital activity was poor, as no detailed structured data relating to diagnoses or procedures were available.

Inspired by DRG-based hospital payment systems in other countries, it was decided to introduce a new hospital payment system to overcome these problems. Using a DRG-like patient classification system was expected to increase cost–effectiveness, limit cost inflation and contribute to a reduction of the ALOS – all while guaranteeing high-quality health care. In particular, using DRGs for hospital payment was intended to reduce multiple diagnostic procedures and to promote a shift from inpatient care to ambulatory care, thus contributing to a reduction in hospital beds (BMGFJ, 2008e). Furthermore, it was hoped that the introduction of a DRG-like system would increase transparency and improve documentation quality (BMGFJ, 2008f).

Today, the primary purpose of the LKF-PCS as part of the LKF framework is to enable activity-based budget allocations to Austrian acute care hospitals. Beyond that, the LKF framework provides a catalogue of diagnoses, an Austrian modification of the World Health Organization's International Classification of Diseases (ICD-10-WHO), and a catalogue of selected procedures; 'selected' to the effect that only expensive and highly frequent procedures are listed. Together with the Austrian Structural Plan for Health, the LKF framework is also used as a planning and steering instrument by stipulating minimum department sizes, staffing standards or volume thresholds as prerequisites for the financing of certain services.

11.2 Development of and updates relating to the LKF-PCS

11.2.1 The LKF-PCS at a glance

The Ministry of Health is the owner of the LKF-PCS and as such responsible for the content, structure, development and maintenance of the system. As already mentioned, the Austrian LKF-PCS is the backbone of the core area (*Kernbereich*) of the LKF framework. The LKF-PCS defines procedure- and diagnosis-oriented case groups (*Leistungsorientierte Diagnosefallgruppen* in German; LDF).

The LKF-PCS classifies each hospital case into exactly one of 979 LDFs. There are two main steps (for details see section 11.3). First, in the event that a patient has undergone at least one grouping relevant procedure listed in the Austrian catalogue of procedures, (s)he is grouped into one of the 209 single medical procedure-based groups (*medizinische Einzelleistungen* in German; MEL). Otherwise, the patient is grouped into one of 219 main diagnosis groups (*Hauptdiagnose-Gruppen* in German; HDG). These groups are similar to base-DRGs, adjacent DRGs, or classes used in other DRG-like patient classification systems (see Chapter 4 of this volume). Second, depending on the patient's characteristics (that is, age, diagnoses or treatments), MEL groups may be split into one of 427 procedure-oriented MEL-LDFs; and HDGs may be split into one of 552 diagnosis-oriented HDG-LDFs.[1]

Each LDF has a specific score that is determined based on information about average costs of treating patients within that LDF (see section 11.4). These LDF scores, together with add-on scores for additional expensive procedures or for stays in specialist departments serve as the basis for hospital budget allocation from SHFs and the PRIKRAF (see subsection 11.5.3).

The steering area (*Steuerungsbereich*) of the LKF framework allows each state to determine hospital budget allocations from its SHF according to state-specific priorities. As each state uses different criteria to adjust hospital budgets, there are 10 different ways of paying hospitals based on the LKF-PCS of the core area: one for each of the nine SHFs, plus one in the nationwide PRIKRAF (Hofmarcher & Riedel, 2001).

11.2.2 Development of the LKF-PCS

In the 1980s, different performance-oriented hospital payment systems were tested with the conclusion that none of them fitted exactly the special needs of the Austrian health care system and that an appropriate legislative framework for documentation standards was still lacking (BMGFJ, 2008f). It was therefore decided to introduce documentation standards for hospitals and to develop an Austrian patient classification system from scratch.

Working in close collaboration with medical experts from various fields, an interdisciplinary team of economists and statisticians developed a system that would be tailored to the specific needs of the Austrian inpatient sector. The result was a precursor version of today's LKF-PCS. Between 1988 and 1990 the system was tested by a sample of 20 hospitals across the country. The outcome was that further development was needed.

Meanwhile, an obligation to document diagnoses was introduced in all Austrian hospitals. Between 1991 and 1996 an Austrian catalogue of procedures was developed by the Ministry of Health, which was the prerequisite for defining procedure-oriented LDFs. Around that time, the potential effects of using the LKF-PCS for hospital financing were calculated for testing purposes. A pilot project in Vorarlberg in 1995 and in Lower Austria in 1996 tested the potential of using the LKF-PCS for hospital budget allocation. The pilot project showed good results as the LKF-PCS seemed to fulfil the aims connected with its introduction (see section 11.3). After final evaluation and further adjustments, the LKF-PCS was introduced within the LKF framework for all acute care hospitals in 1997.

Table 11.3 summarizes some main features of the Austrian LKF-PCS. Since its introduction, the LKF-PCS has undergone annual revisions. However, the Ministry of Health distinguishes years during which revisions are related to 'maintenance' (meaning that only absolutely essential corrections are implemented) from those during which 'amendments' are implemented that imply far-reaching further developments of the system (BMG, 2010). Therefore, the table shows only the three LDF versions resulting from major amendments.

One of the main aspects of annual maintenance work is the introduction of new procedures to keep the system up to date (see section 11.6). In addition, in 2001 the minimum basic data set (MBDS) was extended and the coding of diagnoses was changed to ICD-10-BMSG-2001 (see Table 11.4 in subsection 11.3.1), an Austrian modification of the ICD 10th revision (ICD-10) that was developed together with the German Institute of Medical Documentation and Information (*Deutsches Institut für medizinische Dokumentation und Information* in German; DIMDI).

In 2002, the first major amendment took place. Based on data from 15 reference hospitals, LDF scores, ALOS and trim-points were recalculated for every LDF. LDFs were rearranged or new ones created and new procedures were introduced. Since then, the LDF scores for each LDF consist of a day component and a performance component. The performance component includes costs directly connected to procedures (for example, personnel costs during surgery and medical products) calculated by the reference hospitals' data. The day component includes costs that accrue during the whole hospital stay, such as nursing and hotel costs.

Again, years of minor maintenance revisions followed and in 2006/2007 the LDF scores for day patients were recalculated to discourage unnecessary longer hospital stays. Extra scores for necessary stays in specialist departments and intensive care unit (ICU) were introduced on a per diem basis.

The next major amendment was performed in 2009. As in 2002, all LDF scores, the ALOS and trim-points were recalculated for each LDF, and LDFs were rearranged if necessary. For the calculation of LDF scores, cost data from 20 reference hospitals from 2005 were used. In addition, new procedures were added to the catalogue of procedures, and its structure was revised.

A detailed description of the development has been given by the BMGFJ (2008f).

Table 11.3 LKF-PCS versions

Year	*1997*	*2002*	*2009*
Purpose	DRG-based budget allocation, planning, performance measurement		
DRG system	LKF-PCS Version 1997	LKF-PCS Version 2002	LKF-PCS Version 2009
Data used for development	Cost data from 20 reference hospitals, activity data from all hospitals	Cost data from 15 reference hospitals, activity data from all hospitals	Cost data from 20 reference hospitals, activity data from all hospitals
Number of LDFs	916	842	979
Applied to	Public and non-profit-making acute care hospitals	All acute care hospitals (including those paid through PRIKRAF)	
Included services	All acute inpatient care (including day cases), excluding psychiatric, rehabilitation and long-term care		

Source: Authors' own compilation based on BMGFJ 2008f.

11.2.3 Data used for development and updates of the LKF-PCS

Two main databases are used for updates of the LKF-PCS. First, a hospital activity database is maintained at the Ministry of Health, containing the aggregated information of all MBDS from all hospitals (see Table 11.4). For each admission, hospitals complete the MBDS, which is then sent to the SHFs or the PRIKRAF. There, the data are integrated into a state discharge database, plausibility checks are performed and the data are searched for errors. If necessary, hospitals are asked to correct the data. After approval by the SHF, the data are forwarded to the Ministry of Health.

Second, for the two revisions in 2002 and 2009, detailed resource-consumption data were provided by 20 reference hospitals. The data from these hospitals were merged into a resource-consumption database maintained at the Ministry of Health that contains detailed information for the procedures listed in the catalogue of procedures, including personnel hours spent (by type of personnel and type of treatment), costs for medical consumables and investment costs for large-scale medical equipment. In addition, department-level cost information is available for the calculation of the day component of LDF scores. (For further details, see section 11.4 and subsection 11.5.2.)

Updates of the system rely on information relating to changes in the Austrian catalogue of procedures, which is updated annually. As part of the yearly revisions of the LKF-PCS, the Austrian catalogue of procedures is reviewed for procedures that are used only rarely or no longer fulfil the criteria of the Ministry of Health. After consultation with the SHFs, those procedures are deleted (BMGFJ, 2008c).

11.2.4 Regularity and method of system updates

Revisions of the LKF-PCS are carried out by the LKF team within the Ministry of Health and are divided into two major areas: (1) recalculation of scores for each LDF; and (2) revisions of the LKF-PCS.

LDF scores have been recalculated only twice since the introduction of the LKF-PCS. Recalculations in 2002 relied on data from the year 1999. Recalculations in 2009 were based on data from 2005. As already described, the scores for each LDF comprise two components, which are calculated separately: a performance component related to the direct resource consumption of procedures, and a day component related to hotel costs of keeping a patient in hospital.

Revisions of the LKF-PCS rely on all the types of information described. On a yearly basis, updates (which are almost always related to the inclusion of new procedures) concern only a small number of LDFs, for which the ALOS, thresholds and (if necessary) LDF scores are recalculated (see section 11.6). This is carried out for all LDFs in years of systematic revision. ALOS and thresholds are calculated on the basis of the hospital activity database (BMGFJ, 2008a).

Before a new version of the system comes into effect, simulation calculations are performed to estimate the financial impact for hospitals. No major system amendments are planned before 2013.

11.3 The current patient classification system

11.3.1 Information used to classify patients

The LKF-PCS classifies patients on the basis of information provided in the MBDS that hospitals are required to prepare for every admission. Table 11.4 shows the kind of data that are included in the MBDS.

For the grouping process, only the following data are used as classification variables: (1) procedures, (2) main diagnosis, (3) age classes, (4) secondary diagnoses, and (5) treatment at specialist departments (that is, acute geriatric care, remobilization, palliative departments or neuropsychiatric departments for children and youths).

The procedure catalogue is particularly important for the LKF-PCS and was specifically developed for the purpose of supporting the system. As already mentioned, procedures in the catalogue are called single medical procedures (MELs). Consequently, MEL groups in the LKF-PCS simply summarize the procedure-based groups, similar to base-DRGs in an operation-room partition of a DRG system (see Chapter 4). In contrast to the extensive procedure catalogues used in other countries, the Austrian catalogue of procedures contains only 1500 selected procedures that range from surgical, through cancer treatment, to diagnostic procedures using large-scale equipment. In addition, possible plausibility information is provided for each procedure, such as age, gender, and day-case flag.

The close relationship between the procedure catalogue and the LKF-PCS is also illustrated by the fact that the catalogue indicates a group of expensive and highly frequent procedures that qualify individual cases to be grouped into procedure-oriented LDFs. By contrast, secondary diagnoses and treatment at specialist departments are very rarely used for the classification of patients.

Table 11.4 Content of the MBDS

Administrative data	Admission data • hospital code • admission code and date • type of admission • departments and transfers • discharge date and type	Patient data • date of birth • gender • citizenship • principal residence • insurance or funding body
Medical data	• main diagnosis (ICD-10 BMSG 2001) • any additional diagnoses (ICD-10 BMSG 2001) • any medical services from the catalogue of procedures	
LKF data[a]	• LDF • LDF score • score for outliers • extra scores for ICU stays • extra scores for multiple treatments • scores for specialist departments • total scores	

Source: BMGFJ, 2008f.

[a] Only if required by the respective SHF.

11.3.2 Grouping algorithm

On the basis of information contained in the MBDS (see subsection 11.3.1), every hospital admission is grouped into exactly one LDF. The classification process follows a series of iterative steps that are illustrated in Figure 11.1. Coding and grouping is carried out by medical doctors within hospitals using special software provided by the Ministry of Health.

The objective of the LKF-PCS (as with any other DRG-like patient classification system) is to assign cases into medically meaningful and economically homogeneous groups. In order to do so, the grouping algorithm checks first whether patients were treated in specialist departments (for example, acute geriatric care

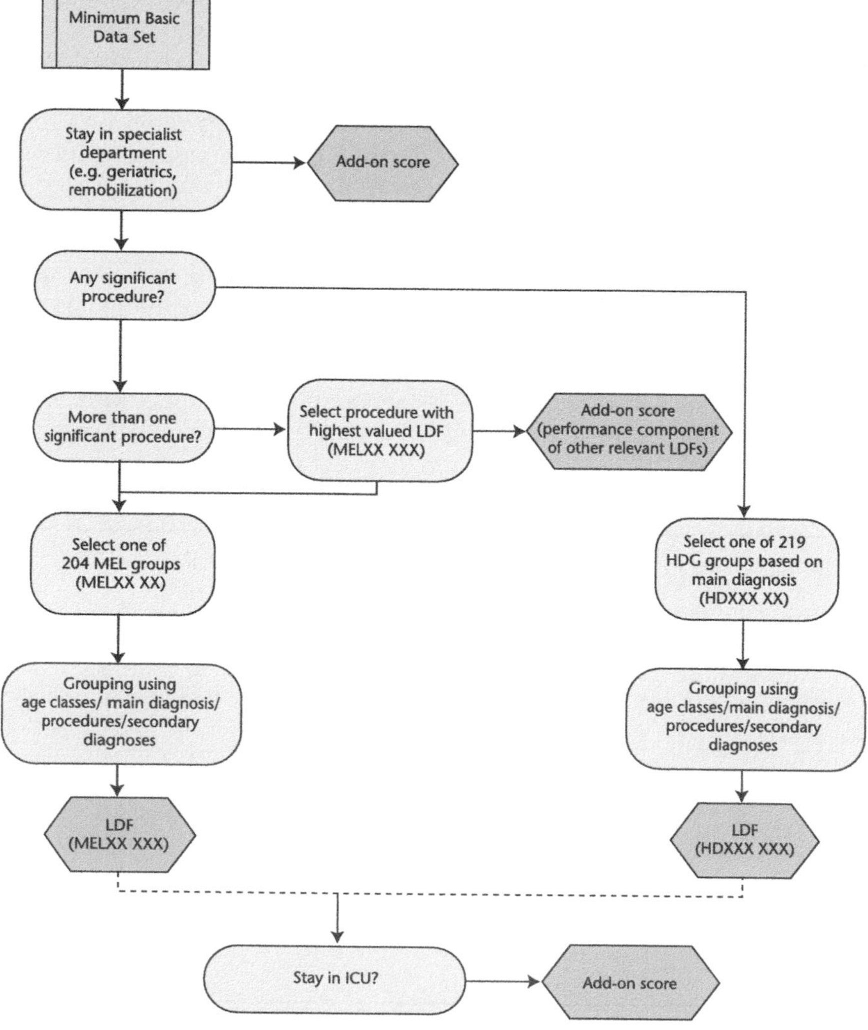

Figure 11.1 LKF grouping process

Source: Based on BMGFJ, 2008e; Grubinger et al., 2010.

or remobilization). If this was the case, the system assigns extra scores based on the number of days spent in these departments. As a second step, the grouping process also checks whether patients have received significant procedures. These are procedures that significantly influence the total costs of the hospital stay. If no such procedures have been carried out, the case is assigned into one of the 219 HDGs on the basis of the main diagnosis. If patients received any significant procedures during the hospital stay, the algorithm checks whether more than one such procedures was performed. If this is the case the procedure and LDF that returns the highest LDF score is selected and add-on scores for all other significant procedures are added, based on the performance component of their LDF. If only one procedure was performed, the case is directly assigned into one of the 204 MEL groups.

Each of the 219 HDG groups and of the 204 MEL groups is characterized by a four-digit number code, which follows a prefix (either 'HDG' or 'MEL'). As a result of the grouping process, HDG groups comprise cases with similar diagnoses, and MEL groups pool procedures that are medically similar and have similar resource-consumption levels. MEL and HDG groups are similar to base-DRGs or classes in other DRG systems. In order to increase economical homogeneity of the final LDFs, MEL and HDG groups are either split into several severity levels according to age classes, principal diagnoses, procedures and secondary diagnoses, or they remain as one group (unsplit). If groups remain unsplit, the letter A is added to the four-digit MEL or HDG code and defines the final LDF. If MEL or HDG groups are split, additional letter codes are assigned (B, C, D). However, the LDF codes are not ordered by resource consumption. The system does not limit the number of splits per MEL or HDG group but subdivides them into as many LDFs as necessary in order to achieve relative homogeneity of resource consumption within each group. In total, there are 979 LDFs in the 2009 LKF-PCS: 427 MEL-LDFs and 552 HDG-LDFs.

After assignment of the final LDF, the system checks whether patients were treated in an ICU and assigns additional per diem points per day of ICU treatment. Four types of ICU exist, with differing per diem scores: intensive monitoring units, and three stages of ICU. Hospitals need approval by the SHF or the PRIKRAF in order to be able to provide ICU treatment. If a patient stays in an ICU, the patient's status has to be documented every 24 hours according to standardized reporting schemes, for example TISS-28, SAPS and TRISS (BMGFJ, 2008a; BMGFJ, 2008d). A minimum score is required to justify ICU stays.

Although the assignment of per diem-based add-on scores is not – strictly speaking – the result of the grouping process, these scores are determined during the grouping process and are an integral part of the Austrian LKF-PCS (BMGFJ, 2008e). Since the LKF-PCS does not use the concept of major diagnostic categories (MDCs) used in other DRG systems, the main diagnosis of procedure-oriented groups is often not checked during the grouping process.

11.3.3 Data quality and plausibility checks

The grouping software, which is available free of charge from the Ministry of Health includes a set of data quality and plausibility checks. The most important plausibility and data quality rules are:

- plausibility of diagnoses and age and gender
- plausibility of procedure and age and gender
- for each procedure, there must be at least one diagnosis
- whether a certain procedure is allowed/possible in a certain hospital.

In each SHF and in the PRIKRAF a data quality group is responsible for carrying out data quality controls at hospitals. Usually, random samples from the hospital activity database are taken and the structured documentation is compared with the patient history documented at the hospital. Questionnaires are used to identify the main problems, such as incorrect main diagnosis, wrong fourth digit of the ICD-10 codes assigned, missing or too many procedures or secondary diagnoses, and so on. Some states apply special algorithms to identify suspicious datasets (Pfeiffer, 2002a). This also allows a data quality profiling of hospitals.

11.3.4 Incentives for up- or wrong-coding

Up-coding is not an issue in Austria, probably because severity levels are rarely based on secondary diagnoses. They are most frequently defined on the basis of relatively objective criteria, such as age, or specific procedures. Since the introduction of the LKF framework, some companies have offered so-called 'optimization' software. However, software has also been developed by the Ministry of Health that allows a certain level of control, if systematic optimization has been used.

In principle, sanctions are possible, if up-coding is found to be an issue. However, thus far hospitals have never been sanctioned, even where misuse has been detected.

11.4 Cost accounting within hospitals

In general, cost accounting within hospitals is not part of the LKF framework and it is not even regulated. Hospitals can therefore implement cost-accounting systems suited to their own needs. However, hospitals financed by SHFs report highly aggregated and standardized data to the SHF. These data include, for example, total costs for consumables (medical and non-medical), energy, fees and administration; the number of full-time equivalents by type of personnel and the respective total costs (reported at department level).

Hospitals that act as reference hospitals for the recalculation of the LDF scores provide data on average resource consumption for procedures. For each procedure, average working time by type of personnel is reported. A distinction is drawn between times for preparation, anaesthesia and actual treatment or surgery. Average costs are reported for 'expensive' medical consumables, such as blood products, implants, prostheses and operation linen. For non-surgical procedures, usage times for large-scale equipment and its costs are reported. These costs include acquisition, depreciation, interest and maintenance (BMGFJ, 2008a). In addition, total costs at the departmental level are reported (including the allocated share of overheads), which are used for calculation of the day component.

11.5 Hospital financing on the basis of the LKF-PCS

11.5.1 Range of services and costs paid through the LKF framework

The LKF framework serves as the reimbursement framework for all hospital stays covered by the SHI in all acute care hospitals (public, private non-profit-making and private profit-making hospitals), including day care and stays in specialist departments, such as acute geriatric care, rehabilitation, palliative departments or neuropsychiatric departments for children and youths. However, payment based on the LKF-PCS does not apply to stays in specialist departments which are financed on a per diem basis. In addition, the SHFs can finance investments as part of their steering activity from within their own budgets. Private profit-making hospitals are financed partly by the LKF-PCS. The PRIKRAF pays directly for those treatments that are listed in the catalogue of procedures covered by the SHI.

Besides financing by the SHFs or PRIKRAF, hospitals also receive payments from various other sources. Treatment of private patients is paid for by private health insurance or out-of-pocket payments by the patients themselves. The federal Government pays a lump sum to university hospitals to cover additional expenses for teaching and research.

11.5.2 Calculation of the LDF scores

The LDF scores are calculated based on the hospital activity data from all hospitals and the resource-consumption data for procedures from the reference hospitals (see subsections 11.2.3 and 11.2.4). As already described, the score of each LDF contains two components: (1) a performance component that includes all resource consumption directly connected to procedures; and (2) a day component which comprises the sum of all remaining costs accruing during the hospital stay.

Performance component

Based on the data for procedures provided by the reference hospitals, the average procedure-related costs for each LDF are determined.

For each procedure the reference hospitals provide the average cost, which is the sum of four categories: (1) personnel costs, which are calculated as working time multiplied by average salary according to type of personnel; (2) costs of expensive consumables, established by multiplying the quantity by the price; (3) large-scale equipment costs; and (4) procedure-related overheads.

Day component

At department level all costs that cannot be allocated to one of the procedures are divided by the total number of bed days, which provides the adjusted costs of a bed day. The day component of an LDF score is then calculated as the average sum of the adjusted costs for each bed day, assuming the ALOS of this LDF.

The ALOS in MEL-LDFs is calculated as a 10 per cent trimmed mean, and as a 20 per cent trimmed mean in HDG-LDFs. In MEL-LDFs, 'outliers' are defined as patients staying longer than the minimum of 1.5*ALOS and the 90th percentile of the length of stay or staying less time than the maximum of 0.3*ALOS and the 10th percentile of the length of stay. In HDG-LDFs, outliers are defined by a slightly different method. Long stays are those longer than the minimum of 1.5*ALOS and the 80th percentile, while short stays are those shorter than the maximum of 0.5*ALOS and the 20th percentile (BMGFJ, 2008e).

Adjustments for outliers

The additional daily score for long-stay outliers is reduced for each following outlier day, but remains stable at the minimum of half of the daily day component. The calculation is carried out as follows (BMGFJ, 2008e):

$$Score\ (x) = max \left\{ DC \times \frac{t}{x}, \frac{DC}{2} \right\}$$

x = number of hospital days (and has to be above the trim-point)
Score(x) = extra points for day x
DC = day component per day
t = trim-point = bound for long-stay outliers

The LDF score of short-term outliers contains the full performance component, whereas the day component is reduced (BMGFJ, 2008e).

$$Score = PC + \frac{(LDF\ score - PC)*\ (x + 1)}{t + 1}$$

x = number of hospital days (and has to be below the trim-point)
Score = reduced LDF score
LDF score = score of the LDF-group
PC = performance component
t = trim-point = bound for short-stay outliers

For 0-day stays, approved treatments in day hospitals are reimbursed in the same way as 1-day stays. 0-day stays with non-approved treatments receive the full performance component but only 10 per cent of the reduced day component calculated for short-stay outliers.

11.5.3 LDFs in actual hospital payment

SHFs allocate the majority of hospital budgets on the basis of LDF scores. As the general rules that apply for determining the LDF score are the same nationwide, these are part of the LKF core area. However, how SHFs make use of this information in order to determine hospital budgets depends on state-specific priorities and is defined in the LKF steering area, which is specific to each state.

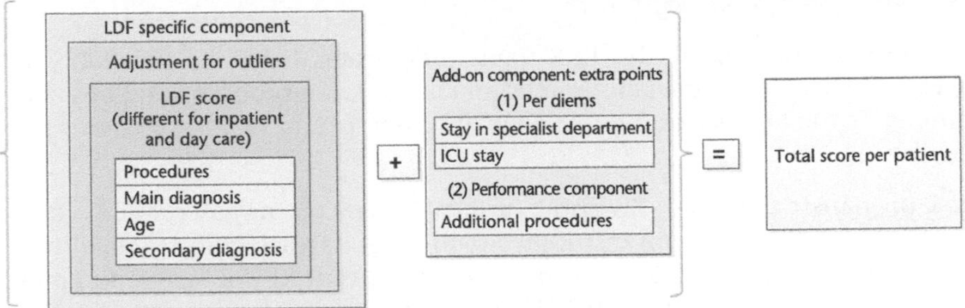

Figure 11.2 Calculation of total LDF score per patient

Source: Based on BMGFJ, 2008e.

LKF core area (Kernbereich)

The LKF core area defines how the LDF score per patient is determined on the basis of the LKF-PCS. Figure 11.2 shows that the total score consists of two main components: (1) the LDF-specific part; and (2) add-on scores for certain services.

Every hospital discharge is assigned to an LDF on the basis of its diagnoses, procedures, and so on (see section 11.3). Each LDF has a specific score which is calculated based on average costs of treatment of patients within that LDF (see subsection 11.5.2). In addition, the LDF score is adjusted for outlier patients, that is, patients with exceptionally long or short lengths of stay. For long-stay outliers, the day component is increased for every day that patients stayed beyond the upper length-of-stay threshold. For short-stay outliers, the day component of the LDF score is reduced for every day that patients were discharged below the lower length-of-stay threshold. For day cases (for which length of stay is 0), the reduction depends on whether day-care treatment is explicitly allowed or not.

Add-on scores are assigned in two ways. Per diem-based add-on scores are given for every day a patient spent in specialist departments (such as acute geriatric care, remobilization, palliative departments or neuropsychiatric departments for children and youths) or in an ICU. Additional procedure scores are added if patients received more than one significant procedure during a hospital stay, as the performance component of an LDF for patients with multiple procedures reflects only the resource consumption of the most complex procedure. Possible reductions apply for multiple treatments on the same day.

As the basis for hospital payment, the sum of all LDF scores of each hospital in a given state is calculated. In addition, the total sum of all LDF scores in a state is calculated and serves as a reference point from which to determine the share of total score provided by a specific hospital. A comparable procedure is used to determine hospital budget allocations to private profit-making hospitals from the PRIKRAF. The main difference is that only one nationwide global budget exists (financed by SHIs) that is distributed to all private profit-making hospitals.

LKF steering area (Steuerungsbereich)

In the steering area of the LKF framework, states have the possibility to determine hospital budgets for public and private non-profit-making hospitals funded by the SHF according to provincial criteria. Four main approaches can be identified.[2]

1. Upper Austria allocates the entire hospital budget on the basis of LDF scores; that is, the SHF budget is distributed to the hospitals according to their share of LDF scores. This is also the case for 98 per cent of the budget in Lower Austria. Only 2 per cent of the SHF budget is allocated according to the hospital type – that is, block grants are made to hospitals depending on structural characteristics of those hospitals, for example according to teaching status or size.
2. In three states, fixed rates are used between the core area and the steering area. Tyrol and Burgenland allocate 70 per cent according to LDF scores. The remaining 30 per cent of the budget is allocated after weighting the LDF scores, depending on the hospital type (for example, LDF scores produced by university hospitals are inflated) or depending on the specific hospital. In Vorarlberg, 15 per cent of the budget is allocated by adjusting LDF scores for higher personnel costs in certain regional areas.
3. Carinthia, Styria and Vienna do not use fixed rates between the core area and the steering area, but weight LDF scores by certain criteria. While Vienna combines personnel costs and additional costs as a factor, Carinthia and Styria weight hospital types by different factors. This means that the LDF scores of each hospital are weighted by a factor and the budget is allocated based on the weighted shares.
4. In Salzburg, financing is divided into two tiers. In the first, 75 per cent of the budget is allocated without weighting and 25 per cent is weighted by a hospital-related factor. A total of 40 per cent of the second tier is based on past deficits and 60 per cent on weighted LDF scores.

11.5.4 Quality-related adjustments

Hospital budget allocations under the LKF framework are not adjusted for quality. However, the Austrian Structural Plan for Health (ÖBIG, 2008) requires minimum standards for certain treatments financed through the LKF framework. For example, there are specifications relating to hospital size, availability of infrastructure and personnel, and minimum volume thresholds.

11.5.5 Main incentives for hospitals

The budgets of the SHFs are distributed mainly according to the amount of LDF scores that hospitals produce in a given year. Therefore, hospitals may try to increase their share of the budget by producing more LDF scores, for example by treating more patients, especially day cases. However, as the LKF hospital budget allocation system operates within a fixed global budget, increased production of LDF scores by one hospital reduces the value of LDF scores and thus the budget available for other hospitals.

Several states were forced to take up counter-measures in order to avoid an uncontrolled growth of hospital activity by defining score budgets for each hospital. If a hospital produces more than the permitted amount of LDF scores, the value of these LDF scores is reduced.

11.6 New/innovative technologies

The inclusion of new technologies into the Austrian catalogue of procedures and the LKF framework follows several predefined steps.

Hospital departments that want to use a specific technology must prepare a request containing a detailed description of the technology and a calculation of costs. Subsequently, the request is submitted by the hospitals and their owners to the respective SHF using a standardized form, which is now based on an Internet platform maintained by the Ministry of Health.[3]

SHFs evaluate the requests and forward them to the LKF team at the Ministry of Health, where medical and economic aspects are assessed. In the event of a positive evaluation, new technologies are preliminarily included in the catalogue of procedures, nationwide, for two years. However, utilization is often restricted to a limited number of hospitals based on certain structural criteria, such as number of beds or hospital types.

In order to assure adequate reimbursement of hospitals, the LKF-PCS is modified by the LKF team. In most cases, new procedures can be assigned to existing MEL groups comprising similar procedures, and the cost of a new procedure is assumed to be similar to the existing ones. If no similar procedures exist, a new LDF can be created and the performance component of the LDF score is estimated based on the cost calculation included in the request for inclusion in the catalogue. Consequently, new technologies are financed through the LKF framework in the same way as any existing procedure, and there are no separate or supplementary payments for new technologies.

After the first and the second years the new technology is evaluated based on medical evidence. For the ultimate inclusion in the catalogue, the respective LDF scores are calculated based on the collected data. If necessary, a new LDF is created (BMGFJ, 2008c).

11.7 Evaluation of the LKF framework in Austria

Ten years after the introduction of the LKF-PCS as the basis for the hospital budget allocation system, an evaluation process was initiated by the Ministry of Health. As part of this evaluation, a group of international experts was contracted to assess the status quo and to propose future developments. Their findings are programmed to have a great impact on the next Article 15a treaties between the states and the federal Government. However, unfortunately, the results have not yet been made public.

11.7.1 Official evaluations

Some research has assessed whether the switch from per diem-based financing to hospital budget allocation on the basis of the LKF-PCS has had an effect on ALOS and hospitalization rates or not (Frick et al., 2001). Other research has focused on the impact that the introduction of the LKF framework has had on health care as a whole (Theurl & Winner, 2007). All authors found that the introduction of the LKF framework had a decreasing effect on the overall ALOS, on top of the long-term trend of declining lengths of stay (Frick et al., 2001, Theurl & Winner, 2007). However, when looking at separate medical disciplines, Frick and colleagues (Frick et al., 2001) showed that only 3 out of 21 disciplines had displayed significant reductions in lengths of stay. Furthermore, they found that in 8 disciplines, hospitalization rates had increased significantly.

Theurl & Winner (2007) came to similar conclusions and showed that 8 out of 20 diagnostic groups (according to ICD-10) had significant declines in ALOS. The authors concluded, 'Our evidence suggests that the Austrian hospital sector has gained a substantial increase in efficiency through the reform of the financing system. This conclusion is also confirmed by the fact that the annual increase of hospital costs declined after the implementation of the LKF1997' (Theurl & Winner, 2007).

In addition, the authors highlight that the introduction of the LKF-PCS could only have a limited influence on shifting inpatient care to ambulatory care, because organizational structures and financing of different health care sectors are highly segmented in Austria. SHI funds do not pay the full costs of inpatient care, contributing only flat fees per member to the SHFs. Consequently, they are not particularly interested in shifts towards outpatient care for which they would be required to cover a higher percentage of the total costs.

Pfeiffer (2002b) has observed that the amount of day-care treatment in hospitals is increasing every year. However, the majority of these cases do not replace inpatient admissions. Instead, they represent a shift from the outpatient to the inpatient sector (Pfeiffer, 2002b) – the opposite of what was intended when the LKF framework was introduced (see subsection 11.1.3). Pfeiffer (2002b) explains this trend with reference to the strict separation of health care in Austria. Beyond that, he finds that there is a missing link in health care provision, highlighted by the example of clinics located between inpatient care and care provided by private physicians.

11.7.2 Authors' assessment

The introduction of the LKF framework was an important improvement in hospital financing in Austria, as hospital budget allocations under the LKF framework are more closely related to hospital activity than under the old per diem system. In addition, hospitals now report detailed activity data, contributing to increased transparency in the hospital sector and improving documentation quality.

Now, 13 years after the introduction of the LKF framework, it still serves its purpose(s). However, reforms are needed that require a consensus by all relevant stakeholders, including the federal Government and all nine states, which is almost impossible to reach. Financial issues are particularly difficult to solve. For example, it remains unclear how SHFs are to be compensated for financing the treatment of patients from other states, or how 'fairness' of budget allocations from the federal Government to the SHFs can be improved.

Other countries, such as France or England have recently updated their patient classification systems, especially in terms of their systematic assessment of secondary diagnoses for the definition of severity levels. In Austria, secondary diagnoses play a very minor role in defining severity levels. Aside from changes in the catalogue of procedures, the classification process as such has not changed.

Although transparency and activity documentation have been improved, research into the hospital sector is rarely carried out. Unfortunately, detailed information – such as hospital activity data or resource-consumption data – is only available to a limited number of people at the federal Government, the states and a group of contracted experts at the Ministry of Health (the LKF team). For researchers outside this circle of people it is very difficult, if not impossible, to obtain hospital activity data. Yet, such research could help to improve health care in Austria.

11.8 Outlook: Future developments and reform

In Austria there is a clear separation between inpatient and outpatient care. In order to improve the continuity of care and to avoid unnecessary hospital admissions, it is necessary to build interfaces. However, there are many obstacles to this, such as the different financing systems for inpatient and outpatient care and varying interests on the part of stakeholders.

Concerning technical issues of the LKF framework and the LKF-PCS grouping algorithm, further extensions and specifications of the catalogue of procedures are necessary, along with updates to diagnosis coding. However, after the major maintenance of the LKF framework in 2009, the system should remain relatively unchanged for the next few years. Future development will include the implementation of plausibility checks in the provided grouping software and specific access criteria for ICUs. Furthermore, how to improve the severity classification will be discussed, along with how to define LDFs that extend beyond individual hospital admissions and include transfers or readmissions of patients.

Currently, the development of a procedure classification system for the outpatient sector is coming to an end, and pilot tests have been initiated (BMG, 2009). This is important, as an outpatient procedure classification is a prerequisite for any attempts to extend the LKF framework to the outpatient sector.

11.9 Notes

1 Figures correct for the 2009 LKF-PCS.
2 Further details can be found in Hofmarcher and Riedel (2001) or in Hofmarcher and Rack (2006).

3 More information can be obtained at the Ministry of Health web site (http://mel.lkf.bmgf.gv.at, accessed 26 June 2011).

11.10 References

BMG (2009). *Dokumentation im ambulanten Bereich – Bericht zur Entwicklung des Leistungskatalogs 2010*. Vienna: Bundesministerium für Gesundheit.

BMG (2010). *The Austrian DRG system*. Vienna: Bundesministerium für Gesundheit.

BMGFJ (2008a). *Handbuch zur Dokumentation in landesgesundheitsfonds- finanzierten Krankenanstalten (Anhang 1) 2004+*. Vienna: Bundesministerium für Gesundheit, Familie und Jugend.

BMGFJ (2008b). *Krankenanstalten in Österreich*. Vienna: Bundesministerium für Gesundheit, Familie und Jugend.

BMGFJ (2008c). *Leistungsorientierte Krankenanstaltenfinanzierung – LKF – Änderungen und Neuerungen im Modell 2009*. Vienna: Bundesministerium für Gesundheit, Familie und Jugend.

BMGFJ (2008d). *Leistungsorientierte Krankenanstaltenfinanzierung – LKF – Medizinische Dokumentation inklusive 17*. Vienna: Rundschreiben. Bundesministerium für Gesundheit, Familie und Jugend.

BMGFJ (2008e). *Leistungsorientierte Krankenanstaltenfinanzierung – LKF – Modell 2009*. Vienna: Bundesministerium für Gesundheit, Familie und Jugend.

BMGFJ (2008f). *Leistungsorientierte Krankenanstaltenfinanzierung – LKF – Systembeschreibung 2009*. Vienna: Bundesministerium für Gesundheit, Familie und Jugend.

Frick, U., Barta, W., Zwisler, R., Filipp, G. (2001). Auswirkungen der leistungsorientierten Krankenhausfinanzierung (LKF) auf die Verweildauern und Hospitalisierungen im Land Salzburg seit 1997. *Gesundh ökon Qual manag*, 6(04):95–104.

Grossmann, B., Hauth, E. (2007). *Verwaltungs- und Pensionsreformen im öffentlichen Dienst sowie Finanzierung des Krankenanstaltenwesens*. Vienna: MANZ'sche Verlags- und Universitätsbuchhandlung.

Grubinger, T., Kobel, C., Pfeiffer, K.P. (2010). Regression tree construction by bootstrap: model search for DRG systems applied to Austrian health data. *BMC Medical Informatics and Decision-Making*, 10:9.

Hofmarcher, M.M., Rack, H-M. (2006). Austria: Health system review. *Health Systems in Transition*, 8(3):1–247.

Hofmarcher, M.M., Riedel, M. (2001). Gesundheitsausgaben in der EU: Ohne Privat kein Staat, Schwerpunktthema. Das österreichische Krankenanstaltenwesen – eines oder neun Systeme? *Health System Watch*, 1/Frühjahr:1–24.

ÖBIG (2008). *Österreichischer Strukturplan Gesundheit 2008*. Vienna: Bundesministerium für Gesundheit.

OECD (2010). *OECD Health Data 2010: Statistics and Indicators*. Paris: Organisation for Economic Co-operation and Development (http://www.oecd.org/document/30/0,3343,en_2649_34631_12968734_1_1_1_1,00.html, accessed 20 August 2010).

Pfeiffer, K.P. (2002a). *Documentation, data quality and continuous observation of the hospital sector*. 18th PCS/E Conference. Innsbruck, Austria. 2–5 October 2002:398–406.

Pfeiffer, K.P. (2002b). Fünf Jahre Erfahrung mit der Leistungsorientierten Krankenanstaltenfinanzierung (LKF) in Österreich, in M. Arnold, J. Klauber, H. Schellschmidt. *Krankenhaus-Report 2001*. Stuttgart: Schattauer Verlag.

Statistics Austria (2010). *Health expenditure in Austria*. Vienna: Statistik Austria (http://www.statistik.gv.at/web_en/static/health_expenditure_in_austria_according_to_the_system_of_health_accounts_1_027971.xlsx, accessed 20 December 2010).

Theurl, E., Winner, H. (2007). The impact of hospital financing on the length of stay: evidence from Austria. *Health Policy*, 82(3):375–89.

Thomson, S., Foubister, T., Mossialos, E. (2009). *Financing health care in the European Union. Challenges and policy responses*. Copenhagen: WHO Regional Office for Europe on behalf of the European Observatory on Health Systems and Policies.

chapter twelve

England: The Healthcare Resource Group system

Anne Mason, Padraic Ward and Andrew Street[1]

12.1 Hospital services and the role of DRGs

12.1.1 The English health care system

The United Kingdom spends about 8 per cent of its gross domestic product (GDP) on health, and 87 per cent of expenditure comes from the public sector (Hawe, 2009). The National Health Service (NHS) is funded by general taxation (80.3 per cent), national insurance contributions (18.4 per cent) and patients' out-of-pocket payments for prescriptions, dental and optometry services (1.3 per cent). Private expenditure constitutes about 13 per cent of total health care expenditure, which is lower than the average (23 per cent) for the countries belonging to the European Union prior to May 2004 (EU15) (Hawe, 2009).

In England, the Department of Health has overall responsibility for the NHS and is under the direction of a politician – the Secretary of State for Health. In 2010, 10 Strategic Health Authorities managed the local NHS, overseeing provision, capacity and quality on behalf of the Secretary of State. Special health authorities, such as the National Blood Authority and the National Institute for Health and Clinical Excellence (NICE), provided national services for the English NHS.

Most NHS services are delivered by public providers. In the primary care sector, general practitioners (GPs) typically work in group practices. Although their income originates from public funds, GPs are effectively self-employed and their practices employ nurses, health visitors and administrative staff. The GP contract was revised in 2004 and pays GPs for the provision of basic services, as well as rewarding GP practices for the achievement of specific 'quality' targets. Some practices also act as purchasers ('Practice-based Commissioners').

In secondary care, hospitals are grouped into legal bodies known as NHS Trusts. These are mostly acute trusts (168) but there are also 73 mental health trusts. These trusts cover around 1600 hospitals and specialist centres.[2] There are also 10 'care trusts' that provide health and social care, and 12 ambulance trusts, which provide emergency and non-emergency patient transport.

12.1.2 Hospital services in England

The number of NHS hospital beds by provider type available in England in 2008/2009 is summarized in Table 12.1. Statistics on the number of beds available in the private sector are not available at a national level.

Acute trusts provide elective and non-elective care, surgical and diagnostic procedures, Accident & Emergency (A&E) services, and some maternity services. Inpatient and outpatient psychiatric services are mostly provided by mental health trusts. Some NHS patients are treated in Independent Sector Treatment Centres, although this amounts to less than 1.5 per cent of elective care patients (Mason et al., 2009).

In 2010, most NHS hospital care was purchased by 152 Primary Care Trusts (PCTs), each of which covered populations of between 300 000 and 350 000 individuals. PCTs can purchase elective services from any hospital or treatment centre in England, including private providers. For services covered by the prospective payment system, known as 'Payment by Results' (PbR), PCTs pay hospitals a fixed price (tariff) for each patient treated. For services not covered by PbR, such as mental health care and high-cost pharmaceuticals, volume-based contracts are agreed between PCTs and hospitals and prices are negotiated locally.

Information on English NHS hospital services originates from two main databases; in both, data relate to a financial year which ends on the last day of the month of March. First, the Hospital Episode Statistics (HES) database comprises activity data, including individual patient records for all inpatient

Table 12.1 Average daily number of available and occupied beds, 2008/2009

Sector	*Available beds (share (%))*	*Occupied beds (share (%))*	*Occupancy (%)*
All ward types	160 254	136 860	85.4
General and acute (acute + geriatric)	122 538	106 142	86.6
– Acute	101 520	86 779	85.6
– Geriatric	21 018	19 363	92.1
Mental illness	26 448	22 793	86.2
Learning disabilities	2 882	2 393	83.0
Maternity	8 386	5 532	66.0
NHS organizations			
Acute trusts	121 448 (76)	103 407 (76)	85
Mental health trusts	29 512 (18)	25 465 (19)	86
PCTs	8 737 (5.0)	7 492 (5.0)	86
Care trusts	116 (0.1)	92 (0.1)	80

Source: Department of Health, 2009a.

admissions, outpatient appointments and A&E attendances. England is unusual in that the recording 'unit' in the HES refers to the time spent under the care of each consultant during the hospital stay. However, these records can be linked to construct a 'provider spell', which corresponds to the usual measure of an inpatient stay, defined as the period between admission and discharge. Second, the NHS Reference Cost database contains provider costs for inpatient spells, outpatient and A&E attendances, psychiatric care, and critical care amongst other specialist services. Reference costs are used as the basis for the PbR tariff (Street & Maynard, 2007b).

Healthcare Resource Groups (HRGs), an English version of diagnosis-related groups (DRGs) are the unit of analysis both for activity and cost. The main focus of this chapter is on HRGs, the classification system used to describe patients admitted to hospital. We outline their development and construction; the uses to which they have been put; how costs are calculated for each HRG; and the use of HRGs for reimbursement. Recent years have also seen the development of classification systems for patients treated in other hospital settings – notably outpatient and A&E departments – and these are addressed briefly.

12.1.3 Purpose of the DRG system

In most countries, the purpose of the DRG system has evolved from benchmarking to reimbursement. The evolution has been similar in England and by the mid-1990s HRGs were being used for three main purposes (Sanderson, 1995).

First, HRGs were used for benchmarking, providing the basis for comparative performance assessment. The (then) National Casemix Office constructed an interactive national database that hospitals could use to assess the average length of stay for their patients compared to the national average or compared to a selective set of hospitals for each HRG. The database could also be used to identify patients with excessive lengths of stay (so-called 'outliers') and to produce specialty-level and hospital-level comparisons.

Second, hospitals were encouraged to use HRGs to assist with internal resource management. HRGs were used to assess the budgetary impact of anticipated changes in the volume and casemix of patients within specialties or clinical directorates, as well as to monitor actual versus expected expenditure.

Third, HRGs were used to inform the contracting process. In the 1990s, hospitals received their income via three main types of contractual arrangement. Block contracts specified payment for a fixed volume of activity; cost-and-volume contracts allowed for payments to be withheld (or made) if volumes fell below (or surpassed) expectations; and cost-per-case contracts involved patient-specific payments. Originally, contracts distinguished patients according to the specialty in which they were treated but, from 1994 onward, increasingly more contracts were specified using HRGs. This required hospitals to undertake HRG-level costing, applying a standardized method of cost allocation (see section 12.4).

In 1997, the incoming Labour Government announced that they would be developing a national schedule of 'reference costs' itemizing the cost of HRGs across the NHS (NHS Executive, 1997). It was intended that, by benchmarking costs in a standardized manner, purchasers would be able to identify and address inefficiency. However, the provision of benchmarking information alone probably did not provide sufficient incentive for hospitals to address cost differentials (Dawson & Street, 2000). In 2002, therefore, the Government published proposals to introduce a prospective payment system, with hospitals receiving a fixed national payment per patient according to the HRG to which they are allocated (Department of Health, 2002). PbR – as these reimbursement arrangements have been called – was introduced for a small number of HRGs in 2003, and coverage has gradually expanded to other HRGs.

12.2 Development and updates of the DRG system

12.2.1 The current DRG system at a glance

All patients admitted to hospital are classified by HRGs, which are clinically similar and resource homogeneous (Anthony, 1993). Allocation is carried out according to which (if any) procedures are received, primary diagnosis, age and level of complications. The current system, known as HRG4 contains about 1400 groups (in 22 'chapters').

Psychiatric inpatient care is not currently covered by HRG4, but the intention is that it will be incorporated in future (Mason & Goddard, 2009). There are also plans to extend the tariff system to a number of other types of care (see subsection 12.8.2). Figure 12.1 provides an overview of HRG4 and Table 12.4 details how HRG4 is used to reimburse inpatient and day-case activity.

Patient-level outpatient activity data have been collected within the HES since 2003/2004 (NHS Information Centre for Health and Social Care, 2009). Attendances are classed by specialty, subdivided by first or subsequent appointment, primary diagnosis, main procedures and interventions, as well as by hospital provider. However, providers are not obliged to submit outpatient data or to code procedures and diagnoses, and data quality is consequently poor (NHS Information Centre for Health and Social Care, 2009). HRGs are used only for outpatient procedures, with other classifications based on specialty. Reimbursement of outpatient activity is not based on HRGs, but differentiated according to whether attendance is a first or follow-up appointment, the number of clinicians seen and by specialty.

Patient-level data on A&E activity were first collected in 2007/2008 and cover attendances at major A&E departments, single-specialty departments, minor injury units and walk-in centres. However, as the submission of records is not mandatory for all providers, the data quality is sometimes poor, as already mentioned in the context of outpatient activity data. In 2009/10 there were 12 tariffs for A&E reimbursement that varied by investigation or procedure cost.

12.2.2 Development of the DRG system

Development of an English version of DRGs first commenced in 1981 when the Department of Health funded a research project to assess the ability of the contemporary version of DRGs in the United States to explain variation in the length of stay of English patients (Coles, 1993). Further research eventually led to the development of the United Kingdom's own categorization system of HRGs, launched in 1991. While DRGs were based on major diagnostic categories (MDCs) that correspond to a single organ system, HRGs were (and remain) more directly related to specialties. They also differ from (historical) DRGs in using local procedure codes, developed by the Office of Population Censuses and Surveys (OPCS), in addition to the International Classification of Diseases (ICD) codes for diagnoses.

As shown in Table 12.2, the first version comprised 534 categories (including 12 undefined categories) but did not cover all acute activity, lacking groups for psychiatry, radiotherapy and oncology (Anthony, 1993). HRG version 2 was released in 1994, with a reduction in the number of categories to 533, including 6 undefined ('U') groups, but also including psychiatric HRGs. Further refinements led to the release of HRG3.1 in 1997, comprising 572 groups and including chemotherapy (Benton et al., 1998). This version remained in use for a number of years, becoming the basis for the reporting and benchmarking of hospital 'reference' cost data (Street & Dawson, 2002). A less-dramatic revision appeared with the release of HRG3.5 in 2003, expanding the number of groups to 610. It was this version that was in place when the Government started to use HRGs explicitly for reimbursement purposes, with the phased introduction of PbR (Department of Health, 2002), which commenced in 2003/2004.

The HRG4 design represents a major development from HRG3.5, and uses ICD-10 (10th revision) diagnoses and OPCS-4.5 procedure codes. It was first used in the 2006/2007 reference cost collection exercise and replaced HRG3.5 as the basis for reimbursement in 2009/2010 (Information Standards Board for Health and Social Care, 2009). HRG4 is designed to evolve year on year, so the number of categories is not constant, containing approximately 1400 groups, only one of which is an undefined category.

HRG4 differs from the previous version in various respects (NHS Information Centre for Health and Social Care, 2008a), as detailed here.

1. HRG3.5 covered only inpatient and day-case activity, but HRG4 covers non-admitted (outpatient) care, emergency medicine and some specialty areas not covered by HRG3.5, such as critical care (NHS Health and Social Care, 2008a).
2. Under HRG3.5, each episode of care generated a single HRG and all elements of treatment were subsumed under this base- (core) HRG. Under HRG4, some (high-cost) elements of treatment are separated from the base-HRG, generating unbundled HRGs that can be reimbursed as additions to base-HRGs. Therefore, one patient can have several HRGs. To qualify for unbundling, there must be at least 600 cases expected annually, or the total annual cost must be at least £1.5 million.
3. HRG4 refines the classification of complications and co-morbidities (CCs) to better reflect variations in severity.
4. This latest version also provides spell-based HRGs that cover the whole stay from admission to discharge (including one or more episodes) to make reimbursement 'fairer'.

Table 12.2 and Figure 12.1 provide an overview of the evolution of the English DRG system.

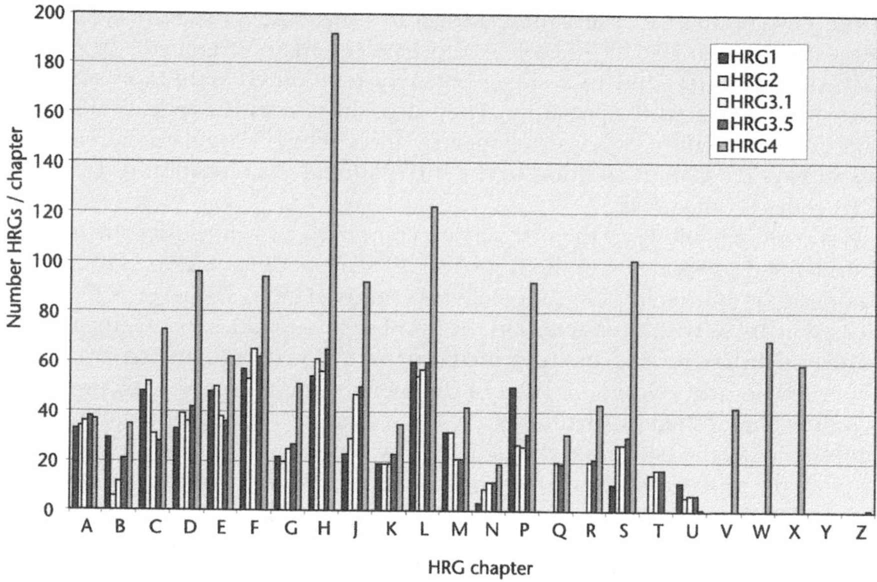

Figure 12.1 Overview of previous and current DRG systems

Sources: Anthony, 2993; Sanderson et al., 1995; NHS Information Centre for Health and Social Care, 2006a, b, 2008b.

Notes:

HRG4 CHAPTERS DEFINITIONS			
A	Nervous system	N	Obstetrics
B	Eyes and periorbita	P	Diseases of childhood and neonates
C	Mouth, head, neck and ears	Q	Vascular system
D	Respiratory system	R	Diagnostic imaging and interventional radiology
E	Cardiac surgery and primary cardiac condition	S	Haematology, chemotherapy, radiotherapy and specialist palliative care
F	Digestive system	T	Reserved for mental health currencies
G	Hepatobiliary and pancreatic system	U	Undefined groups
H	Musculoskeletal system	V	Multiple trauma, emergency and urgent care, and rehabilitation
J	Skin, breast and burns	W	Immunology, infectious diseases and other contacts with health services
K	Endocrine and metabolic system	X	Critical care, high-cost drugs and devices
L	Urinary tract and male reproductive system	Y	Empty
M	Female reproductive system and assisted reproduction	Z	Unbundled

Table 12.2 Evolution of the English DRG system

	1st DRG version	*2nd DRG version*	*3rd DRG version*	*4th DRG version*	*5th DRG version*
Date of introduction	May 1992	August 1994	June 1997	October 2003	In transition [a]
(Main) Purpose	Patient classification	Patient classification	Patient classification	Patient classification	Patient classification
DRG system	HRG1	HRG2	HRG3.1	HRG3.5	HRG4
Data used for development	Adaptation of United States DRGs	Data analysis of groupings	Clinical review to refine for ICD-10. Statistical analysis	Clinical Working Groups refined categories. Statistical analysis	Expert working groups' micro-costing data
Number of DRGs	534	533	572	610	1389
Applied to	Public hospitals	Public hospitals	Public hospitals	Public hospitals / private hospitals or treatment centres treating NHS patients	Public hospitals / private hospitals or treatment centres treating NHS patients
	Acute admissions	Acute admissions	Acute admissions	Acute admissions	Acute admissions Outpatients

[a] The version shown is for 2007/2008.

In evaluating alternative arrangements for the classification architecture, performance has always been judged by considering reductions in variance in length of stay, this being the primary definition of 'resource' for grouping purposes. This reflects the fact that patient-level cost data are not available in England (see section 12.4).

12.3 The current patient classification system

12.3.1 Information used to classify patients

HRGs are standard groupings of clinically similar treatments that use comparable levels of health care resources (NHS Information Centre for Health and Social Care, 2007a). Developed under the auspices of 33 Clinical Working Groups, HRG4 was devised by clinicians, finance specialists, statisticians, health economists, users, as well as the PbR (reimbursement) team and casemix experts.

HRG4 uses a five-character code structure (AANNA). The first two characters represent the chapter/sub-chapter (for example, *BZ* = Eyes and Periorbita Procedures and Disorders). The next two numeric characters represent the HRG number within the chapter (for example, BZ*06*A = Oculoplastics category 2: 19 years and over). The final character (BZ06*A*) signifies the 'split' level applicable to the episode (for example, an age split or a severity split). In general, 'A' codes signify greater resource use than 'B' codes, which in turn signify greater resource use than 'C' codes. An HRG ending with Z indicates that no splits are applied to that HRG. Episodes that cannot be grouped because of data insufficiency or data validation issues are allocated to an 'uncoded' HRG (for example, UZ01Z).

Of the 1390 HRGs within HRG4 (2007/2008 version), 511 are not adjusted by age, gender or any other modifier. Patients are classified within HRGs based on clinical data (diagnoses (ICD-10), procedures (OPCS) and severity (presence and level of CCs)); demographic data (age, gender); and resource use (length of stay). HRGs are not defined by patient weight or by disease stage.

HRG4 uses the latest procedure codes (currently OPCS-4.5) to ensure better specificity of grouping than OPCS-4.2/HRG3.5. The OPCS-4 classification, which was fully implemented across the NHS in 1990, is based on a statistical classification of surgical operations first introduced in the United Kingdom in 1944. The OPCS system is updated annually to reflect modern clinical practice (NHS Information Centre for Health and Social Care, 2007a). HRG4 uses an improved mapping of CCs that modifies HRG assignment to reflect the additional cost of more complex cases. For many HRGs there are three splits to reflect the scale of complexity: 'Without CC', 'Intermediate CC' and 'Major CC'. Where no relevant secondary diagnoses are recorded, the activity will group to the 'Without CC' variant of the relevant HRG, designed to be the lowest resource use category.

12.3.2 Classification algorithm

Clinical Working Groups make judgements on resource homogeneity within HRGs, which are tested on patient-level data. The principal data source is the HES database. The HES comprises individual patient records and all NHS trusts in England routinely provide HES data for every inpatient and day-case patient they treat, so the full dataset comprises about 15 million records each year. Each patient record includes a number of variables containing demographic data (such as age, gender); clinical information (such as diagnosis, procedures performed); type of admission (such as elective, non-elective, day case); and length of stay, which is used as a primary measure of resource use.

A variety of statistical techniques are employed to assist in the optimal design of groupings and to measure statistical coherence. The main analytical approach to the design of HRGs employs Classification and Regression Trees (CARTs) (NHS Information Centre for Health and Social Care, 2007a). This is a non-parametric analysis technique that makes no assumptions about the underlying distribution of values of the predictor variables (length of stay). Thus, CARTs can handle numerical data that are highly skewed. CARTs will use variables contained in the HES, such as procedures, diagnoses, age and so on, to identify HRGs that best differentiate between cases with long or short lengths of stay. These CART analyses are undertaken to support the Clinical Working Groups whenever there is a major review of the HRG system.

Patients are grouped to a single HRG on the basis of several data elements. If these data are missing or invalid, the patient is allocated to an 'uncoded' HRG (UZ01Z). The stages of the algorithm are shown in Figure 12.2 and described in more detail in the remainder of the chapter.

Unbundling is the first step in the grouping process (NHS Information Centre for Health and Social Care, 2007b). Unbundled activity is identified and removed as separate 'unbundled' HRGs (see Figure 12.3). The grouper then ignores these unbundled components when deriving the core HRG for an episode or spell.

Second, a new mechanism has been defined to identify high-resource, complex treatments associated with *multiple trauma* sites. This dominates all other procedure hierarchies and so follows the unbundling step shown at the top of Figure 12.2.

The third step in the grouping process concerns *procedures*. In HRG4, procedures are ranked using a hierarchy based on cost data and clinical knowledge. When several procedures are recorded, a procedure hierarchy list is used to decide which procedure is dominant and should be used to assign the HRG. The procedure hierarchy used for HRG version 3.5 has been extensively updated for HRG4 and now contains 11 bands (from 2 (lowest resource use) to 12 (highest resource use)). In addition, Band 0 identifies procedures that are not valid for HRG assignment (for example, site-of-operation codes) and Band 1 identifies minimal resource-use codes for non-operative procedures (such as injections). If procedures are planned but not carried out, patients are allocated to a bespoke HRG (WA14).

If no procedure is recorded, HRG is assigned by the primary *diagnosis*. This includes respite or convalescent stays, and mental health diagnoses treated by providers not strictly in the mental health care sector. In the 2009 version of HRG4, there are just three mental health HRGs that are differentiated only by age group.

CC splits are a way of incorporating variations in severity and complexity within HRGs. Lists of CC splits are specific to each HRG chapter and are particularly important for the medical HRGs (as these are driven by primary

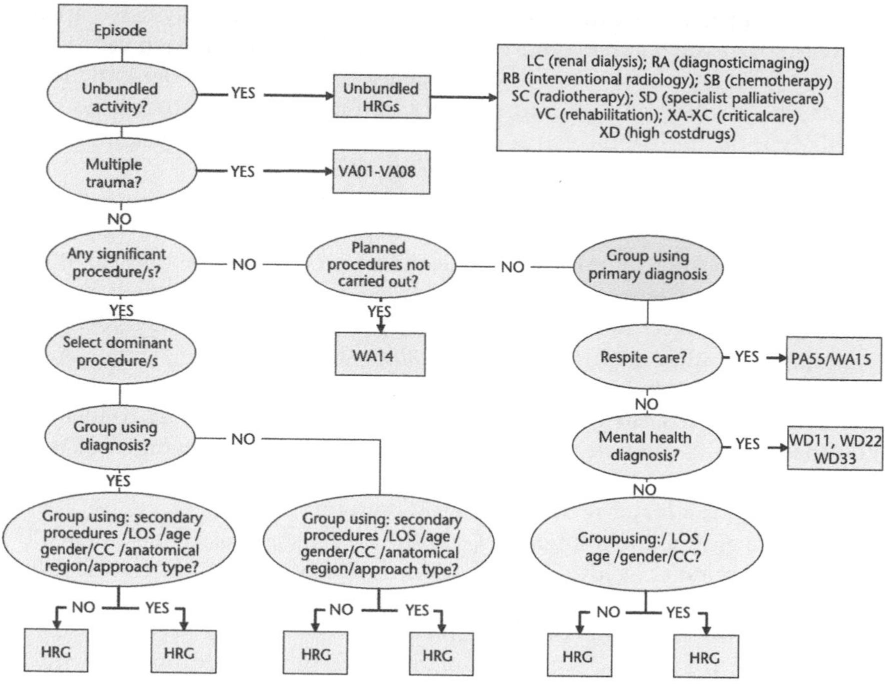

Figure 12.2 HRG4 – Classification flow chart for inpatients

Sources: Dawson & Street, 1998; NHS Information Centre for Health and Social Care, 2007a, b, 2008a.

diagnosis). However, secondary diagnoses can be considered as CCs for both surgical and medical episodes. Depending on their explanatory power in terms of explaining cost variation, some HRGs are also split by secondary procedures, age, gender, length of stay, anatomical region (for digestive system diagnoses or procedures) or approach type (for example, laparoscopic surgery).

12.3.3 Data quality and plausibility checks

HRG4 is updated annually to meet clinical and costing requirements. Continuing formal engagement with clinicians is ensured through the Expert Working Groups and the Clinical Advisory Panel.

Since 2006, all acute trusts in England have received an external clinical coding audit by the Audit Commission, an independent public body responsible for ensuring value for money in the public sector (Audit Commission, 2006). The audit process involves comparing a random sample of patients' case notes with the trust's actual coding (Audit Commission, 2010). The Audit Commission assesses coding accuracy and adherence to national standards for coding and data definitions. An online national benchmarking tool is available to PCTs and trusts so that organizations can compare their performance and identify areas for further investigation.

Unbundled activity	HRG Chapter	Examples	
Renal dialysis	LC	LC01A	Haemodialysis/filtration on patient with Hepatitis B 19 years and over
		LC03A	Peritoneal dialysis on patient with Hepatitis B 19 years and over
		LC04B	Peritoneal dialysis, 18 years and under
Diagnostic imaging	RA	RA01Z	MRI scan, one area, no contrast
		RA08Z	CT scan, one area, no contrast
		RA24Z	Ultrasound scan more than 20 minutes
Interventional radiology	RB	RB01Z	Interventional radiology – category 10
		RB02Z	Interventional radiology – category 9
		RB03Z	Interventional radiology – category 8
Chemotherapy	SB	SB01Z	Procure chemotherapy drugs for regimens in Band 1
		SB11Z	Deliver exclusively Oral Chemotherapy
		SB15Z	Deliver subsequent elements of a chemotherapy cycle
Radiotherapy	SC	SC01Z	Define volume for SXR, DXR, electron or Megavoltage radiotherapy without imaging and with simple calculation
		SC09Z	Prepare for interstitial radiotherapy
		SC29Z	Other radiotherapy treatment
Specialist palliative care	SD	SD01A	Inpatient specialist palliative care, 19 years and over
		SD03A	Hospital specialist palliative care support, 19 years and over
		SD05B	Non-medical specialist palliative care attendance, 18 years and under
Rehabilitation	VC	VC01Z	Assessment for rehabilitation (unidisciplinary)
		VC18Z	Rehabilitation for joint replacement (without treatment episode)
		VC42Z	Rehabilitation for other disorders (without treatment episode)
Critical care (neonatal)	XA	XA01Z	Neonatal critical care intensive care
		XA03Z	Neonatal critical care special care without external carer
		XA06Z	Neonatal critical care transportation
Critical care (paediatric)	XB	XB01Z	Paediatric critical care intensive care – ECMO/ECLS
		XB04Z	Paediatric Critical Care Intensive Care Basic Enhanced
		XB08Z	Paediatric critical care transportation
Critical care (adult)	XC	XC01Z	Adult critical care – 6 organs supported
		XC04Z	Adult critical care – 3 organs supported
		XC07Z	Adult critical care – 0 organs supported
High-cost drugs	XD	XD01Z	Primary pulmonary hypertension drugs band 1
		XD18Z	Bone metabolism drugs band 1
		XD38Z	Antiviral drugs band 1

Figure 12.3 Unbundled activity: Components for unbundled HRGs

Source: Information Centre for Health and Social Care, 2007b.

Notes: ECMO: extracorporeal membrane oxygenation; ECLS: extracorporeal life support.

12.4 Cost accounting within hospitals

12.4.1 Regulation

The *NHS Costing Manual* sets out the mandatory practice of costing to be applied in NHS hospitals (Department of Health, 2009b). Introduced in 1999, it brings a degree of consistency to the production and collection of cost information.

The Clinical Costing Standards Association of England (CCSAE), a working group of costing experts was established to develop clinical costing standards for the acute care sector, while also supporting the implementation of Patient-Level Information and Costing Systems (PLICS) within the NHS. The implementation of PLICS is currently not mandatory.

12.4.2 Main characteristics of the cost-accounting system(s)

All NHS hospitals are required to report their activity and unit costs annually to the Department of Health (Department of Health, 2009b). Unit costs reflect the full cost of provision and include all operating expenses, staff costs and capital costs (both interest and principal), but exclude the costs of teaching and research. Total costs are reconciled to the financial costs of the provider for the previous financial year.

As data on itemized resource use by individual patients are not collected in England, costs are estimated using a top-down approach. Figure 12.4 illustrates the initial and Figure 12.5 the latter stages of this costing exercise (Department of Health, 2009b). The starting point for the costing process is the general ledger. Here, total costs or 'high-level control totals' are established. Costs are calculated on a full absorption basis; that is, all costs are allocated to the services delivered. These costs are allocated and apportioned by maximizing direct charging and, where this is not possible, using standard methods of apportionment matched to the services that generate them.

Aggregate costing figures are then divided into one of three cost categories – direct (D), indirect (I) and overhead (O) costs. Direct costs are those which can be directly attributed to the service(s) that generated them. For instance, the type and amount of nursing staff working in a particular specialty can be estimated with reasonable precision. Costs that cannot be attributed directly must be apportioned by other means. Indirect and overhead costs are pooled in order to do this. These 'cost pools' bring together costs into identifiable groups (for example, wards, pharmacies, theatres) and allow them to be apportioned to the relevant services. Each type of cost pool can be identified as being fixed, semi-fixed or variable. The pooling of costs allows for the calculation of units of activity (for fixed and semi-fixed pools) and time (for variable pools). Within each costing pool, key cost drivers are established. These may include length of stay for time-based ward costs, or event-based costs, such as the number of prostheses used.

For all services not directly attributed to patients, the high-level control totals are analysed by setting, indicating whether the patient was treated as a day case or as an inpatient (elective or non-elective), whether (s)he underwent an outpatient procedure, or was treated in 'other' settings (Figure 12.5).[3] For inpatient and day-case activity, as well as outpatient procedures, costs are further disaggregated into HRGs. To do this, the main HRGs used by the provider are identified within each specialty. These key HRGs should cover at least 80 per cent of cost and activity within each setting. The main conditions

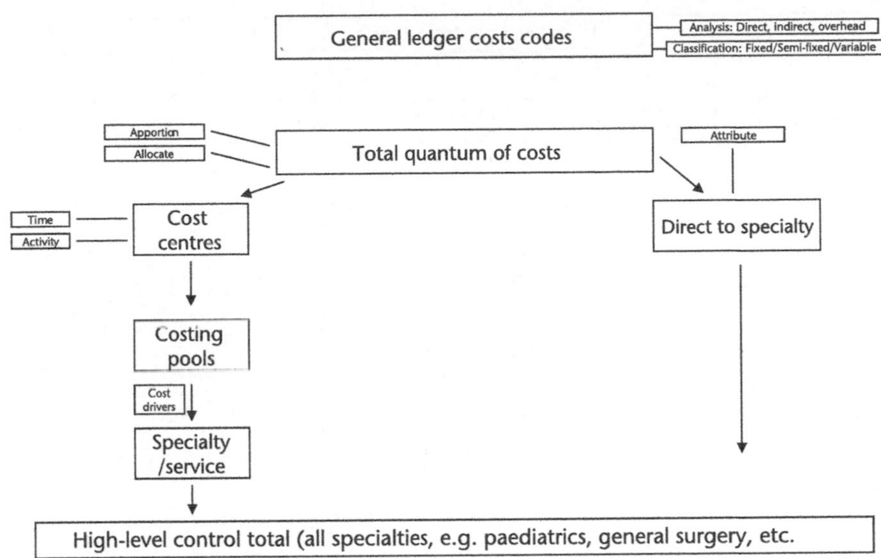

Figure 12.4 English cost-accounting system: Initial stages

Source: Based on Department of Health, 2009b.

or procedures of the provider are then identified within each HRG. A weighted average cost of each HRG is then calculated by:

- multiplying each diagnosis/procedure in a given HRG by the total number of patients for that diagnosis/procedure;
- adding up all the costs of the diagnosis/procedure;
- dividing this total cost by the total number of patients in the HRG.

For each HRG there will be a small number of cases which have an abnormally long length of stay. An upper trim-point is calculated for each HRG: the upper quartile of the length of stay distribution for that HRG plus 1.5 times the interquartile range (Schreyögg et al., 2006). Instead of excluding outlier cases, only excess bed days beyond the upper trim-point are excluded, and a cost per excess bed day is calculated. For clarity, the process of allocating HRGs to elective inpatient activity is illustrated.

The outcome of this cost-allocation process is a cost per HRG (i=1... I) according to the treatment setting (j=1...5) and type of admission. The formula for the cost per HRG in each setting (c_{ij}) is

$$c_{ij} = D_{ij} + \gamma_{ij} I + \varphi_{ij} O, \quad i = 1 \ldots I, \quad j = 1 \ldots 5 \tag{1}$$

where D_{ij} indicates the direct costs attributable to the HRG, and γ_{ij} and φ_{ij} represent, respectively, the shares of indirect and overhead costs attributed to the HRG.

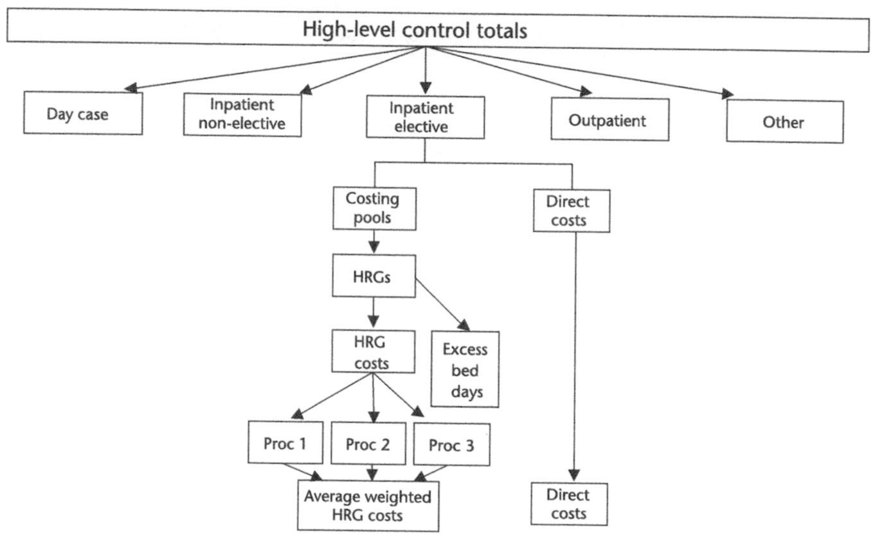

Figure 12.5 English cost-accounting system: Latter stages

Source: Based on Department of Health, 2009b.

12.5 DRGs for hospital payment

12.5.1 Range of services and costs included in DRG-based hospital payments

Phased in since 2003, almost all hospital care in England is reimbursed under the PbR system. PbR tariffs are based on average hospital costs, and include labour, equipment and capital costs. In 2009/2010, HRG4 replaced HRG3.5 as the system underpinning the PbR tariff (with the exception of payment for A&E services). Clinical activity can now be coded more specifically and the increased number of HRGs means that providers can be more fairly reimbursed for the activities they carry out. HRG4 also allows for 'unbundling'. This means that some services now can be priced separately (Figure 12.3).

In 2009/2010, the national PbR tariff was payable for inpatient care (involving admission to hospital), outpatient care and A&E services, and covers almost all hospital activity. Services not covered by PbR included primary care services, community services, mental health services and ambulance services. A full list of exclusions from the tariff is available from the Department of Health web site (Department of Health, 2009c). Although there are no published tariffs for services that are not covered under PbR, prices have been disclosed to support and guide local negotiations (Department of Health, 2009c).

12.5.2 Calculation of DRG prices

The HRG price (tariff) is determined for the year ahead by the Department of Health according to a standard methodology (Department of Health, 2009c).

Details of the tariffs for admitted patients, outpatients and A&E attendances are summarized in Table 12.3. Prices are set based on the average of the costs calculated by all hospitals for each of their HRGs, as detailed earlier in equation 1. The tariff for each HRG and admission type for a given year t, p_{ijt}, is calculated as:

$$p_{ijt} = \pi_i \bar{c}_{ijt-3} \qquad (2)$$

where $\bar{c}_{ij}$ is the average cost for each HRG by admission type across all hospitals. There is a three-year[4] delay between hospitals submitting cost data and these data being converted into prices, hence the $t - 3$ subscript attached to these average costs. To take account of this delay, an inflationary adjustment π_i is made to each HRG. This adjustment is HRG-specific, allowing for inflationary impacts such as clinical guidance and technology appraisals (issued by NICE) that may have occurred in the intervening period.

12.5.3 DRGs in actual hospital payment

Originally, a single tariff was applied to elective patients treated on a day-case and inpatient basis, to encourage providers to move patients to cheaper day-case settings (Street & Maynard, 2007b). From 2009/2010 the same tariff no longer applies to inpatient and day-case care.

A single PbR tariff applies to all providers regardless of geographical location. However, it is argued there are some costs outside the control of hospitals that mean they face higher-than-average overall costs, irrespective of how efficient they are. Thus, to reflect unavoidable cost variations in factor prices, the Department of Health (DH) makes a payment directly to providers based on a single index known as the Market Forces Factor (MFF). This single MFF index is based on three sub-indices – labour, land and buildings. Labour costs for each hospital are based on local variation in wages in the private sector for analogous service sector jobs. The land index is calculated for each hospital in the NHS using data from the Valuation Office on the NHS estate in 2004, and the building index is based on a rolling average of tender prices for all public and private contracts (Miraldo et al., 2008).

The MFF is adjusted periodically by the Department of Health in order to ensure it relates to current, unavoidable cost variations. In 2009, following a review of the staff component of the MFF by the Advisory Committee on Resource Allocation (ACRA), there were changes to how the MFF index was calculated and how it was paid (Department of Health, 2009c). PCTs now pay the MFF payment to providers at the same time as activity payments, whereas the MFF was previously paid directly by the Department of Health. To smooth the impact of this change on provider income, the new index was capped at plus or minus 2 per cent (Department of Health, 2009c).

The MFF can be represented as a hospital-specific adjustment to the tariff, so that, in effect, the price paid per HRG is unique to each hospital k, with:

$$p_{ijkt} = \delta_{kt} p_{ijt} \qquad (3)$$

where δ_{kt} is the MFF adjustment applying to hospital k at time t.

Table 12.3 HRG prices, 2009/2010

	Admitted patients	*Outpatients*	*A&E*
Currency	HRG spell	Attendance by specialty (for procedures: HRGs)	Attendance
Structure	Tariffs for: • electives • non-electives • planned same-day activity (day cases only in 2009/2010) • short-stay elective • short-stay emergencies	Tariffs for: • first attendance • follow-up attendance • multi-professional as well as single professional appointments, for treatment function codes where data are available • Procedures carried out in outpatient setting subject to non-mandatory tariff based on HRGs, with the intention that this activity is covered by the mandatory 'Planned Same Day' tariff in future years • Non-mandatory tariff for outpatient appointments not carried out face to face	Tariffs for: • High-cost attendance • Standard attendance • Combined Minor A&E/Minor Injuries Unit attendance
Specialized service adjustments	• Top-up payment for specialized services for children and orthopaedic activity • Exclusions	• Exclusions	• Not applicable
Outliers	• Long-stay outlier payment triggered at predetermined length of stay (dependent on HRG). Daily rate specific to HRG	• No outlier policy	• No outlier policy
Flexibilities	• Unbundling of care pathway subject to local agreement • Local 'pass through' payments for new technology • Emergency readmissions: local arrangements for determining appropriate reimbursement and criteria	• Unbundling of care pathway subject to local agreement • Local 'pass through' payments for new technology	• Local flexibilities could be applied to support service redesign

Source: Department of Health, 2009c.

Note: Teaching and research are funded entirely separately, and their costs are not included in PbR.

12.5.4 Quality-related adjustments

Following recommendations in *High-quality care for all* (Darzi & Department of Health, 2008), from 2009/2010 all acute trusts publish 'quality accounts' alongside their financial accounts. The Commissioning for Quality and Innovation (CQUIN) payment framework came into effect in April 2009. It allows PCTs to link a specific, modest proportion of providers' income (agreed nationally) to the achievement of realistic locally agreed goals. In 2009/2010, the CQUIN payment framework covered 0.5 per cent of a provider's annual contract income (Department of Health, 2008), increasing to 1.5 per cent in 2010/2011. CQUIN payments are made at monthly intervals, alongside payment of regular income, and adjusted to reflect achievement against contractual goals. The CQUIN framework applies to all patient-related activity, including activity reimbursed as part of the PbR system.

12.5.5 Main incentives for hospitals

The principal aims of PbR are to increase 'throughput' (activity), reduce waiting times, support patient choice and improve efficiency, as well as increasing patient satisfaction while at the same time keeping costs under control (Miraldo et al., 2006). Because hospitals are given a fixed tariff per HRG for the work they carry out, PbR encourages them to cut costs and reduce lengths of stay, thus freeing up capacity to treat more patients. Increasing activity means that patients are treated more quickly, improving access to health care for patients on waiting lists (Mannion et al., 2008). PbR also facilitates choice by encouraging new providers into the market, increasing competition in the field, and improving the mix of care provided by hospitals (Miraldo et al., 2006).

International empirical evidence suggests that the introduction of a prospective payment system can offer providers perverse incentives to improve their financial position. For example, hospitals can engage in 'DRG drift', up-coding patients to more expensive DRGs and resulting in over-reimbursement.

PbR may encourage providers to 'cream-skim' (select less complicated cases) in order to reduce costs. However, the Audit Commission – which now regularly monitors and audits coding performance in English hospitals – found little evidence of systemic gaming or deliberate up-coding: observed coding errors were associated with both positive and negative financial consequences (Audit Commission, 2008).

12.6 New/innovative technologies

12.6.1 Steps required prior to introduction in hospitals

While adoption decisions for most new technologies are made by individual hospitals, NICE also provides guidance to the NHS on health care technologies, public health and clinical practice. The overall aim is to promote good health and prevent and treat ill health (NICE, 2007).

NICE assesses selected new and existing medicines. Almost all newly licensed cancer drugs are appraised by NICE before they are made available routinely to patients by the NHS. The appraisal process can introduce significant delays in patient access, partly due to the assessment process, but also because of stakeholder appeals against NICE's preliminary decisions.

Since January 2002, the NHS has been legally obliged to provide funding and resources in England and Wales for medicines and treatments recommended by NICE's technology appraisal process. This means that when NICE recommends a medicine, the NHS must ensure it is publicly available within three months of the guidance being issued. If a new medicine is not recommended by NICE (perhaps because other options are more cost-effective), it should not be provided routinely by the NHS. However, the Richards report recommended that patients be allowed to pay privately for medicines not funded by the NHS, without losing their entitlement to NHS care that they would otherwise receive (Richards, 2008).

12.6.2 Payment mechanisms

'Pass through' payments are used to fund new and innovative technologies. These apply to new devices, drugs, treatments and technologies or a new application of an existing technology. They give the purchaser the flexibility to make additional payments for higher quality care than the standard care covered by the national tariff. Any such arrangement between a provider and purchaser should be fixed for a maximum of three years, and the price should be agreed in advance and be directly related to the additional cost of the new technology.

Some activity, including some high-cost drugs, devices and procedures are excluded from the PbR tariff, such as magnetic resonance imaging (MRI) scans, cochlear implants, orthopaedic prostheses and chemotherapy. Instead, purchasers and providers agree local prices and local arrangements for monitoring activity.

12.6.3 (Dis-)incentives for hospitals to use new technologies

The financial incentive to the provider to innovate depends on the impact on provider costs, and on whether the innovation improves patient outcomes but increases provider costs (Boyle et al., 2007).

If the innovation is cost-saving in nature, there is a clear incentive to adopt it. If the innovation is more expensive and more effective, the provider may be reluctant to adopt the new technology. To address this disincentive, the price under prospective funding must be adjusted to compensate providers for the additional cost. Technology lags also result in higher costs for providers. When new technologies enter the market, the HRG system will not reflect the costs of adopting them, which is why pass-through payments are used. However, creating economic incentives for health care providers to adopt innovative technologies can lead to a sharp rise in expenditure, diverting resources from other parts of the health system where they might be used to deliver greater health benefits (Schreyögg et al., 2009).

12.7 Evaluation of the DRG system in England

12.7.1 Official evaluation

Since its inception in 2004, various aspects of PbR have been studied, such as the benefits and costs of the policy (Marini & Street, 2006; Miraldo et al., 2006) and its incentives and disincentives (Mannion et al., 2008). The evidence suggests that PbR has generally had a positive impact on hospital activity and efficiency, with no deterioration in the quality of care provided (Table 12.4).

A national evaluation of PbR used mixed methods to assess the effects on hospital behaviour (Farrar et al., 2007). This included the exploration of an appropriate theoretical framework, a series of semi-structured interviews, and an econometric analysis of routine data. The theoretical framework hypothesized that a fixed national tariff would lower unit costs. The interviews revealed positive attitudes toward PbR, despite some scepticism as to whether it would achieve its objectives. The econometric analysis found that unit costs fell with the introduction of PbR, with no adverse effect on the quality of care, suggesting that lower unit costs were the result of efficiency savings. Meanwhile, volume of activity increased, while there was little evidence of a change in coding patterns.

The Audit Commission's evaluation of PbR (Audit Commission, 2008) found broadly similar findings to those of the national evaluation. PbR was associated with increased activity and efficiency in elective care, although PbR itself was not considered to be the principal driver behind these changes. Findings on quality of care were similar to those reported in the national study. The Audit Commission made a number of recommendations on the future development of PbR, including (1) strengthening of the information infrastructure so that providers are more accurately reimbursed for activity carried out; (2) greater flexibility in the national tariff, with a greater scope for unbundling tariff prices into separate components; (3) greater consideration given to the possibility of separate funding streams for capital and quality; and (4) the introduction of some normative tariffs for selected HRGs, whereby the tariff would be based not on average prices but on the costs of higher performing providers (a view also shared by others) (Street & Maynard, 2007a).

12.7.2 Authors' assessment

Despite implementation difficulties (Department of Health & Lawlor, 2006), PbR has been rolled out as the funding mechanism that covers almost all NHS inpatient care in England. Concerns regarding unintended consequences and up-coding have proved largely unfounded and large increases in tariff-funded hospital activity have not materialized. This implies that PbR has not led to widespread financial instability among purchasers (PCTs). This may be because

Table 12.4 Impacts of PbR: Overview of evidence

	Impact of PbR	*Study*
Activity	Proportion of elective care provided as day cases has increased	2007[a]
	'PbR has had a positive effect on activity in elective care. Day cases have increased and the LOS for elective inpatients has fallen.'	2008[b]
	'Other policies have also encouraged increases in activity. We consider that PbR has at most contributed to these positive trends rather than driven them.'	
Unit costs	Unit costs have fallen more quickly where PbR was implemented	2007[a]
Volume of spells	Both Foundation Trusts and non-Foundation Trusts have increased volumes, although these may be linked to other initiatives, such as waiting-time targets, which have also affected the volume of care provided	2007[a]
Efficiency	Improved efficiency through reduction in unit costs with no reduction in quality	2007[a]
Quality	Little change in quality	2007[a]
	The negative impact on quality which some feared has not materialized	2008[b]
DRG coding	Very limited evidence of a change in the pattern of coding	2007[a]
Financial management and information systems	Have encouraged commissioners and providers to strengthen their systems as well as their overall planning	2008[b]
Administrative costs	Estimated to have increased in both hospital trusts and PCTs	2006[c]

Sources: [a]Farrar et al., 2007; [b]Audit Commission, 2008; [c]Marini & Street, 2006.

PCTs have improved their monitoring of provider activity and performance; some have tried to manage demand by investing in initiatives to reduce avoidable hospital admissions (Audit Commission, 2008). However, they have been less successful at restraining the strong incentives that motivate hospitals to undertake more elective activity (Mannion et al., 2008).

HRG4 – the new classification system underpinning the 2009/2010 tariff – has potential for improving the fairness of the payment system. The role of 'unbundling' has been enhanced, and the increased number of categories and greater separation of patients by different complexity levels should, in principle, help to ensure that payments better reflect casemix differences. However, there is a risk that unbundling could lead to increased pressure on budgets, as activities that were previously paid for by a single tariff are now funded separately.

12.8 Outlook

12.8.1 Trends in hospital service or general care delivery

Historically, there has been a trend toward reduced use of inpatient care and toward treating more patients on a day-case basis or in outpatient departments. The development of HRG4 allows greater scope for 'unbundling' elements of care from the base-HRG so that services can be provided in non-inpatient settings where appropriate.

12.8.2 Trends in DRG application/coverage

PbR drives the refinement of HRGs and the development of classification systems in non-hospital settings. The Department of Health has progressively been extending the scope of PbR to cover adult mental health, long-term conditions, preventative services, sexual health, community services, ambulance services and out-of-hours primary care (Department of Health, 2007). In some of these areas, pilot work is under way locally to determine the appropriate units of activity ('categories'). The NHS reference costs already collect cost data for most of these areas, but local costing exercises are also being carried out to test whether the use of tariffs for these 'de novo' categories is feasible, particularly for mental health services (Mason & Goddard, 2009).

Perhaps the most important initiative is the development of 'best practice' tariffs for high-volume areas, with significant unexplained variation in quality of clinical practice and clear evidence of what constitutes best practice (Department of Health, 2009d). In 2010, prices for cholecystectomy, fragility hip fracture, cataracts and stroke were based on the most efficient cost rather than average cost. From 2011/2012, best practice tariffs are to be extended to adult renal dialysis, interventional radiology, transient ischaemic attack, and paediatric diabetes (Department of Health, 2011). This means that DRGs have progressed gradually from a means of classifying activity, then to paying for activity, and now to incentivizing quality and better outcomes for patients. This welcome direction of travel represents the next challenge for policy development and evaluation over the coming decade.

12.9 Notes

1 The authors thank Martine Bellanger (EHESP) and Alexander Geissler (TUB) for helpful comments on an earlier draft. We are responsible for all remaining errors and omissions.
2 More information is available at the NHS Choices web site (http://www.nhs.uk/NHSEngland/thenhs/about/Pages/nhsstructure.aspx, accessed 29 June 2011).
3 'Other' here refers to all other hospital costs that are not part of day-case, inpatient or outpatient activity. It includes community services, critical care services, A&E medicine, radiotherapy and chemotherapy, renal dialysis, and kidney and bone marrow transplantation, for example.

12.10 References

Anthony, P. (1993). Healthcare resource groups in the NHS: a measure of success. *Public Finance and Accountancy,* 23:8–10.

Audit Commission (2006). *Payment by Results Assurance Framework: Pilot Results and Recommendations.* London: Audit Commission.

Audit Commission (2008). *The Right Result? Payment by Results 2003–2007.* London: Audit Commission (http://www.audit-commission.gov.uk/SiteCollectionDocuments/AuditCommissionReports/NationalStudies/The_right_result_PbR_2008.pdf, accessed 29 June 2011).

Audit Commission (2010). *Improving Data Quality in the NHS: Annual Report on the PbR Assurance Programme 2010.* London: Audit Commission.

Benton, P.L., et al. (1998). The development of healthcare resource groups. Version 3. *Journal of Public Health Medicine,* 20:351–8.

Boyle, S., Hutton, J., Street, A., Sussex, J. (2007). *Introducing Activity-Based Funding to Financial Flows between Providers and Commissioners in Northern Ireland. Draft Report for McClure Watters.* York: York Health Economics Consortium.

Coles, J.M. (1993). England: ten years of diffusion and development, in J.R. Kimberley, G. de Pourourville, eds. *The Migration of Managerial Innovation.* San Francisco: Jossey-Bass Publishers.

Darzi, A., Department of Health (2008). *High-Quality Care for All: NHS Next Stage Review Final Report.* London: Department of Health.

Dawson, D., Street, A. (1998). *Reference Costs and the Pursuit of Efficiency in the 'New' NHS.* York: University of York Centre for Health Economics.

Dawson, D., Street, A. (2000). Reference costs and the pursuit of efficiency in the 'new' NHS, in P.C. Smith, ed. *Reforming Markets in Health Care: An Economic Perspective.* Buckingham: Open University Press.

Department of Health (2002). *Reforming NHS Financial Flows: Introducing Payment by Results.* London: Department of Health.

Department of Health (2007). *Options for the Future of Payment by Results: 2008/2009 to 2010/2011.* Leeds: Department of Health.

Department of Health (2008). *Using the Commissioning for Quality and Innovation (CQUIN) Payment Framework.* London: Department of Health.

Department of Health (2009a). *Department of Health Activity Statistics* [web site]. London: Department of Health (http://www.dh.gov.uk/en/Publicationsandstatistics/Statistics/Performancedataandstatistics/Beds/DH_083781, accessed 29 June 2011).

Department of Health (2009b). *NHS Costing Manual 2008/2009.* London: Department of Health (http://www.dh.gov.uk/prod_consum_dh/groups/dh_digitalassets/documents/digitalasset/dh_095858.pdf, accessed 12 July 2011).

Department of Health (2009c). *Payment by Results Guidance for 2009–2010.* Leeds: Department of Health.

Department of Health (2009d). *Payment by Results in 2010–2011: Letter from David Flory, Director General, NHS Finance, Performance and Operations.* London: Department of Health.

Department of Health (2011). *Payment by Results Guidance for 2011–2012.* Leeds: Department of Health.

Department of Health, Lawlor, J. (2006). *Report on the Tariff-Setting Process for 2006/2007.* London: Department of Health.

Farrar, S., Sussex, J., Yi, D. et al. (2007) *National Evaluation of Payment by Results.* Aberdeen: University of Aberdeen Health Economics Research Unit.

Hawe, E. (2009). *OHE Compendium of Health Statistics: 2009.* Abingdon: Radcliffe Publishing.

Information Standards Board for Health and Social Care (2009). *Healthcare Resource Groups 4 (HRG4): Dataset Change Notice 17/2008*. Leeds: Information Standards Board for Health and Social Care.

Mannion, R., Marini, G., Street, A. (2008). Implementing payment by results in the English NHS: changing incentives and the role of information. *Journal of Health Organization & Management*, 22:79–88.

Marini, G., Street, A. (2006). *The Administrative Costs of Payment by Results*. York: University of York Centre for Health Economics.

Mason, A., Goddard, M. (2009). *Payment by Results in Mental Health: A Review of the International Literature and an Economic Assessment of the Approach in the English NHS*. York: University of York Centre for Health Economics.

Mason, A., Street, A., Miraldo, M., Siciliani, L. (2009). Should prospective payments be differentiated for public and private health care providers? *Health Economics, Policy and Law*, 4:383–403.

Miraldo, M., Goddard, M., Smith, P.C. (2006). *The Incentive Effects of Payment by Results*. London: Dr Foster Intelligence.

Miraldo, M., Siciliani, L., Street, A. (2008). *Price Adjustment in the Hospital Sector*. York: University of York:

NHS Executive (1997). *The New NHS: Modern, Dependable*. Leeds: NHS Executive.

NHS Information Centre for Health and Social Care (2006a). *Hospital Episode Statistics 1998/9. Ungrossed Data*. Leeds: NHS Information Centre for Health and Social Care.

NHS Information Centre for Health and Social Care (2006b). *Hospital Episode Statistics 2003/4. Ungrossed Data*. Leeds: NHS Information Centre for Health and Social Care.

NHS Information Centre for Health and Social Care (2007a). *The Casemix Service. HRG4 Design Concepts*. Leeds: NHS Information Centre for Health and Social Care.

NHS Information Centre for Health and Social Care (2007b). *The Casemix Service. HRG4 Guide to Unbundling*. Leeds: NHS Information Centre for Health and Social Care (http://www.ic.nhs.uk/webfiles/Services/casemix/Prep%20HRG4/Guide%20to%20 Unbundling_090213v4.0.pdf, accessed 12 July 2011).

NHS Information Centre for Health and Social Care (2008a). *HRG Version 3.5 & HRG4 Comparative Chapter Analysis: Version No 1.0*. Leeds: NHS Information Centre for Health and Social Care (http://www.ic.nhs.uk/webfiles/Services/casemix/Prep%20 HRG4/HRG%20v3.5%20and%20HRG4%20Comparative%20Chapter%20Analysis %202008.pdf, accessed 11 July 2011).

NHS Information Centre for Health and Social Care (2008b). *The Casemix Service. HRG4 Reference Cost Grouper – Guide to File Preparation*. Leeds: NHS Information Centre for Health and Social Care.

NHS Information Centre for Health and Social Care (2009). *Explanatory Notes: Outpatient Data 2008–2009*. Leeds: NHS Information Centre for Health and Social Care.

NICE (2007). *About NICE Guidance: What Does It Mean For Me? Information for Patients, Carers and the Public – An Interim Guide*. London: National Institute for Health and Clinical Excellence.

Richards, M. (2008). *Improving Access to Medicines for NHS Patients. A Report for the Secretary of State for Health by Professor Mike Richards CBE*. London: Department of Health.

Sanderson, H.F. (1995). The use of healthcare resource groups in managing clinical resources. *British Journal of Hospital Medicine*, 54:531–4.

Sanderson, H.F., Anthony, P., Mountney, L.M. (1995). Healthcare resource groups – version 2. *Journal of Public Health Medicine*, 17:349–54.

Schreyögg, J., Baumler, M., Busse, R. (2009). Balancing adoption and affordability of medical devices in Europe. *Health Policy*, 92:218–24.

Schreyögg, J., Stargardt, T., Tiemann, O., Busse, R. (2006). Methods to determine reimbursement rates for diagnosis related groups (DRG): a comparison of nine European countries. *Health Care Management Science*, 9:215–23.

Street, A., Dawson, D. (2002). Costing hospital activity: the experience with healthcare resource groups in England. *European Journal of Health Economics*, 3:3–9.

Street, A., Maynard, A. (2007a). Activity-based financing in England: the need for continual refinement of payment by results. *Health Economics, Policy and Law*, 2:419–27.

Street, A., Maynard, A. (2007b). Payment by results: qualified ambition? *Health Economics, Policy and Law*, 2:445–8.

chapter thirteen

France: Implementing homogeneous patient groups in a mixed market

Zeynep Or and Martine Bellanger

13.1 Hospital services and the role of DRGs

13.1.1 The French health care system

The French health care system is based on social insurance, with universal coverage. Health care provision relies heavily on private providers. Ambulatory care is mainly provided on a private, and usually solo practice basis. Inpatient care is delivered both by public hospitals and profit-making and non-profit-making private hospitals. Patients can choose freely between public and private providers without necessarily needing a referral.

Compared with most other European countries, the French system is characterized by high levels of spending. France devotes about 11 per cent of its gross domestic product (GDP) to the health sector, which contrasts with an average of 9 per cent in Organisation for Economic Co-operation and Development (OECD) countries (OECD, 2010). In terms of hospital financing, about 91 per cent of total expenditure is financed by the public health insurance funds, while another 5 per cent is paid for by private complementary insurance. Direct contributions from the state amounted to only about 1.3 per cent in 2008 (Fenina et al., 2008).

At the macro level, financial stewardship of the health system is shared between the Government and the health insurance funds. The Government sets annual financial targets to limit the expenditure of the health insurance funds. There are separate targets for the hospital sector, the ambulatory sector and social/long-term care. The hospital sector budget is further divided into two components: one for acute care, which is financed through diagnosis-related group (DRG)-based hospital payment (including hospital care at home), and one for other hospital services (mainly psychiatric and rehabilitative care), with separate objectives for the public and private sectors. The public health insurance funds define the baskets of benefits, regulate the prices of procedures, drugs and devices, and define the levels of co-payment (Mousques & Polton, 2005). The health insurance funds are also in charge of setting tariffs for health professionals in private practice. Doctors working in private hospitals contract with health insurance funds and they are paid according to a negotiated fee-for-service schedule,[1] while those in public hospitals are salaried. The salaries and working conditions of the hospital staff – as well as the prices set for DRGs – are regulated by the Government.

Budget targets for financing the hospital sector are defined by the state for each region. At the regional level, Regional Hospital Agencies (*Agences Régional d'Hospitalisation*, ARH) are responsible for organizing and assuring the quality of hospital care. In 2010 these agencies were replaced by the newly created Regional Health Agencies (*Agences Régionales de Santé*, ARS), which will be responsible not only for acute care but also for prevention, rehabilitation, long-term and social care. Currently, the Government is reforming the governance structure of the health care system in France, shifting the power to the ARS, which will control the resources and define the strategy for hospitals within a given region (Or, 2008). Each hospital (including private ones) will have to sign a contract to define its activity and financing needs. Despite this trend in the shift of power towards local and regional authorities, regions have little responsibility for hospital funding.

13.1.2 Hospital services in France

The hospital sector plays an important role in health care provision in France. One person in six is hospitalized each year, either as an inpatient or on a day-case basis. Hospitals are also significant providers of outpatient care: they account for about 33 million specialist consultations and an estimated 15.5 million emergency visits per year. Figure 13.1 compares the volumes of different types of services provided by hospitals, including psychiatry and rehabilitation care.

With about 4 beds per 1000 inhabitants, hospital bed capacity in France is at a level comparable to the OECD average. Acute care (including day cases and home hospitalizations) accounts for about 16 million cases and is administered by a mixture of public and private facilities (Table 13.1).

Public hospitals represent 60 per cent of all hospitals and 65 per cent of all acute inpatient beds (about 221 000 beds in 2007). These hospitals are obligated by law to ensure continuity of care, which means providing 24-hour emergency care, accepting any patient who seeks treatment and participating in activities corresponding to national/regional public health priorities.

The private profit-making sector represents 25 per cent of all inpatient beds in France, including 46 per cent of surgical beds and over 70 per cent of ambulatory beds (patient places). The market share of private hospitals depends heavily on the type of hospital activity. About 56 per cent of all surgery and a quarter of obstetric care services are provided by private profit-making hospitals. Their

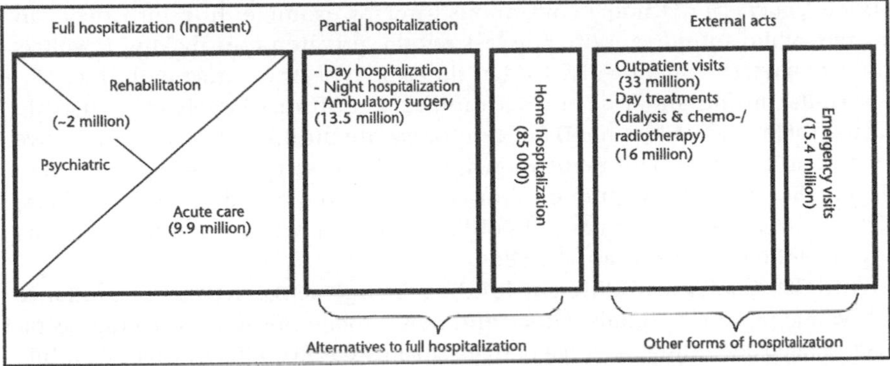

Figure 13.1 Overview of hospital activity in France, 2006

Source: HCAAM, 2009.

market share goes up to more than 70 per cent in some areas of elective surgery, such as eye surgery (cataract in particular), ear surgery and for endoscopies. However, certain complex procedures are carried out almost exclusively by public hospitals, for example in the case of burn treatments (92 per cent) or treatment of patients needing surgery for serious multiple trauma (97 per cent).

Finally, private non-profit-making hospitals specialize more in medium- to long-term care; they represent about 8 per cent of acute care activity. Three quarters of these hospitals have a special agreement with the state and they have the same engagement terms as public hospitals for providing 'public

Table 13.1 Distribution of acute care beds and activity between public and private hospitals, 2007

	Total	*Public*	*Private non-profit-making*	*Private profit-making*
Number of beds	221 990	146 461	19 251	56 278
%	100.0	66.0	8.7	25.4
Surgical beds	88 280	41 307	8 151	38 822
%	100.0	46.6	7.5	45.9
Total hospital stays (episodes, millions)	15.9	8.9	1.3	5.7
%	100.0	56.1	7.8	36.0
of which:				
Surgery	5.6	2.0	0.45	3.1
%	100.0	36.4	7.4	56.2
Medicine	9.1	6.1	0.7	2.3
%	100.0	67.0	7.8	25.2
Obstetrics	1.3	0.9	0.086	0.33
%	100.0	67.6	6.6	25.8
ALOS (days)	4.0	4.9	4.2	2.5

Source: Authors' own compilation based on 2007 data from the French hospital activity database (PMSI).

services', such as (24-hour) continuous care, for example. In return they can receive public subsidies. With the last reform, private profit-making hospitals will also have the opportunity to sign the same type of contract with the ARS.

Hospital profiles in terms of size (number of beds) vary largely by ownership status (Table 13.2). Close to 60 per cent of private profit-making hospitals have fewer than 100 beds. This figure increases to 90 per cent for those specialized in surgery. By contrast, the public sector is characterized by a diversity of profiles, with about 30 per cent of general public hospitals having over 300 beds, while 20 per cent have fewer than 100 beds.

Until 2004/2005, two different funding arrangements were used to finance public and private hospitals. Public and most private non-profit-making hospitals operated according to global budgets, mainly based on historical costs, while private profit-making hospitals were financed through a mixture of per diem and fee-for-service payments. Since 2004, DRG-based hospital payment has been gradually introduced into French hospitals. In public hospitals, the share of all acute care activities financed by the system has progressively increased: from 10 per cent in 2004 to 25 per cent in 2005, reaching 100 per cent in 2008. Private profit-making hospitals have been financed entirely by DRG-based hospital payment since February 2005. However, during a transition period that extends

Table 13.2 Distribution of hospitals by size and ownership status

		No. of hospitals	*< 30 beds (%)*	*30–99 beds (%)*	*100–199 beds (%)*	*200–349 beds (%)*	*350 + beds (%)*
Private profit-making	Establishments for surgical care	171	18	70	12	0	0
	Establishments for medical care	35	14	60	26	0	0
	Establishments for multidisciplinary care	374	3	41	43	13	0
	Total private, profit-making	**580**	**8**	**51**	**32**	**8**	**0**
Private non-profit-making	Establishments for surgical care	12	17	83	0	0	0
	Establishments for medical care	45	24	53	18	2	2
	Establishments for multidisciplinary care	119	6	35	39	16	4
	Total private, non-profit-making	176	11	43	31	11	3
Public	University hospitals	170	0	5	10	18	66
	Local hospitals	355	25	58	15	2	0
	General hospitals	643	1	19	26	23	31
	Total public	1168	8	29	21	16	27
	TOTAL	1924	8	37	25	13	17

Source: Or et al., 2009.

until 2012, national DRG prices are still adjusted to reflect hospitals' historical cost patterns, in order to shelter them from excessive budget cuts.

13.1.3 Purpose of the DRG system

Initially introduced for reporting on hospital activity in France, the DRG classification system has since been used to adjust budget allocations and is now used for hospital payment. The first French patient classification system, *Groupes Homogènes des Malades* (GHM, translated into English as 'homogeneous groups of patients') was introduced in 1986 for a sample of voluntary public hospitals in order to better describe hospital activity. Following the hospital reform measures passed in 1991, collecting/reporting data on hospital activity using GHMs became mandatory for all public hospitals. Increasingly, these data were used to compare hospital productivity and to make adjustments to global budgets. However, during the 1990s, several Ministers of Health still declared that DRG data will never be used for hospital payment.

Providing DRG data only became compulsory for private profit-making hospitals in 1998. It took another six years to use these data as a basis for paying hospitals, which is currently the main purpose of the DRG system. DRG-based hospital payment was introduced in 2004/2005 for acute care services (including home hospitalization), with the following objectives: to improve efficiency; to create a 'level playing field' for payments to public and private hospitals; to improve the transparency of hospital activity and management; and to improve quality of care.

13.2 Developing and updating the DRG system

13.2.1 The current DRG system at a glance

There is one national DRG system in France – GHMs – used as the basis of hospital payment in France since 2004/2005. The system applies to all hospitals (public and private) and all patients (inpatients and day cases), except those treated under psychiatry, rehabilitation and long-term care. Payments received through this system account for 56 per cent of all hospital expenditures (ATIH, 2009).

The current GHM system (version 11) was introduced in January 2009. It defines 2297 GHMs within 26 Major Diagnostic Categories (*catégories majeures de diagnostic*, CMD (MDC in English)), one Pre-MDC group (*catégorie majeure* 27) for organ transplantations and one undifferentiated group for 'sessions' (*séance*), mainly for chemotherapy, radiotherapy or dialysis (CMD 28). Furthermore, it differentiates between 'surgical', 'other procedure', 'medical', and 'undifferentiated' categories. There are 606 base-GHMs, most of which are split into four severity levels.

The institution responsible for developing the GHM patient classification system and calculating prices is the Technical Agency for Hospital Information (ATIH). The ATIH was created in 2002 and is an independent public administrative institution, co-funded by the Government and the national health insurance funds. It includes an advisory committee, involving representatives of public and private health care facilities, which make suggestions based on their experiences of or within the system.

13.2.2 Development of the French DRG system

The initial idea of a French patient classification system dates back to the early 1980s, when the Government decided to introduce global budgets at the hospital level to replace the previously existing poorly regulated per diem system. It was planned to adjust the budgets allocated to hospitals by measuring their clinical activity through the GHMs (Michelot & Rodrigues, 2008).

The initial French GHM classification (tested between 1986 and 1990) was inspired directly from the third DRG version of the United States Health Care Financing Administration (HCFA-DRG) but the GHM system was later modified to include parts of the All-Patient DRG system. The most important modification was the introduction of a specific major category (CM 24) for day cases. In 1996 a National Cost Study (ENC) was set up with data from about 35 voluntary public hospitals in order to calculate French GHM cost weights.

The first GHM version was introduced in public hospitals between 1990 and 1993. Eleven versions have been implemented since then (Table 13.3). In earlier versions of the GHM system, a closed list of secondary diagnoses (inspired from the original Yale list) was used to identify 'significant complications' (CMAs), independent of the principal diagnosis of the patient. However, later versions of the GHM used several lists of 'exceptions' in order to deal with specific cases. Version 9 (2004–2005) introduced a separate list of diagnoses for episodes which are acutely severe/complicated (the aforementioned CMAs).

Version 10 (2006–2008) aimed to improve the classification system, taking into account problems encountered in financing hospitals. In response to requests from the hospital federations and from the Ministry of Health, a number of extra (mostly ambulatory) surgical groups and specific DRGs for non-surgical ambulatory procedures were created.

The current version (11) has seen a major change: the number of GHMs increased almost threefold through the introduction of four levels of case severity applied to most base-GHMs (see Table 13.3). Information on length of stay, secondary diagnoses and old age is now used in a more systematic way in order to improve cost homogeneity of GHMs, especially of medical GHMs. Moreover, day cases can now be identified as a separate group for relevant GHMs and, consequently, the old French specialty 'CM 24' (which was a mixture of day cases and very short stays) was abandoned.

13.2.3 Data used to develop the DRG system

Two different databases have been used to develop the current DRG system. The patient classification system is based on the French hospital activity database (PMSI), which contains information about patient characteristics, primary

Table 13.3 GHM versions used from 1986 to 2009

DRG system	*HCFA-DRG*	*GHM V.1*	*GHM V.2*	*GHM V.3*	*GHM V.4*	*GHM V.5*	*GHM V.6*	*GHM V.7*	*GHM V.9*	*GHM V. 10*	*GHM V.11*
Date	1986–1990	1991–1993	1994	1995	1996–1997	1998–1999	2000–2001	2002–2003	2004–2005	2006–2008	2009 to present
Purpose	Experimentation	Description of hospital activity			Hospital budget allocation				Hospital payment		
Data used for development	Data from voluntary public hospitals	Utilization data from some public hospitals				National utilization data				National utilization data	National utilization data
Number of DRGs	450	480	480	572	582	582	598	598	773 (573*)	784(575*)	2297(606*)
Applied to	Voluntary sample of hospitals, only acute care services	Public hospitals: inpatients and day cases, excluding psychiatry, rehabilitation and long-term care					Public and private hospitals: inpatients and day cases, excluding psychiatry, rehabilitation and long-term care				

*Base GHM in parentheses. For instance, 773 (573) means 573 categories for describing base GHM (combinations of diagnoses/procedures) and 200 to distinguish case severity.

and secondary diagnoses, procedures, and length of stay of treated patients, as well as the GHM to which each patient is assigned. This is a national database covering all public (since 1996) and private (since 1998) hospitals.

The information for calculating DRG cost weights comes from the French hospital cost database (ENCC), which provides detailed cost information for each hospital stay from 70–100 voluntary hospitals. Until 2006 the ENCC covered only public and private non-profit-making hospitals (about 40 in total) representing about 3 per cent of these hospitals. Since 2006, cost information is collected from a set of private profit-making hospitals in order to calculate costs in a comparable way across all hospitals for the ENC. The number of participating hospitals increased slightly between 2006 and 2007 (Table 13.4). At present, the ENCC covers 99 hospitals, representing 13 per cent of total stays.

13.2.4 Regularity and method of system updates

The GHM classification algorithm has been revised continuously since its introduction. Since 2005, the ATIH has introduced a process of regular revisions of the patient classification system in order to take account of changes in medical practice and technology and to adjust for changes in the WHO International Classification of Diseases, 10th revision (ICD-10). Alterations to the system are made on the basis of suggestions from an expert group set up by the ATIH and composed mainly of physicians and statisticians (Patris et al., 2001).

Table 13.4 Number of hospitals and stays included in the National Cost Study[a]

Hospital type	*2006*			*2007*		
	Number of hospitals in data sample[b]	*Number of episodes included*[c]	*Surveyed episodes as percent of all stays (%)*	*Number of hospitals in data sample*[b]	*Number of episodes included*[c]	*Surveyed episodes as percent of all stays (%)*
University hospital	10	512 707	11	13	823 440	17
General hospitals	16	508 520	7	22	718 893	10
Cancer centres	5	268 358	25	7	387 184	36
Private non-profit-making hospitals	11	168 616	15	13	224 590	20
Total public hospitals	42	1 458 201	10	55	2 154 107	15
Private profit-making hospitals	32	628 894	7	44	781 769	9
Total	74	2 087 095	9	99	2 935 876	13

Source: ATIH, 2007b.

Notes: [a] Data samples from 2006 and 2007, which are included in the ENCC 2008 and ENCC 2009. [b] Hospitals for which the data provided fitted the quality standard to calculate costs; [c] Number of episodes contributing to reference cost scale (after trimming procedure).

Information from the PMSI about length of stay, as well as information about costs of treating patients within each GHM from the ENCC are used to assess cost homogeneity of the diagnostic groups and the classification system as a whole. The impact of proposed changes to the classification algorithm is tested using the same data.

GHM cost weights are updated annually by the ATIH on the basis of information from the ENCC. However, there is always a time-lag of two years between the year of the data and the year of the application of prices in hospitals. For example, data relating to hospital costs from the year 2008 were analysed during the year 2009 in order to define the GHM prices to be used for hospital payment in 2010.

13.3 The current patient classification system

13.3.1 Information used to classify patients

Classification of patients into GHMs is based on administrative and clinical information, both of which are available from the standard patient discharge summary (RSS) (see Figure 13.2). Clinical data are reported by physicians and are transmitted to the medical information units (DIMs) of hospitals, where data are processed and checked before a specialized software programme uses the information to select the appropriate GHM.

If a patient was transferred between medical wards during the hospital stay, several departmental discharge summaries (RUMs) are combined into one RSS. Until 2009, the main diagnosis was coded at admission (main diagnosis of first RUM) and any additional diagnoses were coded as secondary diagnoses. In the current GHM version (11), the main diagnosis is assigned by the discharging department (last RUM) and should represent the 'cause' of hospitalization.

Clinical information considered in the classification process includes the main diagnosis and secondary diagnoses coded using the ICD-10 and the procedures coded according to the French classification of procedures (CCAM). In addition, birth weight and age (in days) of neonates are considered. Administrative data that are used to define the severity level of patients include age, length of stay and mode of discharge (death, transfer).

13.3.2 Classification algorithm

Every discharged hospital patient is grouped into exactly one GHM on the basis of information contained in the standard RSS. Figure 13.3 illustrates the grouping algorithm. The first test carried out is to see if the patient's hospital stay corresponded to a 'session' (*séance*) for chemotherapy, radiotherapy or dialysis. If this is the case the patient is classified into a separate CMD (CMD 28), which is divided into 15 GHMs without any severity levels. The next step of the grouping process identifies a type of Pre-MDC group for organ transplantations (*catégorie majeure* 27). Furthermore, 'transversal' cases with multiple trauma or with a diagnosis of AIDS are assigned to specific CMDs (26 and 25).

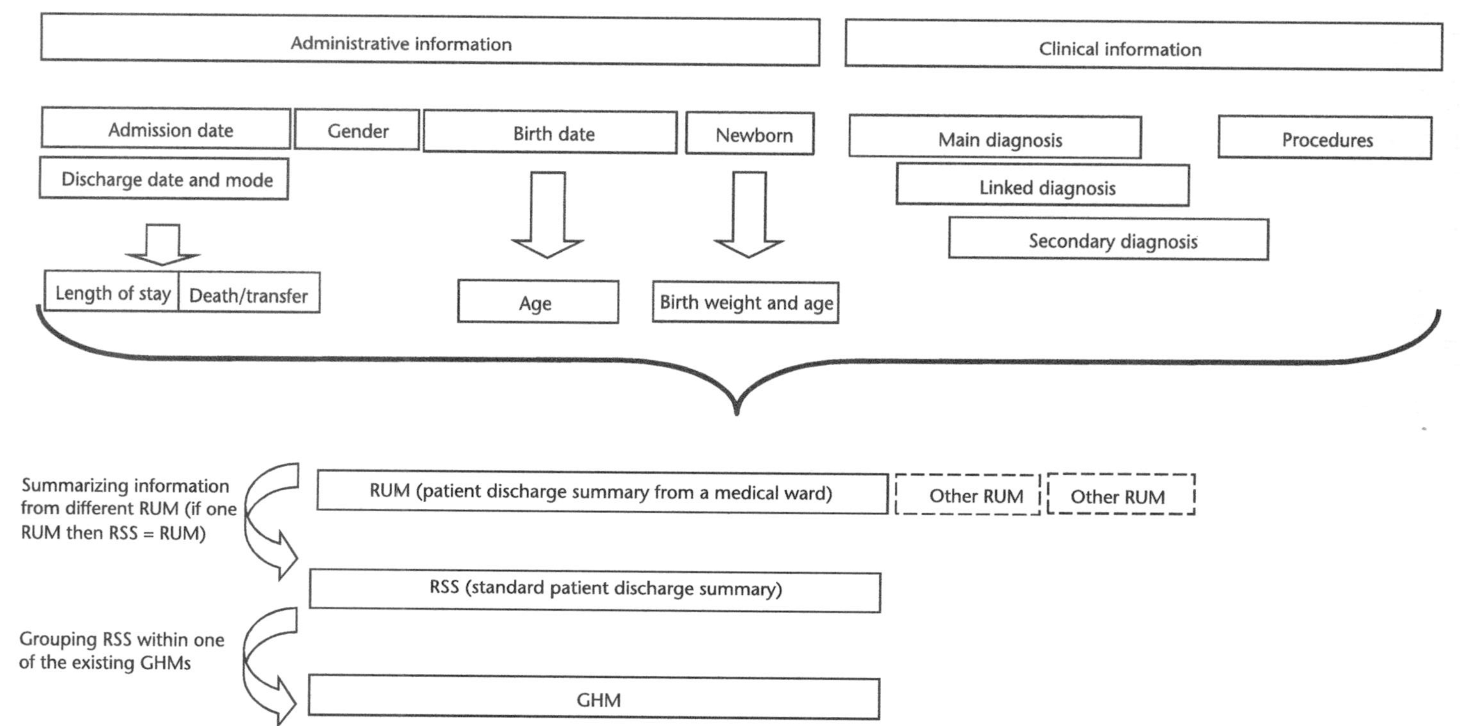

Figure 13.2 Information used for classifying patients into the GHM

Source: PowerPoint presentation prepared in 2009 by R. Cash for Mission T2A.

All other patients are classified into one of 23 mutually exclusive CMDs on the basis of the main diagnosis. Afterwards, the grouping algorithm examines the procedures that were carried out during the hospital stay. Cases with operating room (OR) procedures are classified into a 'surgical' partition. Cases with relevant non-OR procedures are assigned to an 'other procedure' partition. Cases without relevant procedures fall into the 'medical; partition. In certain CMDs, an 'undifferentiated' partition exists, which contains cases that were assigned without testing to establish the type of procedures carried out.

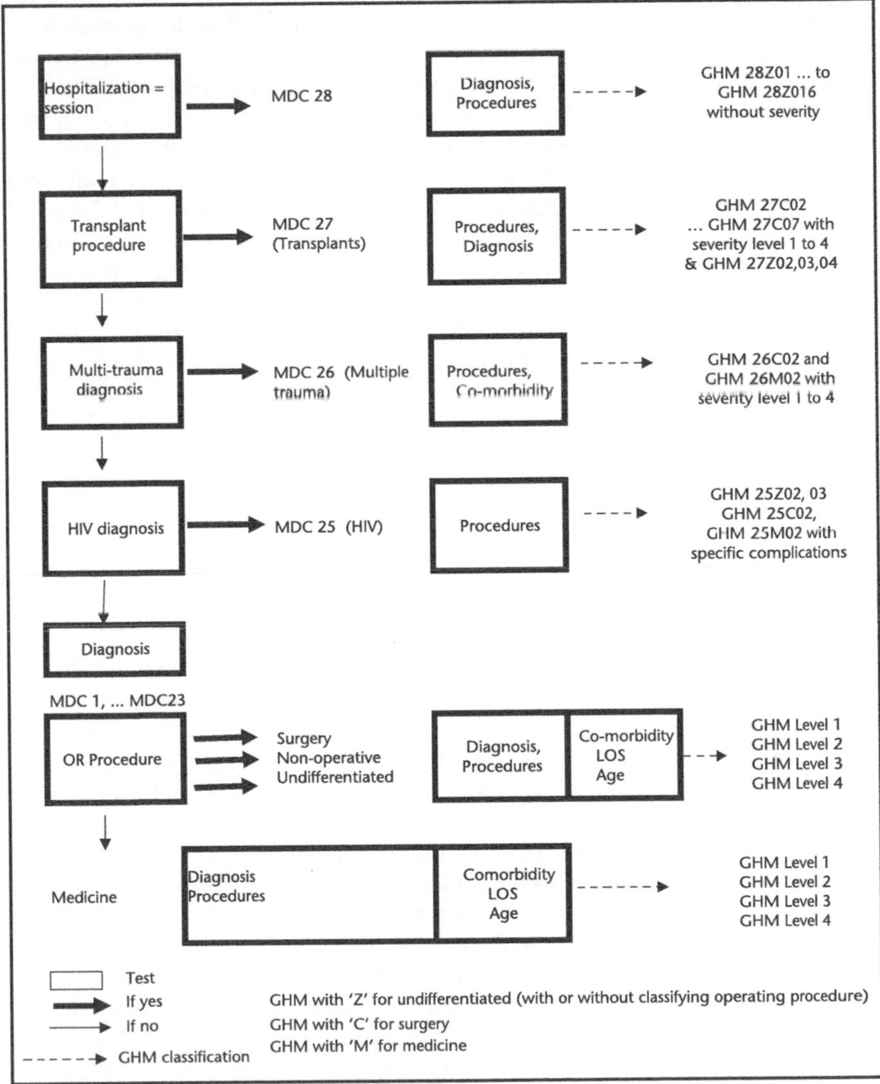

Figure 13.3 GHM classification with level of severity

Source: Adapted from Bellanger & Tardif, 2006.

Within partitions, base-GHMs are selected for a specific combination of main diagnosis and procedures, and often also considering age, complications and length of stay. If several procedures were performed during the hospital stay, the most complicated procedure (in terms of complexity and resource use) determines the classification of patients into base-GHMs. Error-GHMs can be assigned at several stages of the grouping process if inconsistencies exist, for example between diagnosis and patient gender or weight and patient age.

A new feature of the current GHM version (11) is that base-GHMs are systematically split into four levels of severity. Severity levels are defined on the basis of length of stay, age, and secondary diagnoses that represent complications or co-morbidities (CCs). Lists of secondary diagnoses exist that define their level of complexity (levels 2 to 4) and specify excluding conditions (that is, a secondary diagnosis is not considered to be a CC for certain main diagnoses).

Severity level 1 corresponds to cases without any CCs or with a length of stay of less than 3 days. Severity level 2 requires a minimum length of stay of 3 days and level-2 CCs. Severity level 3 requires a minimum length of stay of 4 days and level-3 CCs. Severity level 4 requires a minimum length of stay of 5 days and level-4 CCs. Under certain conditions, patients can be classified into a higher severity level if their age is either below 2 years or above 69 (or even 79) years. In addition, death is also used within the system as a marker of case severity. If the length of stay is more than 3 days, and the patient died during hospitalization, a case without CCs can be reclassified from level 1 into level 2. The idea is to give hospitals sufficient resources to cover the extra costs of dealing with death, but it is not clear what the implications are for the quality of care.

In addition, for some base-GHMs (for example, cataract surgery, for which day surgery is a recognized practice), an additional group is created to classify cases involving ambulatory surgery, previously coded as CM 24.

13.3.3 Data quality and plausibility checks

DIMs within hospitals carry out internal controls to analyse the plausibility of data. To this end, the ATIH provides them with a specific program (DATIM) that checks consistency between length of stay, type of admission, CCs and severity levels. In addition, the ATIH provides to each hospital reference means and standard deviations (from a comparable group of hospitals), as well as an index of outlier cases. The physicians within the DIM can use this information to check and correct the data before validating the database.

External data quality and plausibility checks are performed at the regional level by the ARH and the health insurance funds. The ATIH provides information to support external controls for hospitals with too many 'outlier cases'. The principal objective of external controls is to identify 'unjustified' billing of services and up- or wrong-coding. In 2006, more than 150 000 hospital stays in about 530 hospitals (one third of all hospitals concerned) were inspected: over 60 per cent of inpatient stays (and more than 80 per cent for ambulatory episodes) had some kind of coding error or inconsistency in the procedures billed (CNAM, 2006). The controls also revealed that use of innovative medications (financed separately, on top of the DRG price) was not justified in about 30 per cent of cases.

If up-coding or incorrect coding is detected, hospitals must reimburse payments received. In addition, hospitals may have to pay high financial penalties of up to 5 per cent of their annual budgets. The revenue recovered from these controls amounted to €24 million in 2006. The number of controls doubled for the year 2007, but results are not yet available.

13.3.4 Incentives for up- or wrong-coding

Since classification of patients into GHMs determines hospital revenues, strong incentives exist for hospitals to 'optimize' their coding practices. In 2006, a year after the introduction of DRG-based payment, external controls from health insurance funds demonstrated that a large number of hospitals either intentionally up-coded patients or inadvertently classified them into incorrect GHMs. The up-coding of ambulatory consultations as day cases appeared to be a real problem (CNAM, 2006). Therefore, the Ministry of Health issued a decree in 2007 describing those procedures that should not be coded as day cases. Between 2005 and 2008, the share of inpatient stays without any CCs decreased significantly in all hospitals, which could indicate DRG creep (see Chapter 6).

13.4 Cost accounting within hospitals

13.4.1 Regulation

The recommended hospital cost-accounting model is called 'analytical accounting', which is essentially a top-down accounting model distributing current consumption of resources into various cost groups (Ministry of Health, 2007). Since 1992, all hospitals participating in the ENC must provide data according to this model. In 2007, in order to harmonize cost-accounting methods for private hospitals joining the database, common accounting rules were defined by a decree (Circulaire DHOS 2007/06/27). The rest of the public and private hospitals use a far less detailed accounting system than the analytical one.

13.4.2 Main characteristics of the cost-accounting system

Hospitals participating in the joint ENC use a combination of top-down and bottom-up cost accounting, with elements of both gross-costing and micro-costing (see Chapter 5) (Bellanger & Tardif, 2006). Participating hospitals must be able to provide patient-level information regarding all procedures performed and relating to direct charges for certain specific drugs and medical devices, blood, external laboratory tests and fees for private physicians.

Preparing the hospitals' cost accounts for the analysis requires excluding all expenditure related to activities that are not reimbursed through the GHMs (for example teaching, research, psychiatry, rehabilitation, intensive care, neonatology, physicians' fees in private hospitals), and excluding the costs of high-cost drugs and medical consumables that can be directly attributed to patients. All remaining costs are distributed into a number of cost centres.

In order to calculate costs per hospital stay, unit costs of cost centres are determined and allocated to patients on the basis of easily identifiable allocation criteria. Total costs of each hospital stay are broken down into three main components: medical costs, overheads and capital costs. *Medical costs* include: (1) direct charges, which can be directly attributed to a patient, such as specific drugs and medical devices, blood, outpatient tests and fees for private physicians; (2) costs at direct cost centres – that is, clinical costs at the ward level (for example medical and non-medical staff, drugs, materials and running costs of hospital wards, equipment and maintenance), which are allocated to patients on the basis of length of stay in the hospital ward; and (3) medico-technical costs (such as anaesthesia, surgery, laboratory, radiology, pharmacy, including the running costs of these departments). Since patient-level consumption of these services (relating, for example, to the number of imaging tests or surgical procedures) is recorded by hospitals, it is possible to allocate costs to patients on the basis of services consumed and imputed costs per service at medico-technical cost centres.

Overhead costs include general administration, as well as and management and support services such as laundry, catering, sterilization, pharmacy and hospital hygiene. *Capital costs* include rental of buildings, interests, depreciation of buildings, and taxes. Overheads and capital costs are allocated to patients on the basis of calculated per diem costs. Despite this common methodology, the cost components may not always cover exactly the same cost items in public and private hospitals.

13.5 DRGs for reimbursement

13.5.1 Range of services and costs included in GHM-based hospital payment

Since 2008, all acute care activity in public and private hospitals is financed on the basis of GHMs (see Figure 13.4). Pilot tests to include psychiatric care and rehabilitative care services into GHM-based hospital payment are planned to start in 2011.

Currently, GHM prices differ for public and private hospitals, since they include different cost categories and are based on historical costs in each sector (Table 13.5). The tariffs for public hospitals cover all costs linked to a stay (including medical personnel, tests and procedures), while those for private hospitals do not cover medical fees of doctors (paid for by fee-for-service payments) and the cost of some technical equipment, paid for by a specific allocation to concerned hospitals (*forfeit haute téchnicité*). Until 2010, certain medical devices were billed separately by private hospitals, while they were included in the DRG pricing in public hospitals. The objective is to harmonize cost- and tariff-calculation methods between the two sectors by 2012.

Since 2008, capital costs (equipment, financial and building costs) are included in GHM prices. Hence, hospitals are expected to fund capital investments from these revenues. However, some (unmeasured) part of capital costs is financed through specific funding streams to help public hospitals to finance weighty investment plans imposed by recent hospital reforms. This means that

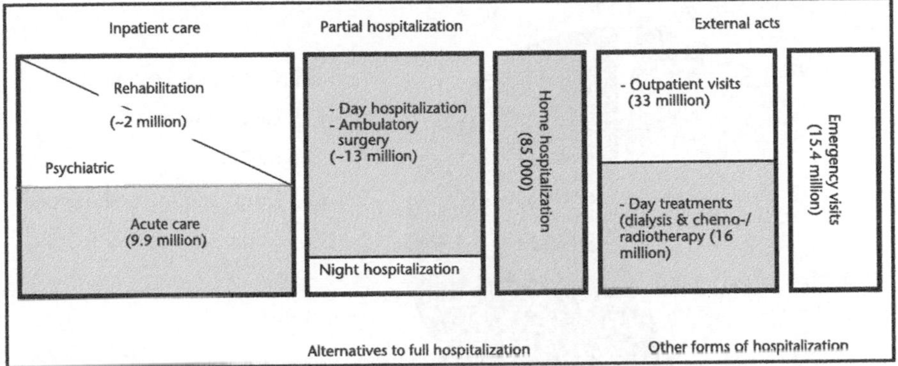

Figure 13.4 Range of services included in the GHM-based hospital payment system

Source: HCAAM, 2009.

the part of the capital costs covered by GHM prices is not completely transparent (Cour des comptes, 2009).

In 2008, payments made through GHM-based hospital payment represented about 56 per cent of hospital expenditure budgets (which amount to €67 billion). The overall payments made for 'missions of general interest' (MIGAC)[2] represented about 10 per cent of the public hospital budget, but there are large variations between hospitals according to their size, ownership status, and so on. Additional payments for expensive drugs and medical devices represent on average about 6 per cent of hospital expenditure, while annual remuneration for providing specific services such as intensive care, emergency care, and organ transplants corresponds to 1.5 per cent of total hospital expenditure (see Figure 13.5). Global budgets are used for the financing of rehabilitative, psychiatric and long-term care and account for about 27 per cent of all hospital expenditure.

13.5.2 Calculation of reference costs and prices

Average costs per GHM (reference costs) are calculated from the ENC separately for public and private hospitals (ATIH, 2007a).

Table 13.5 Cost categories included in GHM prices for public and private hospitals, 2010

Hospitals	*Public*	*Private, profit-making*
Cost categories	*Included in DRG price*	
Payment for physicians including social charges	Yes	No
Payment for other medical staff	Yes	Yes
Investment in technical equipment	Yes	25%
Expensive drugs and devices from a closed list	No	No
All medical material, devices, drugs	Yes	Yes
Infrastructure/Overheads	Partly	Yes

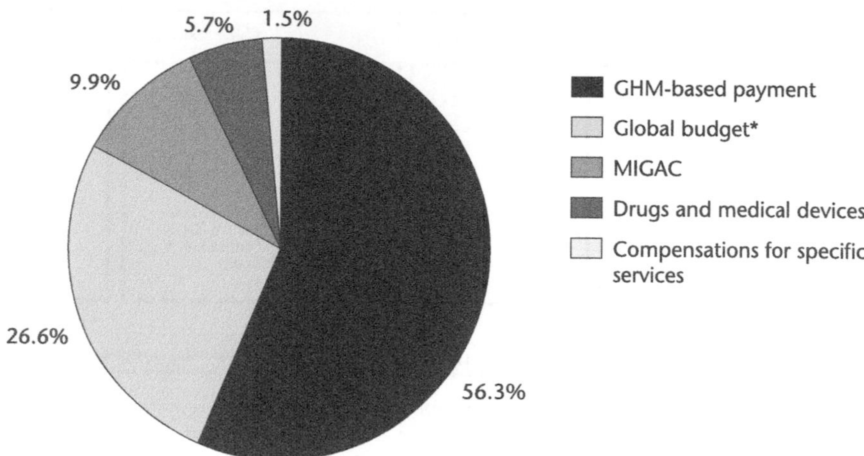

Figure 13.5 Breakdown of total hospital expenditure, 2008

Source: Adapted from ATIH, 2009

* Revenues for rehabilitative, psychiatric, and long-term care.

Using as a basis information relating to costs of individual patients, outlier cases are detected for each GHM through two different 'trimming' procedures: the first on length of stay and the second on costs. Trimming by length of stay is applied only to those GHMs for which the severity level is 1. This involves excluding all GHMs for which length of stay is longer than: [average length of stay (ALOS) × 2.5].

On average, 0.7 per cent of all public hospital stays and 0.4 per cent of all private hospital stays are trimmed from the ENCC on this basis (ATIH, 2009). In rare cases, this is followed by a second stage of trimming based on cost data. However, according to the ATIH, only 92 stays were discarded in 2007 during the cost data part of the trimming process.

Given that the ENCC does not cover all hospitals, but just a small group, costs per GHM are weighted by the type of hospital. For the public sector, five types of hospitals are defined: general hospitals producing fewer than 16 000 episodes per year; those producing more than 16 000 episodes; teaching hospitals; cancer centres; and private non-profit-making hospitals. The ALOS, the ALOS in wards that provide services related to reanimation, and the average number of procedures performed by type of hospital are used to weight average costs per GHM obtained from the ENCC. For private profit-making hospitals, the ALOS for the sector – as well as the ALOS in reanimation/intensive care (when relevant), together with the average number of procedures – are used as weighting variables.

The reference costs are used to compute 'raw' tariffs per GHM given the total budget for GHM-based payments (per sector). The actual prices per GHM are determined by the Ministry of Health, taking into account the budget envelope (expenditure target) for the acute care sector and other political priorities. The result is a macro-level price/volume control mechanism: if the growth in total volume of activity exceeds the target for the inpatient sector, GHM prices are reduced. In 2009 the ATIH noted that GHM prices were modified to adjust for the increase in MIGAC budgets, the growth of expenditures for additional payments on expensive drugs and the evolution of activity volumes and national priorities (for cancer treatment and palliative care). However, it is not clear how these different elements changed the prices of different GHMs. Consequently, it is not possible to predict the evolution of GHM prices from one year to another.

13.5.3 DRGs in actual hospital payment

National GHM prices are set annually. They differ between public and private hospitals since they do not cover the same cost items (see subsection 13.5.1) but they are not affected by hospital size or teaching status.

Hospital payment is adjusted for extreme cases. An upper and a lower threshold are calculated for each DRG in order to identify cases with extremely long or extremely short lengths of stay. The GHM tariff applies to episodes with a length of stay between these limits (inliers). For long-stay outlier cases, hospitals receive GHM-specific surcharges (Tariff EXH) for every day that the patient stayed above the upper length-of-stay threshold. Similarly, if patients are discharged earlier than the lower length-of-stay threshold, the DRG payment is reduced by per diem-based deductions (Tariff EXB). The lower threshold is used to discourage providers from discharging patients earlier than clinically appropriate. These low/high length-of-stay limits are not always the same for public and private hospitals.

Currently, the national DRG prices are weighted with a hospital-specific 'transition coefficient' calculated for each hospital from its own historical costs/prices. The transition coefficients aim to avoid large changes in hospital budgets from one year to another. The objective is for the coefficients within public and private sectors to converge to '1' by 2012. A regional index is also applied to hospitals in the Parisian area and those in overseas French territories, where labour costs are higher.

The initial proposition to introduce one DRG price for public and private hospitals in 2012 has been delayed to 2016 because of the strong reactions from public hospital federations. However, experimentation with selected DRGs is expected over the period 2011–2012.

As already mentioned (see subsection 13.5.1), hospitals receive additional payments for certain services, drugs and medical devices, and if applicable for teaching and research. Budget envelopes for public missions (MIGAC) are distributed by the ARH according to nationally defined rules. The growing size of the MIGAC budgets is currently an issue of concern, as the decision regarding the amount of these budgets seems to be political rather than evidence based.

13.5.4 Quality-related adjustments

There is no specific adjustment for quality of care. GHM payments do not vary according to differences in outcomes. The only GHM-related measure against inappropriate early discharge (as a dimension of quality) is the use of per diem-based deductions below the defined lower length-of-stay threshold(s).

Otherwise, quality-related programmes, such as developing infection control programmes, are negotiated and financed through specific allocations from the ARH as part of the MIGAC budget envelope.

At the same time, with the introduction of GHM-based payment, there has been quite substantial work – led by the Ministry of Health and the High Health Authority (HAS) – towards developing indicators to better monitor care quality in hospitals. A battery of indicators measuring care process and structure/organization quality – which has been tested and validated in a small number of voluntary hospitals – will be generalized over the period 2011–2012. Surprisingly, however, outcome indicators such as standardized mortality rates, readmission and/or complication rates are not part of that battery of indicators and they are currently not monitored routinely.

13.5.5 *Main incentives for hospitals*

The principal incentives provided by GHM-based hospital payment are to increase activity and to improve efficiency. Because hospitals are paid a fixed tariff per GHM, they are incentivized to reduce length of stay and to treat more patients. However, since GHM prices are reduced if activity exceeds the target for the inpatient sector, hospitals do not know whether increasing activity in a given year will always lead to an increased income in the next year. Since it is impossible to predict the evolution of GHM prices from one year to another, it is not clear how much incentive there is for hospitals to increase productivity.

The most obvious perverse incentive for hospitals is for up-coding or wrong-coding (see subsection 13.3.4). Other possible perverse incentives – such as engaging in patient selection and cream-skimming – are seen to be less of an issue for public hospitals since, by law, they cannot select their patients and have to provide a comprehensive package of care.

13.6 New/innovative technologies

The effect of DRG-based hospital payment on development and introduction of cost-increasing innovative technologies in hospitals (see Chapter 9) has been a major preoccupation in France, where access to new therapies (particularly in cancer treatment) remains one of the most generous in Europe (De Pouvourville, 2009).

Ultimately, the patient classification system and/or GHM prices are updated in order to reflect the higher costs for innovative drugs and technologies. However, two financing mechanisms exist to encourage the development and utilization of cost-increasing innovative drugs and technologies during the early stages of introduction to hospitals, as detailed here.

1. Additional payments are made for a certain number of expensive innovative drugs and medical devices, for which a list is defined at the national level. These are funded on the basis of a maximum standard price. Total expenditure on these drugs and devices increased by 37 per cent between 2005 and 2007, reaching €2.4 billion in 2008.

2. The development of innovative technologies is funded by a specific budgetary allocation within the global budget envelope of MERRI (*Missions d'enseignement, de recherché, de reference et d'innovation* – teaching, research, recourse and innovation). These payments are to cover the general cost of innovation-related activities, as well as specific innovative technologies on an experimental basis (such as artificial hearts, new-generation ear implants, and so on). Within this budget, there are specific separate payments to ensure quick access to innovative drugs which have not yet been authorized to be marketed called 'temporary access for treatment' (ATU). ATUs can be requested for one patient or a group of patients. The Agency for Safety of Medical Products (AFSSAPS) examines the request(s) and decides thereon after consultation with medical experts. The authorization and funding for ATUs is for one year, but can be renewed. The duration of the individual ATU corresponds to the duration of the treatment.

13.7 Evaluation of the GHM system in France

13.7.1 Official evaluations

Several public bodies have recently evaluated specific aspects of GHM-based hospital payment in France. The Evaluation Committee set up by the Ministry of Health published a report about the financial effects of the hospital payment reform in September 2009 (DREES, 2009). According to the report, the financial situation of private hospitals has improved since the introduction of GHM-based hospital payment, while that of public hospitals has deteriorated. In 2007, one in three public hospitals was in deficit, with a total budget deficit of about €500 million. The report points out that it has been difficult for the public hospitals to reduce their costs, despite a slight increase in their activity.

The report also examined the organizational changes in hospitals through a survey of 800 hospitals and found that efforts have been concentrated on modifying the structure of hospital activity (through transfers, hospital mergers, and so on) rather than on trying to improve efficiency. There has been little change in medical and human resource management. Finally, the report points out the incoherence between the incentives provided by GHM-based hospital payment and regional health plans aimed at ensuring a needs-based distribution of hospital resources. Currently, the development of the regional health plans is disconnected from financial planning and often ignores the financial constraints faced by hospitals.

In 2009, the Auditor's Office (*Cour des comptes*), within the framework of its annual evaluation of public accounts, presented an evaluation of GHM-based hospital payment. The major conclusion of the report was that it had not improved efficiency in the hospital sector. The report suggests that (1) GHM-based hospital payment has become a very opaque mechanism of cost control for managers and local regulators; and (2) the measurement and follow-up of hospital resources (revenues) is insufficient. For example, it is not possible to establish how hospital revenues (from public health insurance, patients and private complementary insurance) have evolved with respect to their production/activity.

The report also questions the incomprehensible nature of the price/volume control mechanism, which makes it very hard for hospitals to predict their income. Furthermore, it severely criticizes the ambiguous process for fixing prices, given that it is not always clear what is included in the price and what is not.

Furthermore, the Auditor's Office report estimated that within the hospital inpatient budgets, the categories which are not included in DRG prices escalated between 2005 and 2007: the expenditure for expensive drugs and medical devices increased by 37 per cent and other daily supplementary payments by 21 per cent, against an average of a 4 per cent increase in DRG prices.

13.7.2 Authors' assessment

To date, GHM-based hospital payment in France appears to fall short of achieving its stated objectives in terms of improving efficiency, transparency, fairness of funding, and quality.

Cost data are not available to identify efficient providers, to facilitate an understanding of the differences in medical practices and to monitor changes in behaviour of various actors. In terms of productivity improvement, it is not clear to what extent the rise in ambulatory activity represents an increase in efficiency, and to what extent this is due to up- or wrong-coding or to oversupply of services. Quality indicators – such as readmission and avoidable mortality rates – are not available either.

In addition, the macro-level volume/price control mechanism appears to be counterproductive. It creates an extremely opaque environment for hospitals, whereby they cannot predict their income based on their activity. Prices are set (progressively) independently of costs, which encourages health care facilities (especially private ones) to opt for less expensive care/therapies.

In order to achieve expected benefits in terms of efficiency and quality, it is important to improve the monitoring and transparency of the GHM system (methods used for cost/price calculations, data on individual providers, and so on), as well as expenses alongside the GHM payments, which are still allocated through an opaque mechanism. Furthermore, a contractual approach – giving individual providers clear volume and quality signals – could improve efficiency.

13.8 Outlook: Future developments and reform

It is intended to introduce GHM-based hospital payment for other hospital services which are currently financed through global budgets: namely rehabilitative and psychiatric care. The construction of a DRG scale for psychiatric care has proved to be difficult. The Ministry of Health (along with the ATIH) has been developing a DRG system for rehabilitative care, using more or less the same logic as that applied in inpatient care. The Ministry aims to test this classification system in a number of hospitals on a voluntary basis in 2011/2012.

13.9 Notes

1 These costs are not accounted for in the hospital sector budget, but are included in the ambulatory sector.
2 Missions d'intérêt général et de l'aide à la contractualisation: Missions of general interest and assistance with contracting, including payments for education, research and public health programmes.

13.10 References

ATIH (2007a). *Modalités de calcul du référentiel national de coûts 2007. Données ENCC 2007.* Lyon: Agence Technique de l'Information sur l'Hospitalisation (http://www.atih.sante.fr/openfile.php?id=2585, accessed 4 July 2011).

ATIH (2007b). *Principaux résultats issus des données de coûts ENCC 2007.* Lyon: Agence Technique de l'Information sur l'Hospitalisation (http://www.atih.sante.fr/openfile.php?id=2586, accessed November 2010).

ATIH (2009). *Manuel des GHM, version 11.* Lyon: Agence Technique de l'Information sur l'Hospitalisation (http://www.atih.sante.fr/index.php?id=000250002DFF, accessed 4 July).

Bellanger, M., Tardif, L. (2006). Accounting and reimbursement schemes for inpatient care in France. *Health Care Management Sciences*, 9:295–305.

CNAM (2006). *Contrôles et lutte contre les abus et les fraudes.* Paris: Caisse National d'Assurance Maladie (http://www.securite-sociale.fr/institutions/fraudes/fraude.htm, accessed 4 July 2011).

Cour des comptes (2009). *La Securité Sociale, chapitre 7, La mise en place de la T2A : Bilan à mi-parcours.* Paris: Cour des comptes (February).

DREES (2009). *Rapport d'activité du Comité d'évaluation de la T2A, septembre 2009.* Paris: Direction de la recherche, des études, de l'évaluation et des statistiques, Ministère du Travail, de l'Emploi et de la Santé.

Fenina, A., Geffroy, Y., Duée, M. (2008). Les comptes nationaux de la santé en 2007. *Etudes et Résultats*, 655:1–8.

HCAAM (2009). *Note sur la situation des établissements de santé, Avril 2009.* Paris: Haut Conseil de l'Avenir de l'Assurance Maladie.

Michelot, X., Rodrigues, J.M. (2008). DRGs in France, in J.R. Kimberly, G. de Pouvourville, T. D'Aunno, eds. *Globalization of Managerial Innovation in Health Care.* Cambridge: Cambridge University Press.

Ministry of Health (2007). *Guide méthodologique de la comptabilité analytique hospitalière.* Paris: Ministère de la santé (éditions mise à jour 1997, 2004, 2007).

Mousques, J., Polton, D. (2004). Sickness funds reform: a new form of governance. *Health Policy Monitor*, October (http://hpm.org/survey/fr/a4/3, accessed 4 July 2011).

OECD (2010). *OECD Health Data 2010: Statistics and Indicators.* Paris: Organisation for Economic Co-operation and Development.

Or, Z. (2008). Changing regional health governance in France. *Eurohealth*, 14(4):7–8.

Or, Z., Renaud, T., Com-Ruelle, L. (2009). *Les écarts des coûts hospitaliers sont-ils justifiables? Réflexions sur une convergence tarifaire entre les secteurs public et privé en France.* Paris: Institut de Recherche et Documentation en Economie de la Santé (IRDES Working Paper 25).

Patris, A., Blum, D., Girardier, M. (2001), A change in the French patient classification system. *CASEMIX Quarterly*, 34:128–38.

de Pouvourville, G. (2009). Les hôpitaux français face au paiement prospectif au cas: la mise en ouvre de la tarification à l'activité. *Revue Economique*, 60(2):457–70.

chapter fourteen

Germany: Understanding G-DRGs

Alexander Geissler,
David Scheller-Kreinsen,
Wilm Quentin and Reinhard Busse

14.1 Hospital services and the role of DRGs in Germany

14.1.1 The German health system

A key characteristic of the German health care system is the sharing of decision-making powers between the 16 *Länder* (states), the federal Government and statutory civil society organizations. Moreover, Bismarckian principles dominate statutory health insurance (SHI), that is, important competences are legally delegated to membership-based, self-regulated organizations of payers and providers.

In the most important pillar of the German health care system, the SHI, sickness funds, their associations and associations of SHI-affiliated physicians have assumed the status of quasi-public corporations. These self-regulated corporate structures operate the financing and delivery of benefits covered by SHI within a general legal framework. They are based on mandatory membership and internal democratic legitimization. They have the power and a duty to define benefits, prices and standards (at federal level) and to negotiate horizontal contracts to manage and sanction their members' behaviour (at regional level). The vertical implementation of decisions made at superior levels is combined with strong horizontal decision-making and contracting among the legitimate stakeholders involved in the various sectors of health care.

The corner-stone of health service provision in Germany is the fifth book of the German Social Law (SGB V). The SGB V separates the provision of outpatient and inpatient services. Planning, resource allocation and financing are undertaken completely separately in each sector. Beyond the established decision-making organizations, other organizations have been given formal rights to contribute to decision-making bodies by consultation (for example, nurses and allied health professions), participation and proposals (for example, patient organizations) or by becoming a decision-making and financing partner in the process (for example, private health insurance for case-based payments in hospitals).

Financing

Germany spends about 10.4 per cent of gross domestic product (GDP) on health care, with the three main sources being statutory health insurance (57.5 per cent of total expenditure on health), private health insurance (9.3 per cent) and out-of-pocket spending (13.5 per cent) (DESTATIS 2009; data for 2007).

Since 2009, health insurance has been mandatory in Germany, while previously it was only mandatory for around 75 per cent of the population (while de facto over 99.5 per cent were covered). About 86 per cent of the German population are covered by SHI and 10 per cent are privately insured (with the remainder falling under special provisions). Premiums in private health insurance are risk related. One can opt for insurance under this type of health insurance if the earned income passes a certain threshold (€49 950 per year or €4162.50 per month in 2010) for three consecutive years. The SHI system is based on wage-related contributions (since 1 July 2009: 14.9 per cent on gross income up to a threshold of €3750 per month).

14.1.2 Hospital services in Germany

In Germany one can distinguish between three different types of hospital ownership. Almost half of all beds are found in public hospitals. In terms of the remaining capacity, ~35 per cent is provided by non-profit-making hospitals and ~16 per cent by private profit-making hospitals, which have increased their share since the beginning of the 1990s. Table 14.1 summarizes the key statistics for the German hospital sector.

Planning and ensuring hospital capacities

In the inpatient sector, the reimbursement of hospitals follows the principal of 'duality' introduced with the Hospital Financing Act (KHG) in 1972. This means that hospitals are financed from two different sources: investments in infrastructure are covered directly by state budgets, while operating costs are reimbursed by sickness funds and private health insurance.

Each of the 16 state governments is responsible for maintaining hospital infrastructure. The main instruments used to do so are the so-called 'hospital requirement plans', which are set by the state governments after input by the respective hospital federation and the sickness funds. They specify hospital capacity and the range of services to be delivered across all hospitals within a state, as well as within individual hospitals.

The self-governing bodies – namely, provider associations and sickness funds – are responsible both for providing substantive detail to the provisions of the laws defining the framework of hospital financing, and for the continual

Table 14.1 Key hospital figures by size and ownership, 2007

Size and type of ownership	*Hospitals (overall)*	*Beds*	*Beds per 100 000 inhabitants*	*Occupancy*	*Cases*	*Cases per 100 000 inhabitants*	*ALOS**
	Number (share in %)	*Number (share in %)*	*Number*	*%*	*Number*	*Number*	*Days*
Hospital size in beds	**2 087 (100)**	**506 954 (100)**	**616**	**77.2**	**17 178 573**	**20 883**	**8.3**
< 49	407	7 572	9	64.9	210 028	255	8.5
50–99	264	19 354	24	73.3	529 579	644	9.8
100–149	302	36 995	45	74.2	1 108 285	1 347	9.0
150–199	208	35 903	44	74.8	1 179 137	1 433	8.3
200–299	326	79 578	97	76.1	2 612 288	3 176	8.5
300–399	203	69 613	85	77.4	2 361 352	2 871	8.3
400–499	131	58 258	71	77.6	1 953 598	2 375	8.4
500–599	96	52 545	64	77.1	1 870 325	2 274	7.9
600–799	64	43 654	53	78.8	1 564 800	1 902	8.0
> 800	86	103 482	126	80.7	3 789 184	4 606	8.0
Public hospitals	**677 (32.4)**	**250 345 (49.4)**	**304**	**79**	**8 697 755**	**10 573**	**8**
under private law	380	133 957	163	77.5	4 804 914	5 841	7.9
under public law	297	116 388	141	80.5	3 892 841	4 732	8.8
- legally dependent	161	54 319	66	79.5	1 755 576	2 134	9.0
- legally independent	136	62 069	75	81.4	2 137 266	2 598	8.6
Non-profit-making hospitals	**790 (37.9)**	**177 632 (35.0)**	**216**	**75**	**5 970 324**	**7 258**	**8**
Private hospitals	**620 (29.7)**	**78 977 (15.6)**	**96**	**76**	**2 510 494**	**3 052**	**9**

Source: Bölt (2010), with modifications.

development of the German diagnosis-related group (G-DRG) system. The G-DRG system applies to all hospitals, irrespective of ownership status, and all patients (except rehabilitation and psychiatric, psychosomatic or psychotherapeutic patients), regardless of whether or not they are members of the SHI system, have private health insurance, or are self-funding patients (Tuschen & Trefz, 2004). DRGs cover all clinical departments with the exception of institutions or facilities providing psychiatric care, psychosomatic medicine, or psychotherapy services. For these services the 2009 Hospital Financing Reform Act (KHRG) mandated the German self-governing bodies to develop and introduce a prospective payment system by the year 2013, which is to be based on per diem payments adjusted for patient characteristics and procedures.

Range of activities and services in the hospital sector

German hospitals concentrate on inpatient care because sectoral borders are still strict compared with the practice in other countries. Legally, hospitals still mainly provide inpatient services. Ambulatory care, including emergency care, is provided by the regional physicians' associations and their office-based physicians. Only university hospitals have formal outpatient facilities, officially for research and teaching purposes, while in most other hospitals, head physicians need to be authorized by the physicians' association if they (as individuals – and not the hospital as an institution) want to provide ambulatory services.

Activity levels for day surgery and ambulatory pre- and post-hospital care have increased. Since 2004, hospitals have been granted additional competences to provide services to outpatients that require highly specialized care on a regular basis. Also, participation in integrated care models (which require a contract between a sickness fund and providers from different sectors) offers new opportunities to become active in ambulatory care if their partners on the providers' side also include ambulatory care providers.

Nevertheless, hospital care remains clearly separate from outpatient care delivered by general practitioners (GPs) or specialists (Figure 14.1). A typical episode of care starts with a referral including patient's case history and preliminary diagnosis from a GP (or an office-based specialist) to a hospital and ends with a discharge or a transfer back to the GP (or specialist). Diagnostics (such as tests for cancer) are carried out in outpatient as well as inpatient settings.

Relationship with third party payers

As outlined above, the principle of 'dual financing' means that hospitals receive funds for infrastructure from the state governments, while operating costs are covered via DRGs by the sickness funds. Reimbursement for such costs is, to a certain extent, limited by volumes which are negotiated between every hospital accredited in the hospital plan and the sickness funds. If a hospital treats more cases than negotiated, the DRG reimbursement rate is reduced by a certain percentage (and vice versa – it is increased if the number of treated cases is lower).

Long-term infrastructural assets require a case-by-case grant application by each individual hospital. State governments distinguish between grants for

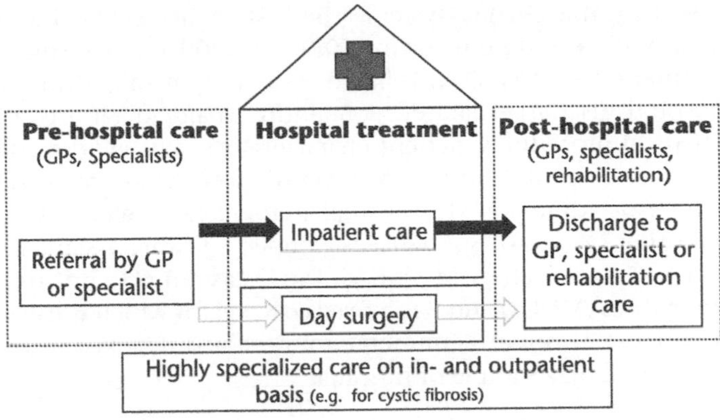

Figure 14.1 Typical episode of care across sectoral borders

construction of hospitals and initial procurement or replacement of other assets. According to the KHG, a hospital acquires a legal claim to subsidy only as long as it is included in the 'hospital plan' of the respective state. Inclusion in the hospital plan also means that flat-rate grants for short-term assets (3–15 years economic life) can be granted. In practice, infrastructural hospital investments are mainly determined by the budgetary situation of the states and by political considerations. If a hospital is not included in a 'hospital plan' it cannot make a claim for state investment financing. The share of public investment in hospitals has decreased continuously since the early 1990s.

14.1.3 Purpose of the DRG system

The introduction of the G-DRG system sought to achieve several objectives. First, the primary motive for fundamentally reforming the old reimbursement system based on budgets with per diem charges as the unit for reimbursement was to achieve a more appropriate and fair allocation of resources by utilizing DRGs. Related goals were to facilitate a precise and transparent measurement of the casemix and the levels of services delivered by hospitals. Moreover, it was assumed that efficiency and quality of service delivery in the hospital sector would increase due to the improved documentation of internal processes and increased managerial capacity. As a consequence, a moderate contribution to cost-containment based on a reduction of length of stay and bed capacity was presumed (Braun et al., 2007).

14.2 Development and updates of the DRG system

14.2.1 The current DRG system at a glance

The national G-DRG system was introduced in 2003, based on the Australian Refined Diagnosis-Related Groups (AR-DRG, version 4.1). Outpatient services are not covered by the G-DRG system. The system has evolved so that the number of groups increased from 664 in 2003 up to 1200 in 2010. The procedure to assign treatment cases to a DRG is based on a grouping algorithm using the inpatient hospital discharge dataset, containing: major diagnosis and other diagnoses, medical procedures, patient characteristics (age, gender and weight of newborns), length of stay, duration of ventilation, reason for hospital discharge and type of admission (for example, emergency, referral from GP or transfer from other hospital). Specialized 'grouper' software assigns these data to a particular DRG (see section 14.3). Each DRG is assigned to one of 25 major diagnostic categories (MDCs) and has a fixed cost weight which is calculated by the Institute for the Hospital Remuneration System (InEK) based on average costs as documented by a sample of hospitals.

14.2.2 Development of the DRG system

In 2000, the Statutory Health Insurance Reform Act paved the way for the G-DRG system. It represented the most significant reform of the German hospital sector since the system of 'dual financing' was introduced in 1972 by the KHG. The reform defined the fundamental features of the G-DRG system for case-based reimbursement of inpatient services. However, under this provision, the self-governing bodies at the federal level (that is, the Federal Association of Sickness Funds, the Association of Private Health Insurance, and the German Hospital Federation) were mandated to select (by June 2000) and then to introduce a DRG-based reimbursement system themselves. As a guiding principle they were required to ensure that the system would be guided by universal and uniform application, performance orientation and case payments, taking account of disease severity and case complexity. In June 2000 the German self-governing bodies decided to use the AR-DRG system as the foundation for the G-DRG system.

Four phases can be distinguished in the G-DRG introduction process (Figure 14.2): first, the *preparation phase*, from 2000 until 2002, in which the selected AR-DRG system was adapted to the German hospital environment in two major steps, as detailed here.

1. The Australian procedure codes based on the WHO's International Classification of Diseases ICD-9-CM (clinical modification) were transformed to the German procedure classification codes (OPS) and the ICD-10-WHO diagnosis codes were modified to the ICD-10-GM (German modification) by the German Institute for Medical Documentation and Information (DIMDI).
2. A cost-accounting system for calculating Germany-specific relative cost weights was developed by the InEK. The institute was founded for this purpose by the self-governing bodies. In 2001 a small set of hospitals tested the Australian grouper. The results were discussed in 2002 and requirements for a German system were derived. By the end of 2002 the first version of the G-DRG system had been prepared. For this early version, approximately 100 hospitals (of ~1800 acute hospitals falling under the DRG system) voluntarily shared their cost data with the InEK to calculate cost weights. Version 1 of the G-DRG system included 664 DRGs in the Case Fee Catalogue.

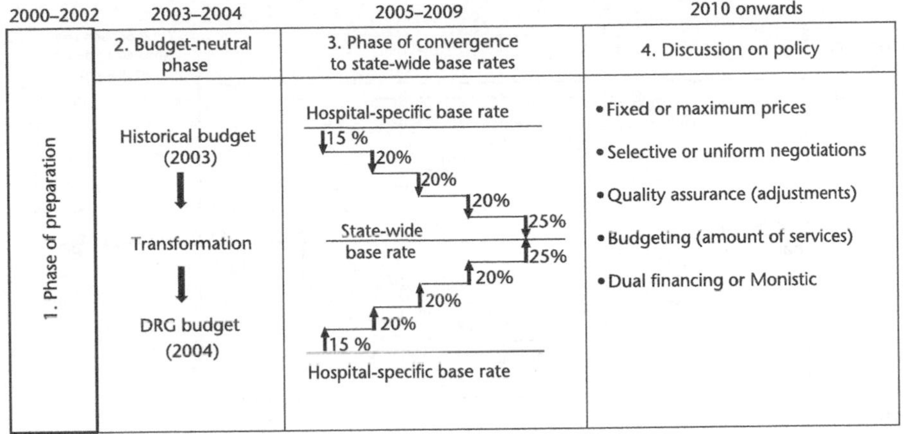

Figure 14.2 Phases involved in introducing DRGs in Germany

Source: Neubauer & Pfister, 2008, with modifications.

The second phase from 2003 until 2004 was the introduction of DRGs. This phase was called the *budget-neutral phase*, as hospitals were receiving the budgets as negotiated previously. The only difference was that the reimbursement units were no longer per diem charges, but were the DRGs instead. In 2003, hospitals could voluntarily group their patients using G-DRGs (incentivized by the option to be able to negotiate higher budgets), then in 2004 they were mandated to do so. In order to change from a budget based on per diem payment to one based on DRGs, it was necessary to transform the historically developed budgets into 'DRG budgets' ('revenue budgets'). This involved defining cost categories within 'DRG budgets' as additional activities by hospitals which continued to be reimbursed differently (for example, psychiatric services, teaching of nursing students).

Whereas until 2002 the budget was based on the agreed number of patient days to calculate the per diem charge, the budget in 2003/2004 was based on its casemix (that is, the number of relative weights for all patients) to give the hospital-specific base rate. For the first time in the German hospital sector, hospital efficiency became visible as it became apparent which hospitals with a high base rate (due to budgets set comparatively high for the patient casemix) produced the same services comparatively less efficiently than those with low base rates. 'Casemix' and the 'casemix index' (CMI) have become common terms in comparing hospitals. The casemix is equal to the sum of the cost weights of all DRGs for a specified time period. The average case weight or so called CMI is calculated by dividing the casemix by the total number of cases. The CMI is thus equal to the average DRG cost weight for a particular hospital and is an important indicator of the costliness of cases treated by a particular hospital. Small rural hospitals typically have CMIs of well below the average of 1, while university hospitals may have CMIs above 1.5.

During the third *phase of convergence* from 2005–2010, hospitals' individual base rates converged to state-wide base rates (one for each of the 16 *Länder*). As a starting point, state-wide base rates were negotiated for the first time in 2005.

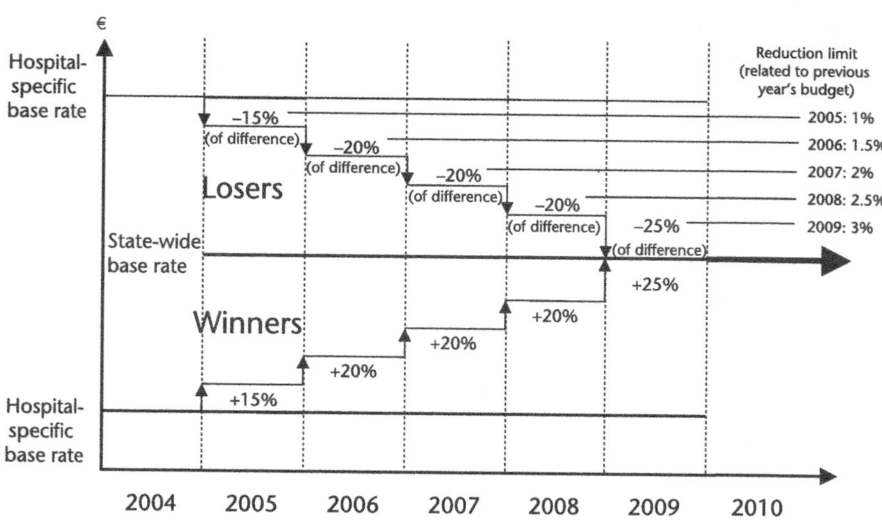

Figure 14.3 Phase of convergence

Source: Neubauer & Pfister, 2008, with modifications.

These were used as a yard stick for the base rates of all hospitals in that state. While hospital budgets (or rather revenue budgets) were still negotiated and used to calculate hospital-specific base rates, the actual base rate used for each hospital diverged year by year from the (calculated) hospital-specific base rate to approach the state-wide base rate. In 2005, the individual base rate was determined by 15 per cent of the difference to the state-wide base rate, in 2006 by 35 per cent (15 per cent plus 20 per cent), and so on, until in 2009 it was meant to reach the state-wide base rate (Figure 14.3).

Initially, hospital-specific base rates varied considerably from ~€2200 (mostly minor hospitals in rural areas) up to ~€3200 (for major hospitals in urban areas), which to some extent reflected historical differences in their reimbursement negotiations (Friedrich et al., 2008). As the G-DRG system does not account for organizational characteristics – such as size, differences in input prices or the teaching status of a hospital – the convergence of the base rate put high-cost hospitals under significant pressure to lower costs.

To make the reform politically more acceptable, resulting losses of the negotiated budget were limited, initially to 1 per cent in 2005 (compared to 2004), but then increasing up to 3 per cent in 2009 (compared to 2008). As a result, not all hospitals with initially high hospital-specific base rates had reached the state-wide levels by 2009. In 2010, however, there was no safety net for losses so that the state-wide base rates were applied to all hospitals (and hospital-specific base rates consequently ceased to exist) (Figure 14.3).

With the fourth phase from 2010/11 onwards, further modifications of the G-DRG system are planned. Among them are:

- From 2010 onewards, a nationwide base rate will be calculated by the InEK. Until 2014 state-wide base rates should converge towards a target corridor of 2.5% above and 1.25% below this rate.

- The 2009 KHRG gave the state governments the opportunity to include the investment costs in the cost calculation of the DRGs. This would result in some states having a single payer approach to hospital reimbursement. Currently, however, it is not clear how the money paid by the states for hospital investment will be channelled into the system.
- Psychiatric services will also be reimbursed by a DRG-like system. This will probably differ from the rest of the system by being a combination of length of stay and resource intensity; that is, the case weights will be calculated on a per diem basis.

Table 14.2 summarizes the main characteristics of the G-DRG system and changes over time. Two developments stand out: (1) the sample for calculating cost weights was substantially increased. Since 2004, an increasing number of major and university hospitals with severe and rare cases have participated; (2) the number of DRGs and supplementary fees (mostly used for the reimbursement of high-cost drugs) increased dramatically as new DRGs were added and existing ones were split.

14.2.3 Data used for the development and updates of the DRG system

Three types of information are important for the development of the G-DRG system: (1) adequate coding of clinical data, both to further develop the grouping system and to facilitate precise reimbursement that takes account of individual patient characteristics (reimbursement of individual hospitals); (2) cost data to calculate cost weights; and (3) information on medical innovations that allows regular updates of fee catalogues.

To calculate cost weights, the InEK relies on retrospective cost and performance data collected in German hospitals (Table 14.2 and Figure 14.4). All German hospitals are obliged to provide hospital-related structural data (relating to type of hospital, ownership, number of beds, number of trainees, labour and total costs) and case-related performance data (regarding diagnoses, procedures, reason for admission, date of discharge) on an annual basis (§21 Hospital Remuneration Act (KHEntG)) to the Data Centre.

Additionally, hospitals can participate voluntarily in the sample used to calculate cost weights (section 14.4). In order to do so, they must provide patient-level cost data, submitted to the InEK. To achieve uniform and comparable cost data, the InEK has developed a standardized cost-accounting system based on a 'Calculation Handbook' (InEK, 2007). Each year up to the end of March the hospitals must deliver all datasets of the previous year to the Data Centre (operated from 3M Medica). After data checks (see subsection 14.3.3), the InEK receives the data before 1 July in order to develop the Case Fee Catalogue for the following year. For example, the G-DRG system for 2010 is based on retrospective cost and structural data from the 2008 calendar year, while 2009 was used to check the data on plausibility and recalculate the cost weights.

The third type of information is needed for the introduction of new diagnostic and treatment options within the OPS, maintained and developed by the DIMDI (subsection 14.2.2). The DIMDI has developed a process by which institutions such as the InEK, the Federal Office for Quality Assurance (BQS)

Table 14.2 Main facts relating to the G-DRG system

Year	*2003*	*2004*	*2005*	*2006*	*2007*	*2008*	*2009*	*2010*
DRGs total	**664**	**824**	**878**	**954**	**1 082**	**1 137**	**1 192**	**1 200**
Inpatient DRGs total	**664**	**824**	**878**	**952**	**1 077**	**1 132**	**1 187**	**1 195**
- valuated (B2*)	642	806	845	912	1 035	1 089	1 146	1 154
- unvaluated (D1*)	22	18	33	40	42	43	41	41
Range of cost weights: min.-max.(rounded)	0.12–29.71	0.11–48.27	0.12–57.63	0.12–65.70	0.11–64.90	0.11–68.97	0.12–78.47	0.13–73.76
Day care DRGs total	**0**	**0**	**0**	**2**	**5**	**5**	**5**	**5**
- valuated (B2*)	0	0	0	1	1	1	1	1
- unvaluated (D3*)	0	0	0	1	4	4	4	4
Supplementary fees	**0**	**26**	**71**	**83**	**105**	**115**	**127**	**143**
- valuated (C1*)	0	1	35	41	59	64	74	81
- unvaluated (D2*)	0	25	36	42	46	51	53	62
Hospitals participating in cost data collection	**125**	**144**	**148**	**214**	**263**	**249**	**251**	**253**
- excluded for data quality	9	0	0	0	38	28	33	28
- actual	116	144	148	214	225	221	218	225
- included university hospitals	0	12	10	9	10	8	10	10
- number of cases available for calculation	633 577	2 825 650	2 909 784	3 531 760	4 239 365	3 900 098	4 377 021	4 539 763
- number of cases used for calculation after data checks	494 325	2 395 410	2 283 874	2 851 819	2 863 115	2 811 669	3 075 378	3 257 497
R^2 all cases	0.4556	0.5577	0.6388	0.6805	0.7072	0.7209	0.744	0.7443
R^2 inlier	0.6211	0.7022	0.7796	0.7884	0.8049	0.8166	0.8345	0.843

Source: Based on data from InEK annual reports.

* Hospital reimbursement according to Figure 14.6

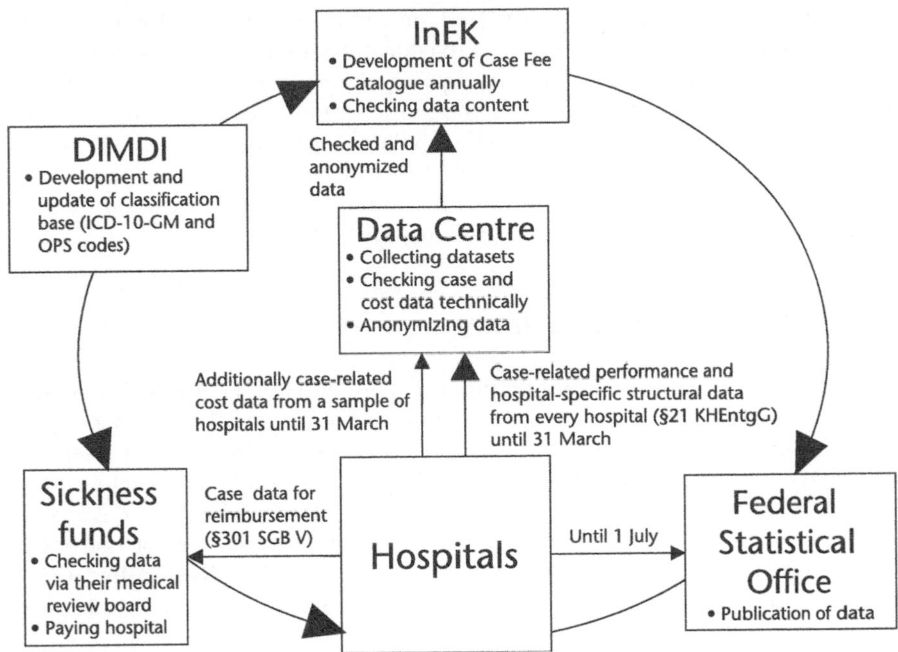

Figure 14.4 Types of data used for reimbursement and further development of the G-DRG system

(see subsection 14.5.4) and other professional (medical) associations can submit suggestions to be considered for classification (both within the OPS as well as within the ICD-10-GM). All proposals are discussed and evaluated and further refined in different working groups. Successful proposals result in a new or modified code. Both the OPS and the ICD are updated annually. New technologies are incorporated sequentially and appended to existing medical coding catalogues (see section 14.6).

The InEK is obliged to take the latest medical knowledge into account when developing the DRG catalogue. Therefore, the InEK developed a proposal process (structured dialogue) whereby medical experts are asked to contribute their knowledge from clinical practice in order to refine certain DRGs. After collecting the suggestions from clinicians, the InEK carries out statistical analysis to prove the proposals empirically. About 37 per cent of the proposals that were able to be tested empirically (410 out of 700) were implemented to the G-DRG 2010 version (InEK, 2009a).

14.3 The current patient classification system

14.3.1 Information used to classify patients

Diagnoses and medical procedures are the most important information used to assign patients to a certain G-DRG. The ICD-10-GM is used to code diagnoses. To code procedures, the OPS is used to assign a specific code to most procedures.

Although the OPS originally contained procedure codes only for inpatient surgical interventions, it has been used to code both these and general inpatient medical procedures since 2004 and thus plays a key role in the implementation of DRGs. Since 2005, ambulatory surgical procedures have also been included in the OPS; it is thus also used in the ambulatory care sector, in which many such surgical procedures are carried out. In addition to its role in the G-DRG system, the OPS is designed to facilitate quality assurance (see subsection 14.5.4) and the uptake of new technologies (see section 14.6).

14.3.2 Classification algorithm

A simplified version of the grouping process is presented in Figure 14.5. In cases with extremely high resource consumption, certain procedure codes (for example, transplantation) determine the DRG directly. The DRGs in this category are referred to as 'Pre-MDC' DRGs. For all others, the major diagnosis determines the classification into one of 25 MDCs, numbered 1 to 23 (with 18 and 21 each split into A and B). Essentially, an MDC corresponds to diseases of the body system comparable to the classification in ICD. While all DRGs relating to the 'Pre-MDC' start with an A, the 25 MDCs use a starting letter between B and Z, for

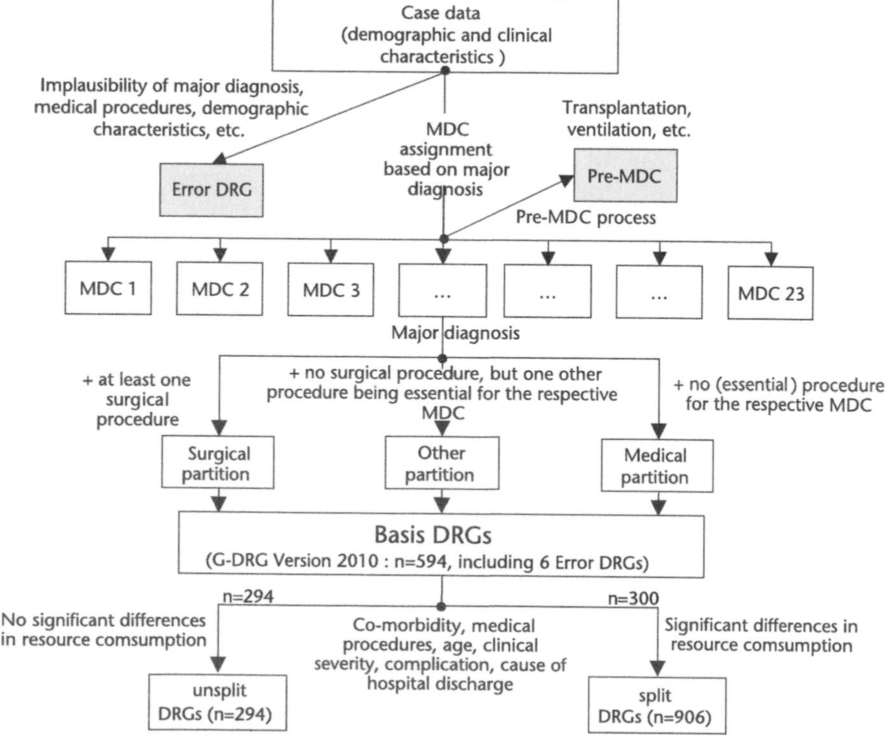

Figure 14.5 G-DRG grouping algorithm

Source: Updated and modified from Schreyögg et al., 2006.

example, MDC 1 (Nervous system) = B or MDC 14 (pregnancy, childbirth and puerperium) = P.

After this step, data on the type of procedure are used to assign a case to a 'base-DRG', which is a group of closely related diagnoses and procedures that have not been subdivided according to criteria such as co-morbidities or patient age. Within each MDC, base-DRGs have a two-digit number, which also shows the 'partition' of the DRG, with 01 to 39 for surgical DRGs (for example, B01–B39 for diseases of the nervous system with surgery), 40 to 59 for DRGs with other important procedures which are essential for the DRG, and 60 to 99 for other DRGs. Since the 2005 system, the strict partitioning has been relaxed in MDC 5 (Circulatory System) and MDC 8 (Musculoskeletal System and Connective Tissue) so that DRGs above 39 can also contain surgical procedures. Base-DRGs may be split into separate DRGs based on additional criteria, thus reflecting different degrees of resource consumption. A case is subsequently assigned to its final DRG (which is either a base-DRG that has not been split, or one of at least two – but usually more – as a result of splitting) using information such as co-morbidities, procedures and patient characteristics on the one hand, and cost data on the other. If a base-DRG is not split, the fourth digit (again a letter) is a Z, for example, B01Z, while split DRGs use A, B, C and so on in descending order of resource intensity, such as B02A > B02B > B02C.

14.3.3 Data quality and plausibility checks

Cost data

Initially, the Data Centre (see Figure 14.4) checks the cost datasets for formal and technical errors. As part of this process the file compatibility and data encryption, as well as the existence of service and cost data in every dataset are validated. Cases without DRG relevance (such as psychiatry) are excluded. Next, the InEK conducts three further steps consisting of economic and medical plausibility checks. First, minimum and maximum costs per module (such as costs of the clinical staff per day, total cost of the hospital) and the ratios between modules (such as costs of the cost centre 'anaesthesia' < costs of the cost centre 'operating room') are given an economic check. Second, adherence to the German DRG classification codes (ICD-10-GM and OPS) is given a medical check, and third, coherence between economic and medical information is checked (for example, the costs per case of a hip replacement must reflect the material cost of implants; if radiology procedures are reported, the costs must be part of cost centre 9 'radiology', see Table 14.3). In 2009, after these data plausibility checks, 3 257 497 out of 4 539 763 records were available (~72 per cent) for the calculation (InEK, 2009a). The datasets that remain serve as the basis for determining the cost weights and trim-points.

Clinical data

For reimbursement purposes, every hospital must deliver case data (§301 SGB V) to the sickness funds, mainly comprising clinical data (diagnoses, procedures), demographic data (age, gender) and administrative data (dates of admission, surgery and discharge). The coding quality of these data is regularly checked by the regional medical review boards of the sickness funds. They evaluate the assignment of cases to DRGs and their respective service utilization (§275 SGB V; §17 KHG). In order to do so, they send teams to randomly selected hospitals which have to disclose their medical and coding practices. In instances where unintended up-coding is revealed, the hospitals must reimburse the sickness funds for the respective revenues that they gained through up-coding. If it is demonstrated that hospitals intentionally used up-coding as a means to increase profits, then in addition to their reimbursement fee they are required to make a penalty payment equal to the sum of their reimbursement fee. In 2009, 12 percent of all hospital cases (~1.7 million cases) were audited by the sickness funds, resulting in average claw-back amounts of about €850 per audited case (MDS, 2011).

14.3.4 Incentives for up- or wrong-coding

Up-coding, wrong-coding

The revenues of a German hospital depend on the number and value of the services delivered. This may incentivize hospitals to encode more or higher reimbursed services than actually delivered. The medical review board of the sickness funds tries to detect this up- or wrong-coding by reviewing individual cases which are randomly selected, as already described.

Cream-skimming or cherry-picking

Adverse selection is contrary to the function and maintenance mission of hospitals, especially in rural areas. As the Case Fee Catalogue is updated annually to reflect current costs for inpatient treatments, it represents a systemic (inherent) method to prevent cherry-picking as cost weights differ from one year to the next. This approach makes it impossible to predict DRG contribution margins for certain treatments in the long run and reduces incentives to adjust capacities accordingly, especially as the delivery of specific hospital services often depends on special infrastructure and may require organizational change.

Inappropriate early discharge

The risks of early discharge in order to cut costs have been well documented ever since DRG systems were first introduced. The G-DRG system tries to avoid early discharge by the application of two major instruments. First, the annual update of the Case Fee Catalogue and the recalculation of cost weights and trim-points for the reimbursement of outliers (section 14.5) are designed to reduce incentives for early discharge by reimbursing adequately for expensive services, as well as deducting payments for short-stay outliers. Second, readmissions for the same cause within 30 days after discharge are reimbursed by the original DRG (§2 Case Fee Agreement (FPV) 2010) and receive no additional funds. This approach financially penalizes inappropriate early discharge (at least if it leads to readmission).

14.4 Cost accounting within hospitals

14.4.1 Regulation

Cost accounting within hospitals is neither obligatory nor directly regulated in Germany. However, the introduction of the G-DRG system required medical and cost-controlling systems to be implemented in order to control for their resource consumption and the level of services delivered. Medical accounting is a separate administrative unit in nearly every hospital in Germany. Medical controllers (mostly physicians with further education in coding) examine hospital cases in terms of correct coding to avoid a review by the sickness funds and to maximize revenue. In addition, patient-level cost accounting is increasingly applied to monitor cost structures and sources of resource waste. In order to calculate cost weights, the InEK established a sample of hospitals that voluntarily collect patient-level cost data (InEK, 2009a). Only hospitals that can deliver cost data to a standard defined by the InEK (in the Calculation Handbook) are eligible to participate. The extra effort is reimbursed via an additional fee, which consists of a lump sum and a variable amount related to the number of delivered cases and their data quality. In 2008 the InEK spent €9 million to compensate hospitals for their additional efforts.

14.4.2 Main characteristics of the cost-accounting system

In this section we focus on hospitals that follow the cost-accounting standards specified by the InEK, as the cost-accounting characteristics of other hospitals do not affect DRG calculation and differ widely. The participating hospitals must meet certain cost-accounting standards. They must calculate costs per case according to the full cost method, using actual costs. This means that all DRG-related costs must be taken into account when calculating the costs of DRG treatment cases. The actual costs are derived from the hospitals' audited annual accounts. Accordingly, the reference period for calculating costs per case is an entire calendar year. The intention is that participating hospitals use step-down cost accounting. However, if this is not feasible they are also allowed to use a mixed calculation (using step-down cost accounting, with gross- (or top-down) costing as a second option), or even make use of a kind of gross-costing when necessary. When calculating costs per case, the only costs to be taken into consideration are those that arise due to the performance of the DRG-related services. The following cost elements are excluded:

- extraordinary expenses and expenses relating to other periods;
- investment costs;
- core business expenses, insofar as these are not related to general inpatient services (for example, costs of scientific research/teaching and costs of psychiatric and outpatient services are excluded);

- taxes, charges, insurance for operational sections of the hospital that do not provide general inpatient services, as well as tax on profits;
- specific and long-term allowance for bad debts;
- interest payable, insofar as this is not related to capital loans;
- imputed costs (for example, hospital building).

The process of calculating costs per case is based on a modular approach, which is detailed in Table 14.3 (InEK, 2007). It entails arranging each set of case-related data in the calculation according to cost-element groups and cost-centre groups. Aggregating costs across cost-element groups and cost-centre groups makes it possible to identify the costs per patient or per patient group (DRGs).

14.5 DRGs for reimbursement

14.5.1 Range of services and costs included in DRG-based hospital payments

Figure 14.6 outlines the inpatient reimbursement components used in Germany. In the Case Fee Catalogue for 2010, there are 1155 DRGs with national uniform cost weights (B2), 45 DRGs without national cost weights (D1 & D3), and 143 supplementary fees (C1 & D2) (see Table 14.2). The DRGs without national cost weights (D1 & D3) are individually negotiated with each hospital as they were excluded from the DRG national cost weights because their sample size was insufficient for calculation, or their cost variance was too large. G-DRGs are intended to cover medical treatment, nursing care, the provision of pharmaceuticals and therapeutic appliances, as well as board and accommodation.

Supplementary fees cover certain complex or cost-intensive services, and/or very expensive drugs. The supplementary fees are used due to a lack of sufficient data for calculating costs for certain DRGs, and the limited appropriateness (in terms of reflecting actual costs incurred) of the current cost weights (InEK, 2009a). These supplementary fees are generally calculated in a uniform manner across Germany. Since the introduction of supplementary fees in 2004, their number has increased from 26 to a total of 143 individual fees in 2010. These include 81 supplementary fees, whereby the amounts were fixed at the national level in the 2010 DRG Case Fee Catalogue (C1). The other 62 treatment services were included in a sub-list of supplementary fees in the Case Fee Catalogue that are to be negotiated on a hospital-by-hospital basis (D2).

In addition, the contracting parties are authorized to negotiate additional reimbursement by means of case-based or per diem remuneration for highly specialized services if it can be proved that the service in question cannot yet be appropriately reimbursed through DRGs or supplementary fees. There are also a number of surcharges which are negotiated between the contracting parties and are especially relevant for hospitals that are using new and innovative treatment options. For instance, it is possible to negotiate surcharges for innovative diagnostic and treatment procedures (E1; see section 14.6) and even to exclude certain special facilities and hospital departments completely from the G-DRG system, financing them instead through individually negotiated fees (for further

Table 14.3 G-DRG modular costing approach

	Cost-element groups									
	*Labour**			*Material†*					*Infrastructure‡*	
Cost- Centre Groups	*1*	*2*	*3*	*4a*	*4b*	*5*	*6a*	*6b*	*7*	*8*
Hospital units with beds	1.1	1.2	1.3	1.4a	1.4b	-	1.6a	1.6b	1.7	1.8
1: Normal ward	2.1	2.2	2.3	2.4a	2.4b	2.5	2.6a	2.6b	2.7	2.8
2: Intensive care unit	3.1	2.3	3.3	3.4a	3.4b	-	3.6a	3.6b	3.7	3.8
3: Dialysis unit										
Diagnostic and treatment areas	4.1	-	4.3	4.4a	4.4b	4.5	4.6a	4.6b	4.7	4.8
4: Operating room	5.1	-	5.3	5.4a	5.4b	-	5.6a	5.6b	5.7	5.8
5: Anaesthesia	6.1	-	6.3	6.4a	6.4b	-	6.6a	6.6b	6.7	6.8
6: Maternity room	7.1	-	7.3	7.4a	7.4b	7.5	7.6a	7.6b	7.7	7.8
7: Cardiac diagnostics/therapy	8.1	-	8.3	8.4a	8.4b	8.5	8.6a	8.6b	8.7	8.8
8: Endoscopic diagnostics/therapy	9.1	-	9.3	9.4a	9.4b	9.5	9.6a	9.6b	9.7	9.8
9: Radiology	10.1	-	10.3	10.4a	10.4b	10.5	10.6a	10.6b	10.7	10.8
10: Laboratories	11.1	11.2	11.3	11.4a	11.4b	11.5	11.6a	11.6b	11.7	11.8
11: Other diagnostic and therapeutic areas										

Key: *1 = Labour costs of the other medical staff; 2 = Labour costs of the nursing staff; 3 = Labour costs of the administrative and technical staff
†4a = Drug costs; 4b = Drug costs (individual costs/actual consumtion); 5 = Costs of implants and grafts; 6a = Material costs (without drugs, implants and grafts); 6b = Material costs (individual costs/ actual consumption, without drugs, implants and grafts
‡ 7 = Medical infrastructure costs; 8: Non-medical infrastructure costs.

Source: InEK, 2007, with modifications.

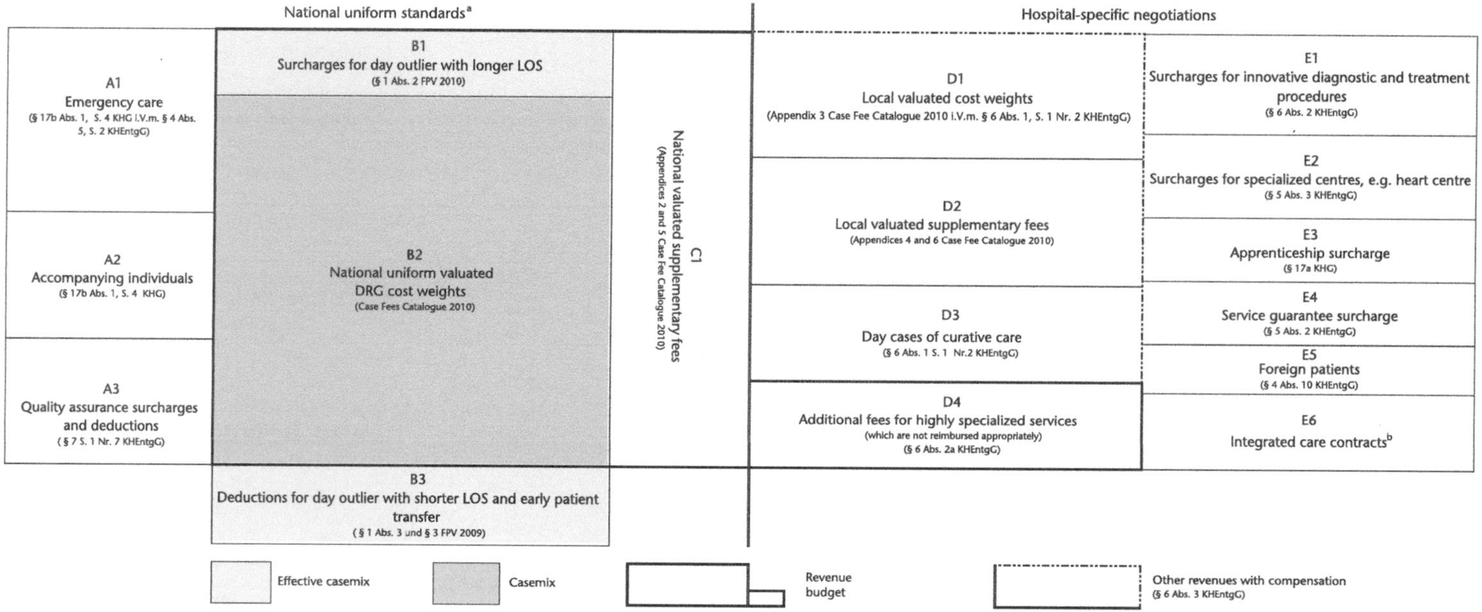

Figure 14.6 Reimbursement components of inpatient care in Germany

Source: Updated and modified from Schreyögg et al., 2006.

Notes: [a] Exception: classification as a special facility (FPVBE 2009)†; [b] Only reimbursement of the additional integrated care service which is not covered by the hospital budget (§ 140d Abs. 4 SGB V)

† Case Fee Agreement for special facilities (FPVBE), updated annually.

details, including the function of the revenue budget, see Busse and Riesberg, 2004)). Including other reimbursement components, for example for individuals accompanying patients (A2) or quality assurance (A3), all reimbursement components besides the uniformly weighted DRGs (B1–B3) currently account for approximately 20 per cent of the total reimbursement for non-psychiatric inpatient care. This remains so even though the political aim is to reimburse hospitals solely through uniformly weighted DRGs.

14.5.2 Calculation of DRG prices/cost weights

In the G-DRG system cost weights are calculated, which define a relationship between the different DRG groups according to resource intensity. Using this framework, the price for the reference treatment group with cost weight 1.0 is equal to the base rate (average costs) and the prices for all other DRGs are calculated by multiplying the DRG cost weight attached to each DRG with the price set for the reference DRG cost weight of 1.0. The cost weight of each DRG group reflects the resource consumption relative to the reference DRG, which adjusts prices for resources.

Trimming methods

The InEK applies a mathematical trimming method to account for extreme cases (InEK, 2004). Because DRG systems attempt to translate inpatient cases into medically coherent and cost-homogeneous groups, outliers are excluded for the calculation of cost weights. The term 'inlier' denotes cases that are treated within a length-of-stay interval. This is demarcated by a low trim-point and a high trim-point, between which the average treatment cases are located (Figure 14.7). Therefore, after data have been refined with plausibility checks, the average costs of inlier cases are determined for each DRG. To determine the

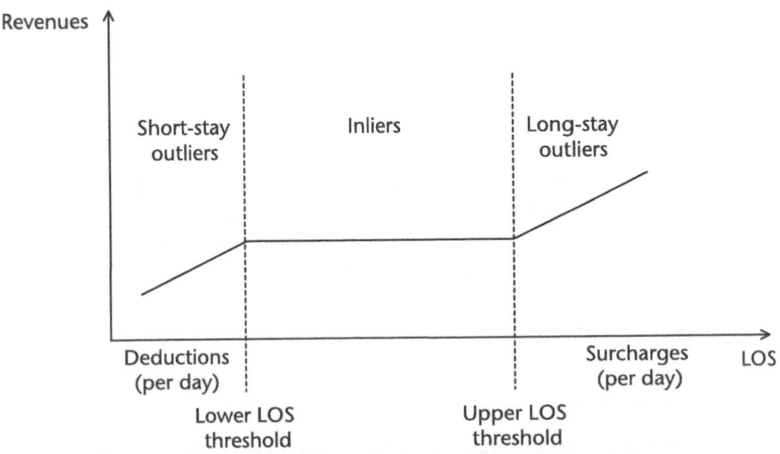

Figure 14.7 Deductions and surcharges related to the length of stay

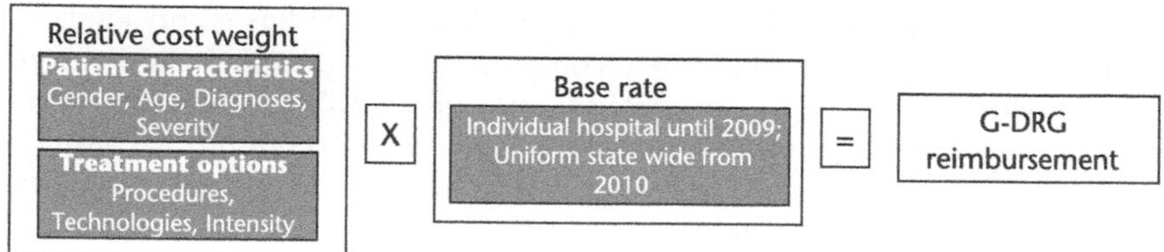

Figure 14.8 Components of G-DRG reimbursement and G-DRG implementation

cost weight for each DRG, the average costs of inlier cases for the DRG in question are divided by the reference value for the respective year. The reference value, defined as the arithmetic mean costs of all inlier cases, is calculated as the sum of DRG-relevant costs (section 14.4.2) divided by the sum of the effective casemix across Germany. The reference value used to develop the Case Fee Catalogue 2010 was €2619.10 (InEK, 2009a).

14.5.3 DRGs in actual hospital payment

The conversion from cost weights into actual reimbursement rates is given by multiplying the applicable base rate by the DRG specific cost weight (Figure 14.8). The calculation of cost weights is described in subsection 14.5.2.

14.5.4 Quality-related adjustments

The current G-DRG-system does not adjust reimbursement for quality. As reimbursement is based on average treatment costs, hospitals with a higher-than-average cost level are incentivized to cut expenditure. This can adversely affect quality as hospitals may reduce quality without incurring reimbursement penalties. To address incentives to increase profits without consideration of quality implications, the legislator introduced regulatory measures, such as mandatory quality reports, external quality assurance, quality management system(s) (QMS) and minimum volume thresholds (§137 SBG V).

Quality reports

In 2002, the Case Fees Act (FPG) introduced hospital quality reports to simplify comparisons between hospitals and to support physicians and sickness funds in advising patients regarding elective hospital treatments. Since 2005, hospitals have been obliged to submit quality reports every second year following a structure mandated by a directive of the Federal Joint Committee (G-BA). The reports are available publicly, online.

External quality assurance

Since the SHI Reform Act of 2000, hospitals have been obliged to participate in an external and comparative quality assurance programme developed by the

BQS. This programme surveys treatment-related quality indicators and compares them nationally. From 2001 to 2009, the BQS has published an annual quality report detailing the results of the hospitals, which are not named. The BQS methodology has been criticized because of the extra effort involved for hospitals to obtain data which are not part of routine datasets. From 2010 onwards, the AQUA-Institute for Applied Quality Improvement and Research in Health Care is charged with further developing and implementing the external quality assurance programme.

Quality management systems

In 1999 the legislator introduced §135a of the SGB V, obliging hospitals to launch and further develop a QMS. Hospitals have a free choice of which kind of QMS they set up. Therefore, a wide range of different QMS from simple (Cooperation for Transparency and Quality in Health Care) to more sophisticated (Joint Commission) systems were introduced across Germany. However, most patients are not able to distinguish between different quality certificates, which led to confusion instead of clarification on the part of patients.

Minimum volume thresholds

In addition to the quality reports, the FPG enacted an ordinance for defining minimum volumes as thresholds to deliver certain (particularly elective) services whereby the outcome is related to the volume of services delivered. In order to determine these services, the G-BA is charged with developing a catalogue that defines the minimum number of delivered services per physician or hospital (Velasco-Garrido & Busse, 2004). Hospitals which do not reach the required volume of services may not deliver the service. Since 2004, the catalogue has contained six elective services (with the annual minimum number per hospital shown in parentheses): liver transplantation (20), kidney transplantation (25), complex procedures on the oesophagus (10), complex procedures on the pancreas (10), stem cell transplantation (25) and knee replacement (50).

14.5.5 Main incentives for hospitals

Under the G-DRG system, hospitals are generally not incentivized to improve their medical outcomes (see subsection 14.3.4). However, within the G-DRG framework, hospitals are incentivized to create and implement a system that controls costs in order to fulfill their budgetary obligations.

14.6 New/innovative technologies

14.6.1 Steps required prior to introduction in hospitals

In Germany, most medical innovations are first introduced in the inpatient sector, because inpatient facilities may employ any technology that has not been excluded explicitly by the G-BA. The G-DRG system was designed, at least in theory, to be always current, and classification and reimbursement rates are updated each year. However, as already outlined, a certain time-lag – and thus a financing gap – is nonetheless inherent in the system, because both the G-DRG classification and the reimbursement rates are based on retrospective data. The time-lag may represent an important hurdle in the uptake of new technologies. To address this deficit, legislators introduced the so-called New Diagnostic and Treatment Methods Regulation (NUB) as part of the 2005 KHEntG. The NUB Regulation has two key objectives: first, to bridge the above-mentioned financing gap by providing for extrabudgetary, non-DRG payments for new technologies and, second, to use the data generated during this time-lag period to expedite the process for including these technologies in the regular system of G-DRG reimbursement. The NUB Regulation sets up three important regulatory hurdles that a new technology must clear before it can be included in the regular system of G-DRG reimbursement: (1) a hospital wishing to employ – and receive appropriate reimbursement for – a new medical technology must first apply to the InEK; (2) if the hospital's application is accepted, it must successfully negotiate with the sickness funds to receive NUB reimbursement for its use of the technology; and (3) the technology must ultimately be included in the regular system of G-DRG reimbursement (Henschke et al., 2010).

Applying to the InEK

A hospital wishing to employ and receive NUB reimbursement for a new medical technology must apply to the InEK for permission to enter into contractual negotiations with the sickness funds. The technology does not need to have an OPS code. The hospital's application is assessed based on the following criteria: (1) benefits to patients; (2) groups of patients who will be treated using the new technology; (3) any additional labour and material costs associated with the new technology; and (4) the reason why the costs of the new technology are not adequately covered by the current G-DRG system.

Successfully negotiating NUB reimbursement with the sickness funds

An accepted application does not guarantee that a hospital will be reimbursed for the use of a new technology. Before NUB reimbursement (E1 in Figure 14.6) can take place, the hospital must negotiate a contractual agreement with the sickness funds concerning the size of the payments to be made. If the technology in question does not have an OPS code, the hospital may negotiate contracts for two types of NUB reimbursement: additional payments, or full payments. NUB reimbursement for a technology without an OPS code represents a preliminary step towards inclusion in the regular system of G-DRG reimbursement and is represented in Figure 14.9 as the box labelled 'Accepted NUB application (without OPS)'. The arrows show prototypical pathways towards complete integration in the system.

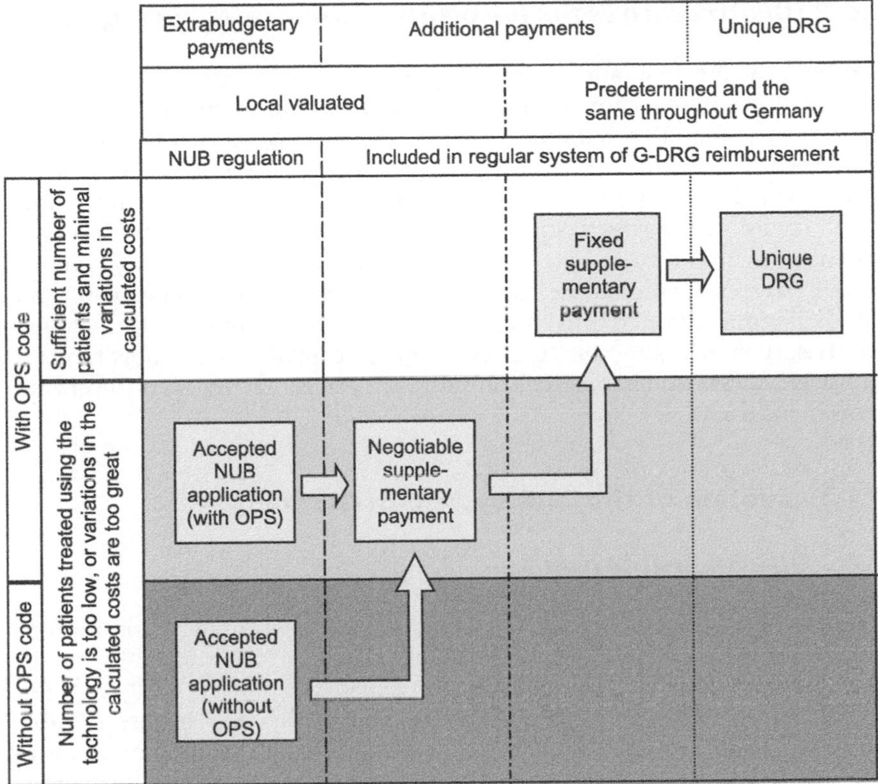

Figure 14.9 Prototypical regulatory pathways for introducing new technologies into the regular system of G-DRG reimbursement

Source: Henschke et al., 2010.

Inclusion in the regular system of G-DRG reimbursement

The lowest stage of integration within the regular system of G-DRG reimbursement is the so-called local valuated supplementary fee (D2 in Figure 14.6). These payments are made in addition to DRG payments if the use of a certain technology does not yet justify creating a unique DRG or a national valuated supplementary fee (C1 in Figure 14.6). The decision to include a technology in this category is made by the InEK. The local valuated supplementary fee has an important advantage over NUB reimbursement: once a technology has been included in the category of local valuated supplementary fees, any hospital in Germany may enter into negotiations with the sickness funds to determine the exact level of this payment. In contrast, when InEK accepts an application for NUB reimbursement, only the hospital that applied may enter into negotiations with the sickness funds; all other hospitals must apply with the InEK separately. Finally, the last stage of integration into the regular system of G-DRG reimbursement is the formation of a unique DRG.

14.6.2 (Dis-)incentives for hospitals to use new technologies

Hospitals will use new and innovative technologies if they are adequately reimbursed or are of major research interest. The NUB methodology enables hospitals to use, and be reimbursed for, new technologies that are generally more expensive than those included in the regular Case Fee Catalogue. As such, being accepted for NUB reimbursement represents a preliminary step towards the full inclusion of a new technology in the regular G-DRG system. However, a recent study found that most German hospitals do not receive any revenue via NUB payments, while those receiving NUB payments only generate 0.3 per cent of revenue through this short-term payment instrument (DKI, 2009). Moreover, the negotiation process between the hospitals and sickness funds is tedious and does not guarantee a minimum payment in the event of unsuccessful negotiations (Henschke et al., 2010).

14.7 Evaluation of the DRG system in Germany

14.7.1 Official evaluation

The corporatist partners (Federal Association of Sickness Funds, Association of Private Health Insurance, German Hospital Federation) are obliged by law to ensure adequate research is undertaken to evaluate the impact of DRGs on the provision of, as well as the quality of care (§17 KHG, para. 8). The research also addresses DRGs' effects on other supply sectors, such as rehabilitation or long-term care (transfer of services out of the hospital). To introduce evaluation activities, the corporatist institutions invite tenders for research assignments. They also assign responsibility to the InEK for evaluating hospital-related structural and case-related performance data (§21 datasets, see subsection 14.2.3). The first results of the evaluation were intended to be published in 2005, but the corporatist partners have yet to meet their legal obligations. To date, only the InEK has reported its analysis of the §21 data annually. As a first step in December 2008, the corporatist partners appointed a private institute (IGES Institute) to conduct the mandatory evaluation. Preliminary results of this evaluation indicate that the intended aims of the G-DRG system introduction will be achieved and that most of the negative consequences of prospective payment systems have not occurred (IGES, 2010). In addition, to obtain a preliminary short-term evaluation, the Federal Ministry of Health developed a qualitative questionnaire for the corporatist institutions and other important stakeholders in 2007. Results indicate a broad acceptance of the G-DRG system. However, the increased documentation effort and the increased system complexity were criticized.

In addition, several research groups and institutions have examined the effects of the G-DRG system on hospital reimbursement and service quality. During the introduction, the adequacy of reimbursement for inpatient services was evaluated (in particular by the DRG Research Group, University Hospital Münster). Through this process, shortfalls were identified in reimbursement relative to the resource consumption of medical services (delivered in certain departments, for example oncology, rheumatology or dermatology), which led to an increased number of DRGs and supplementary fees (see Table 14.2, subsection 14.2.2). Furthermore, the effects of DRGs on quality were examined in a study published in 2009 by the Centre for Quality and Management in Health Care, which is a facility of the physicians' chamber in Lower Saxony. The study found no evidence of adverse effects, such as cream-skimming or inappropriate early discharge. Other studies suggest that quality of care improved or was not substantially affected, due to better organized care since the introduction of DRGs (Sens et al., 2009).

14.7.2 Authors' assessment

As with every case payment system, the G-DRG system has strengths and weaknesses – the main ones are summarized in Table 14.4.

The increased transparency due to more precise documentation of hospital services is one of the main strengths that has been identified. Based on the annually summarized §21 datasets, a structured summary of services delivered and patient characteristics in German hospitals is undertaken.[1] Another advantage is the (increased) compliance of hospitals in supporting the G-DRG system, which involves an accurate mapping of resource consumption and a stepwise introduction process (see subsection 14.2.2). Indeed, hospitals have been obliged to use G-DRGs since 2004, but weak cooperation on the part of the hospitals is likely to have extended the introduction process. With the incorporation of cost data from universities and other large hospitals in 2005, even more complex services were available for consideration by the InEK for developing the Case Fee Catalogue. Because of larger proportions of hospitals delivering cost data, the system is now widely accepted. The use of G-DRGs for reimbursement must also be highlighted. As every coded case is equivalent to an invoice, the hospitals are strongly incentivized to code correctly in order to avoid a review of their invoices by the sickness funds (see section 14.3.3). This improves the coding quality and leads to a more accurate characterization of delivered hospital services in Germany.

Despite these strengths, there are also some weaknesses and areas in need of improvement. First, indicators of the quality of inpatient treatment are not incorporated. Therefore, the level of reimbursement is unrelated to the quality of service provision. Different approaches to incorporating quality of care

Table 14.4 Strengths and weaknesses of the G-DRG system

Strengths	*Weaknesses*
Transparency and documentation	No quality adjustments for reimbursement
Compliance of hospitals	No reflection of different input prices
Reimbursement tool	Uniform accounting system but no full sample of hospitals
Precision	Increasing complexity with number of DRGs

aspects in reimbursement – such as pay for performance (P4P) – have been discussed in Germany, but due to a lack of evidence on effectiveness and cost–effectiveness from other countries that have introduced P4P systems in recent years, there is skepticism about its appropriateness in the German context (Lüngen et al., 2008). Moreover, the development of quality indicators that can easily be collected as part of routine data is still in progress (Busse et al., 2009). Therefore, the connection between quality and reimbursement will be one of the major topics for the further development of the G-DRG system.

Second, the InEK calculates the Case Fee Catalogue with the assumption that hospital input prices do not differ across Germany and all hospitals are working under the same conditions. All cases are summarized and handled as if they were treated in the same hospital. This 'one hospital' approach prevents the consideration of hospital-specific (structural) costs within the reimbursement system. Yet, current research shows that structural differences which are not controllable by the hospitals affect their costs (Busse et al., 2008). Hence, hospitals with higher costs due to structural differences are at risk of inadequate reimbursement.

Third, the sample size of the hospitals delivering cost data could be extended in order to increase the statistical power of the cost weight calculation. With the cost-accounting scheme of the InEK as a standard (see subsection 14.4.2), more hospitals and datasets can easily be incorporated. The resulting uniform accounting system across Germany would simplify efficiency comparisons and benchmarking projects.

A known threat of DRG systems is increasing complexity with an increasing number of DRGs. With the current G-DRG system incorporating 1200 groups and several additional payments, every hospital needs to employ specialized staff for coding purposes (see subsection 14.4.1). This additional effort must be weighed against the advantages for the individual hospital and the whole system.

14.8 Outlook: Future developments and reform

14.8.1 Trends in hospital service or general delivery

There is a general trend towards concentration on selected specialties, which is an indirect result of the introduction of the G-DRGs. This has been associated with increasing hospital market penetration by (profit-making) hospital chains, and the reduction of overall capacities, which forced hospitals to specialize or to accept across-the-board cuts in resources (Leclerque & Robra, 2009). Moreover, regulatory reform of the SGB V (sections §115b, §116b, §140) provides hospitals with more freedom to offer outpatient services and to shift the boundaries between inpatient and outpatient care. A general trend is therefore the establishment of so-called 'Medizinische Versorgungszentren' (Care Centres), which try to achieve clinical as well as economic benefits through integrated care models and economies of scale (Neubauer & Minartz, 2009).

14.8.2 Trends in DRG application/coverage

In recent years the G-DRG has been characterized by two trends with regard to patient classification:

1. refinement of the grouping algorithm inherited from the AR-DRG system, especially the development of a hierarchy of sub-groups below the level of the MDCs;
2. reflection of complex treatments and repetitive surgical procedures in DRG weights; this implied greater use of procedures for defining DRGs and weighting them (Roeder et al., 2008).

Another trend is preparation for the introduction of case payments for psychiatric services/care in Germany. The latter will build on the experiences of the G-DRG system, but will most likely be an independent system that will operate totally separately. We therefore do not discuss this in any further detail here.

14.8.3 Future developments and reform

The main future development activity can be distinguished in two fields: financing and regulation, and the design implications of the G-DRG system.

Financing and regulation

There is a long-standing debate in Germany about hospital financing. Critics argue that the dualistic hospital financing structure leads to inefficient investment decisions (Felder et al., 2008). While this claim is controversial, it is widely accepted that the level of public investment in hospitals is no longer appropriate to meet infrastructural needs. Between 1993 and 2005, public investment in hospitals declined by 3 percent while adjusting for inflation (Augurzky et al., 2007). During the same period, economic pressures, documentation and performance requirements increased due to the introduction of the G-DRG system. Competitive pressures will further increase and hospitals will be even more dependent on adequate investment. Many policy-makers and researchers therefore argue that German hospital financing should follow the principle of monistic financing, that is, sickness funds should cover operating costs as well as investment in infrastructure (capital costs). Often this proposal is linked to demands to liberalize the regulation of prices and the benefits catalogue for the inpatient sector, which are currently strictly defined by collective decision-making. Large sickness funds argue that regulators should define benefits and prices only for acute and emergency services, while for elective procedures provision and prices should be negotiated between hospitals and payers (AOK BV, 2009).

G-DRG system design implications

As outlined in this case study, the G-DRG system is characterized by increasing differentiation, as the grouping of hospital services by diagnosis and procedures is constantly refined to ensure adequate resource allocation. This constant refinement nevertheless also has ambiguous consequences, such as the emergence of DRGs with a very low number of cases, decreasing stability of the payment regime as parameters constantly change, as well as increasing complexity (Roeder et al., 2008). In addition, DRGs are often no longer homogeneous in a medical sense. As a consequence, their use is increasingly limited to reimbursement purposes, as their application in quality monitoring, treatment pathways and so on is no longer appropriate (Roeder et al., 2008, p. 37). The G-DRG system may therefore need to find adequate solutions for financing specialized treatments that are as yet not adequately represented in specific DRGs. One way to achieve this may be to increase reliance on extrabudgetary, non-DRG payments for new technologies (namely, the 'NUB' approach).

14.9 Note

1 The summary for the latest available data year (currently 2008) is published on the InEK web site via an Access database and is publicly accessible (albeit in German only) (www.g-drg.de, accessed 10 July 2011).

14.10 References

AOK BV (2009). *AOK-Positionen zur Gesundheitspolitik nach der Bundestagswahl 2009*. Berlin: AOK-Bundesverband (http://www.aok-bv.de/politik/reformaktuell/index_01540.html, accessed 14 November 2009).

Augurzky, B., Engel, D., Krolop, S. et al. (2007). *Krankenhaus Rating Report 2007 – Die Streu trennt sich vom Weizen*. Essen: RWI.

Bölt, U. (2010). Statistische Krankenhausdaten: Grund- und Kostendaten der Krankenhäuser 2007, in J. Klauber, M. Geraedts, J. Friedrich, eds. *Krankenhaus-Report 2010*. Stuttgart: Schattauer.

Braun, T., Rau, F., Tuschen, K.H. (2007). Die DRG-Einführung aus gesundheitspolitischer Sicht. Eine Zwischenbilanz, in J. Klauber, B.P. Robra, H. Schellschmidt, eds. *Krankenhaus-Report 2007*. Stuttgart: Schattauer.

Busse, R., Riesberg, A. (2004). *Health Care Systems in Transition: Germany*. Copenhagen: WHO Regional Office for Europe on behalf of the European Observatory on Health Systems and Policies.

Busse, R., Nimptsch, U., Mansky, T. (2009). Measuring, monitoring, and managing quality in Germany's hospitals. *Health Affairs*, 28(2):w294–w304.

Busse, R., Schreyögg, J., Smith, P.C. (2008). Variability in healthcare treatment costs amongst nine EU countries – results from the HealthBASKET project. *Health Economics*, 17(1 Suppl.):1–8.

DESTATIS (2009). *Statistisches Jahrbuch 2009*. Wiesbaden: Statistisches Bundesamt Deutschland.

DKI (2009). *Anspruch und Realität von Budgetverhandlungen zur Umsetzung medizintechnischer Innovationen. Gutachten des Deutschen Krankenhausinstituts (DKI) im Auftrag des Bundesverbandes Medizintechnologie (BVMed)*. Düsseldorf: Deutsches Krankenhausinstitut.

Felder, S., Fetzer, S., Wasem, J. (2008). 'Was vorbei ist, ist vorbei': Zum Übergang in die monistische Krankenhausfinanzierung, in J. Klauber, B.P. Robra, H. Schellschmidt, eds. *Krankenhaus-Report 2007*. Stuttgart: Schattauer.

Friedrich, J., Leclerque, G., Paschen, K. (2008). Die Krankenhausbudgets 2004 bis 2006 unter dem Einfluss der Konvergenz, in J. Klauber, B.P. Robra, H. Schellschmidt, eds. *Krankenhaus-Report 2007*. Stuttgart: Schattauer.

Henschke, C., Bäumler, M., Weid, S., Gaskins, M., Busse, R. (2010). Extrabudgetary ('NUB') payments – a gateway for introducing new medical devices into the German inpatient reimbursement system? *Journal of Management and Marketing in Healthcare*, 3(2): 119–33.

IGES (2010). *DRG Impact Evaluation According To Section 17b Paragraph 8 Hospital Financing Act*. Berlin: IGES Institute.

InEK (2004). *Abschlussbericht zur Weiterentwicklung des G-DRG-Systems für das Jahr 2005*. Siegburg: Institut für das Entgeltsystem im Krankenhaus gGmbH.

InEK (2007). *Handbuch zur Kalkulation von Fallkosten Version 3.0*. Siegburg: Institut für das Entgeltsystem im Krankenhaus gGmbH.

InEK (2009a). *Abschlussbericht zur Weiterentwicklung des G-DRG-Systems für das Jahr 2010*. Siegburg: Institut für das Entgeltsystem im Krankenhaus gGmbH.

InEK (2009b). *Verfahrenseckpunkte: Anfragen nach § 6 Abs. 2 KHEntgG (Neue Untersuchungs- und Behandlungsmethoden) für 2009*. Siegburg: Institut für das Entgeltsystem im Krankenhaus gGmbH.

Leclerque, C., Robra, B.R. (2009). Einführung, in J. Klauber, B.R. Robra, H. Schellschmidt, eds. *Krankenhaus-Report 2008/2009*. Stuttgart: Schattauer.

Lüngen, M., Gerber, A., Lauterbach, K.W. (2008). Pay for Performance: Neue Impulse für den Wettbewerb zwischen Krankenhäusern? in J. Klauber, B.P. Robra, H. Schellschmidt, eds. *Krankenhaus-Report 2007*. Stuttgart: Schattauer.

MDS (2011). *Abrechnungsprüfungen der MDK in Krankenhäusern sind angemessen, wirtschaftlich und zielführend. Zahlen und Fakten der MDK-Gemeinschaft*. Essen: Medizinischer Dienst des Spitzenverbandes Bund der Krankenkassen e.V.

Neubauer, G., Minartz, C. (2009). Zentrierte Versorgung – Ziele und Optionen, in J. Klauber, B.R. Robra, H. Schellschmidt, eds. *Krankenhaus-Report 2008/2009*. Stuttgart: Schattauer.

Neubauer, G., Pfister, F. (2008). DRGs in Germany: introduction of a comprehensive, prospective DRG payment system by 2009, in J.R. Kimberly, G. de Pouvourville, T. D'Aunno, eds. *The Globalization of Managerial Innovation in Health Care*. Cambridge: Cambridge University Press.

Roeder, N., Bunzmeier, H., Fiori, W. (2008). Ein lernendes Vergütungssystem – Vom Budgetierungsinstrument zum deutschen Preissystem, in J. Klauber, B.P. Robra, H. Schellschmidt, eds. *Krankenhaus-Report 2007*. Stuttgart: Schattauer.

Schreyögg, J., Tiemann, O., Busse, R. (2006). Cost accounting to determine prices: how well do prices reflect costs in the German DRG system? *Health Care Management Science*, 9:269–80.

Sens, B., Wenzlaff, P., Pommer, G., von der Hardt, H. (2009). *DRG-induzierte Veränderungen und ihre Auswirkungen auf die Organisationen, Professionals, Patienten und Qualität*. Hanover: Zentrum für Qualität und Management im Gesundheitswesen, Einrichtung der Ärztekammer Niedersachsen.

Tuschen, K.H., Trefz, U. (2004). *Krankenhausentgeltgesetz: Kommentar*. Stuttgart: Kohlhammer.

Velasco-Garrido, M., Busse, R. (2004). Förderung der Qualität in deutschen Krankenhäusern? Eine kritische Diskussion der ersten Mindestmengenvereinbarung. *Gesundheits- und Sozialpolitik*, 58(5/6):10–20.

chapter fifteen

Ireland: A review of casemix applications within the acute public hospital system

Jacqueline O'Reilly, Brian McCarthy and Miriam Wiley[1]

15.1 Hospital services and the role of DRGs in Ireland

15.1.1 The Irish health care system

Health care expenditure in Ireland experienced unprecedented growth during the late 1990s, increasing by almost 80 per cent in real terms between 1997 and 2002 (Nolan, 2005; Wiley, 2005; McDaid et al., 2009). Growth in expenditure has remained strong in subsequent years and total current health expenditure was in excess of €19 billion in 2008 (McDaid et al., 2009; Brick et al., 2010). About four fifths of total (current and capital) health expenditure was publicly funded in 2007, up from three quarters in 1997 (McDaid et al., 2009; OECD, 2009; Brick et al., 2010). Private health expenditure from out-of-pocket payments and private health insurance accounted for the remainder (Brick et al., 2010). In 2007, public health expenditure accounted for 7.2 per cent of gross domestic product (GDP) (8.5 per cent of gross national product, GNP) (McDaid et al., 2009).[2]

This period of expenditure growth was followed by fundamental structural reform. The health system was previously organized according to a regional structure. However, this decentralized structure created tensions between national health policy objectives and local service delivery (Brennan, 2003; Prospectus, 2003; McDaid et al., 2009). Consequently, the Health Service Executive (HSE) was established in January 2005 to focus on service delivery and management at national level, while the Department of Health and Children (DoHC) was charged with devising policy and strategy, thereby effecting a separation of operation and management from policy-making. Since October

2009 the Integrated Services Directorate within the HSE oversees the primary care and acute hospital sectors – a task that was previously divided between the Primary, Community and Continuing Care Directorate and the National Hospitals Office (HSE, 2010d).

The unusual public/private interaction in Irish health care means that acute public hospitals can provide private services. Private practice within public hospitals is generally constrained to beds designated for private patients, which amount to approximately 20 per cent of all acute public hospital beds nationally.[3] Consultants in acute public hospitals may – depending on their employment contract – be permitted to treat private patients up to a maximum of 20–30 per cent of their complexity-adjusted workload (Brick et al., 2010). Public hospitals and consultants face different payment mechanisms for public and private patients, which have been criticized for incentivizing the treatment of private patients (Nolan & Wiley, 2000; Colombo & Tapay, 2004; Brick et al., 2010; O'Reilly & Wiley, 2010; Ruane, 2010). Given the relatively low number of private hospitals and the paucity of readily available private sector data, what follows focuses on the acute public hospital sector.[4]

There are three main categories of entitlement to access health care services in Ireland (see Table 15.1). Eligibility for a medical card is largely determined on the basis of income (McDaid et al., 2009).[5] GP visit cards are also allocated on the basis of income, with the income threshold being 50 per cent higher than that for medical card holders (Brick et al., 2010). In 2009, medical card holders and GP visit card holders comprised 33.2 per cent and 2.2 per cent of the population, respectively (DoHC, 2010a). The remainder of the population (approximately 65 per cent in 2009; Brick et al., 2010) do not qualify for a medical card or a GP visit card. About 46 per cent of the population in 2009 held supplementary private health insurance, which mainly covers acute hospital services (Brick et al., 2010). A further 5 per cent held both a medical card and private health insurance (Brick et al., 2010).

15.1.2 Hospital services in Ireland

In 2010, 52 acute public hospitals provided day-case, inpatient, outpatient and emergency department (ED) services to public and private patients (Brick et al., 2010; HSE, 2010c). All of these public hospitals receive funding from the HSE on a global budget basis (McDaid et al., 2009; Brick et al., 2010). Annual global budgets are determined on an historic basis, with some adjustment for, *inter alia*, inflation, pay adjustments and one-off funding. A subset of these public hospitals (39 in 2010; HSE, 2010a) participate in the National Casemix Programme under which their global budgets are prospectively adjusted using diagnosis-related groups (DRGs) (see subsection 15.5).

In addition to funding public hospitals, the HSE also directly operates 34 acute public hospitals (Brick et al., 2010; ESRI-HRID, 2010). The remaining public hospitals are typically owned and operated by voluntary organizations (for example, religious orders) (Robbins & Lapsley, 2008; McDaid et al., 2009). A small number of acute public hospitals provide specialist services (such as maternity, paediatric and orthopaedic care). Table 15.2 provides a breakdown of

Table 15.1 Health care charges for public and private patients

	Public patient		*Private patient*
	Medical card holder	*Non-medical card holder (including GP visit card holder)*	
GP visits	Nil	Charge determined by GP Nil for GP visit card holder	Charge determined by GP
Prescription medicines	50c charge per prescription item up to maximum of €10 per family per month[a]	Free above €120 out-of-pocket payment per month No charge for certain long-term illnesses/ conditions	
Public hospitals			
ED	Nil	€100 unless referred by GP or subsequently admitted to hospital[c]	
Outpatient department	Nil	€100 unless referred by GP or subsequently admitted to hospital[c] No charge for repeat attendances	
Day case/ inpatient	Nil[b]	Daily hospital charge of €75 (up to a maximum of €750 in any 12 consecutive months)[b]	Daily hospital charge as per public patients plus a hospital maintenance charge and consultant fees[d]

Sources: Adapted from Brick et al., 2010; Citizens Information Board, 2011.

Notes: [a]From 1 October 2010; [b]Additional charges may be levied on long-stay patients; [c]Rates effective from 1 January 2009; [d]The hospital maintenance charge is a per diem charge, which varies according to the type of treatment (inpatient or day case), accommodation (private or semi-private bed) and hospital (DoHC, 2009b); For 2011, this charge ranges from €193 for day care in district hospitals to €1017 for private accommodation in certain hospitals, such as regional hospitals (Citizens Information Board, 2010).

public hospitals by their size, ownership and type and Table 15.3 reports the changes in hospital beds and activity between 2000 and 2008.[6]

15.1.3 Purpose of the DRG system

The DRG system in Ireland has a number of national applications. First, following a recommendation of the Commission on Health Funding (1989), the DRG system has been used since 1993 to adjust acute public hospitals' budgetary allocations for the complexity of their casemix and their relative performance. Second, under a renegotiated contract (effective from September 2008), the outputs of the national casemix models are used to adjust hospital consultants' day-case and inpatient activity for complexity and to take account of their involvement in each case (HSE, 2008). Third, DRG data feed into *HealthStat*, a

Table 15.2 Distribution of hospitals by number of beds, ownership and type, 2008

Number of beds	*HSE*			*Public voluntary*			*Total (HSE and public voluntary)*		
	General	*Special*	*Total*	*General*	*Special*	*Total*	*General*	*Special*	*Total*
<100	5	4	9	2	1	3	7	5	12
100–<200	5	1	6	2	4	6	7	5	12
200–<300	10	0	10	2	2	4	12	2	14
300–<400	5	0	5	0	0	0	5	0	5
400–<500	0	0	0	0	0	0	0	0	0
500–<600	3	0	3	1	0	1	4	0	4
≥600	1	0	1	4	0	4	5	0	5
Total	**29**	**5**	**34**	**11**	**7**	**18**	**40**	**12**	**52**

Source: Adapted from Brick et al., 2010.

Notes: Data on psychiatric beds were not available for four hospitals; Bed data relate to the average number of beds available and include both day-case and inpatient beds.

Table 15.3 Summary of hospital activity and beds, 2000 and 2008

	2000			*2008*			*% change 2000–2008*
	Number	*%*	*Rate per 1000 population*	*Number*	*%*	*Rate per 1000 population*	
Hospital beds							
Day-case beds	721	5.8	0.2	1 697	12.2	0.4	135.4
Inpatient beds	11 704	94.2	3.1	12 182	87.8	2.8	4.1
Total beds	*12 425*	*100*	*3.3*	*13 879*	*100*	*3.1*	*11.7*
Discharges							
Day-case discharges	273 677	34.3	72.2	771 145	56.3	174.4	181.8
Inpatient discharges	525 181	65.7	138.6	597 449	43.7	135.1	13.8
Total discharges	*798 858*	*100*	*210.8*	*1 368 594*	*100*	*309.5*	*71.3*
Beds days							
Day case	273 677	7.5	72.2	771 145	17.2	174.4	181.8
Inpatient	3 371 089	92.5	889.6	3 700 959	82.8	836.9	9.8
Total bed days	*3 644 766*	*100*	*961.8*	*4 472 104*	*100*	*1 011.3*	*22.7*
Acute inpatient ALOS (days)[a]	*5.0*	–	–	*4.6*	–	–	*–8.0*
ED attendances	*1 211 279*	–	*319.6*	*1 150 674*	–	*260.2*	*–5.0*
Outpatient attendances	*1 996 474*	–	*526.8*	*3 288 917*	–	*743.7*	*64.7*

Sources: ESRI-HPID, 2007; DoHC, 2009a, 2010a; ESRI-HRID, 2010.

Notes: These data relate to hospitals that participated in the Hospital In-Patient Enquiry (HIPE); All acute public hospitals (apart from one) and a small number of long stay hospitals participated in HIPE in 2008; HIPE data collection has changed over the period (see, for example, ESRI-HRID, 2008b); [a]Acute inpatients are inpatients with a length of stay of 30 days or less.

HSE initiative to monitor and assess performance within the acute public hospital sector (HSE, 2010b). In addition, the DRG system has been (and continues to be) used to inform the planning and reconfiguration of acute hospital services.

15.2 Development and updates of the DRG system

15.2.1 The current DRG system at a glance

The Australian Refined Diagnosis-Related Group (AR-DRG) system was adopted in Ireland in 2005 for classifying day-case and inpatient activity (excluding non-acute psychiatry, geriatric care and rehabilitation) (ESRI-HRID, 2008a). The current version of AR-DRGs (Version 6.0) was introduced in Ireland in January 2009. For the 2010 casemix budgetary adjustment, a patient classification system specifically designed for the HSE – Treatment-Related Groups (TRGs) – was used for the first time to group outpatient attendances. There is currently no grouper for ED attendances in Ireland. The remainder of this chapter will focus on the day-case and inpatient casemix models. The HSE's National Casemix Programme is responsible for developing these models and combining the required cost and activity data from hospitals. The AR-DRG algorithm is outlined in section 15.3.2.

15.2.2 Development of the DRG system

Since DRGs were introduced in Ireland in the early 1990s, 10 classification systems have been used for inpatient and day-case activity (see Table 15.4). These classification systems are discussed in greater detail in the remainder of this section.

Inpatient classification systems

Between 1992 and 2002, the United States Health Care Financing Administration (HCFA)-DRGs, together with Maryland cost/service weights, were used to group

Table 15.4 Overview of inpatient and day-case classification systems used in Ireland

Data year[a]	*Inpatient classification system*		*Day-case classification system*	
	System	*Version*	*System*	*Version*
1992–1993	HCFA	9	No grouper	
1994–1998		12	DPG procedural grouper	
1999–2001		16		
2002			DG procedural grouper	
2003–2004	AR-DRG	5.0		
2005–2008		5.1	ADRG	5.1
2009 to date		6.0		6.0

Note: [a]Data year refers to the year(s) in which the discharge activity took place.

inpatients in Ireland (see Table 15.4). During this period, updates to the grouper were driven by revisions to the clinical coding scheme (International Classification of Diseases 9th revision – Clinical Modification, ICD-9-CM) in Ireland. The HCFA classification had a maximum of two severity levels – with or without complications.

Recognizing the need to update the clinical coding scheme to ICD-10, the DoHC commissioned a review of alternative grouping schemes in 2003 (Aisbett et al., 2007). As part of this review, several groupers were evaluated against a range of criteria, including vendor support, and international use and recognition. The review recommended the adoption of an unmodified version of the AR-DRG Version 5.0 grouper.

For 2003 and 2004, it was necessary to use a coding map to convert clinical data coded in ICD-9-CM to ICD-10-AM (10th revision, Australian Modification) for diagnoses and to the Australian Classification of Health Interventions (ACHI) for procedures.[7] However, since 2005, all Hospital In-Patient Enquiry (HIPE) data have been coded using unmodified versions of ICD-10-AM and ACHI (see Murphy and colleagues (2004) on adopting these coding schemes).

Table 15.5 demonstrates key differences between the four DRG systems used to group inpatients in Ireland since 1999. Compared to previous classifications, AR-DRGs have a slightly higher number of groups, more severity levels, and can be applied to day cases as well as inpatients.

Table 15.5 Key facts on DRG systems used in Ireland since 1999

	HCFA-DRG Version 16	*AR-DRG*		
		Version 5.0	*Version 5.1*	*Version 6.0*
Year of introduction	1999	2003	2005	2009
Data year	1999–2002	2003–2004	2005–2008	2009 to date
Number of groups	511	665	665	698
Sub-classification	None	ADRG (399)	ADRG (399)	ADRG (399)
Maximum severity levels	2	4	4	4
Birth weight	Not used	Required		
Type of cases included	Inpatient only, excluding non-acute psychiatric care, geriatric care and rehabilitation	Inpatients and day cases, excluding non-acute psychiatric care, geriatric care and rehabilitation		
Number of MDCs	25	24[a]	24[a]	24[a]
Number of participating public hospitals	32 (2002)	32 (2004)	39 (2008)	39 (2009)

Sources: Based on information from HCFA (undated); see also Commonwealth Department of Health and Ageing, 2002, 2004, 2008; National Casemix Programme, 2010a.

Note: [a]Includes Pre-MDC.

Day-case classification systems

In Ireland, a day case is characterized by a patient being admitted electively and discharged on the same day, as planned. The National Casemix Programme was extended to include day-case activity in the mid-1990s. The first day-case classification system – the Day Patient Grouper (DPG) – was developed by the DoHC, based on similar United States groupers (Table 15.4). The DPG defined 73 groups, differentiated mainly on the basis of principal procedure coded in ICD-9-CM. Cases without procedures were grouped into a single medical day-case group. In 2002, the DPG was replaced by the Day Grouper (DG), which was also developed by the DoHC and comprised 169 groups. Like its predecessor, the DG was predominantly driven by the principal procedure, although diagnoses were also used in some cases to determine the group.

With the introduction of AR-DRGs in Ireland, day cases and inpatients could be included in the same classification system. Under the AR-DRG classification scheme, Adjacent DRGs (ADRGs) are used to group day cases (see subsection 15.3.2).[8] Unlike the procedural-based DPGs and DGs, the AR-DRG classification for day cases incorporates more information than simply the principal procedure.

15.2.3 Data used for development and updates of the DRG system

The AR-DRG classification system from Australia, which was adopted in Ireland, was developed in the late 1990s by the Australian Casemix Clinical Committee (ACCC). To update the AR-DRG system, the ACCC relies on Australian clinical and cost data, as well as on input from Australian health professionals (Commonwealth Department of Health and Ageing, 2008).

Irish cost/service weights are determined by modifying Australian cost/service weights using Irish data from the hospital costing file. The costing file is based on hospitals' Annual Financial Statements (AFSs) and consists of specialty-level hospital cost data for inpatients and day cases.[9]

Data on day-case and inpatient activity for the DRG system and the National Casemix Programme are obtained from the HIPE system, which is the only national source of administrative, demographic and clinical information on discharges from acute public hospitals in Ireland. Since 1990, the Economic and Social Research Institute (ESRI) has been responsible for all aspects of managing this database.

15.2.4 Regularity and method of system updates

The AR-DRG grouper classification is updated every two years in Australia in conjunction with the update of the ICD-10-AM classification. Since their adoption in Ireland, the clinical coding and AR-DRG classifications have been updated every four years (only twice so far – 1 January 2005 and 1 January 2009).[10] To date, therefore, Ireland has adopted every second version of the AR-DRG classifications.

15.3 The current patient classification system

15.3.1 Information used to classify patients

In Ireland, administrative, demographic and clinical data from the HIPE database are used to group hospital discharges into AR-DRGs (see subsection 15.2.3).[11]

Administrative and demographic data

Relevant administrative data include admission and discharge dates, discharge destination (for example, home, transfer to rehabilitation), and length of stay. Demographic variables consist of date of birth, age in years/days, and gender. Three further variables (non-acute length of stay, leave days, and mental health legal status) are required by the grouper, but are not available in Ireland and, consequently, are set to their default values.

Clinical data

Since January 2009, clinical data are coded in the HIPE using the sixth edition of ICD-10-AM, which contains the ACHI classification for procedures. Two sets of coding standards apply: the Australian coding standards and the complementary Irish coding standards. The grouper requires a principal diagnosis and can accept up to 29 additional diagnoses and up to 30 procedures.[12] Resource-consumption information – such as length of stay in an intensive care environment – is implicit in the coded procedures used in the grouper.

15.3.2 Classification algorithm

Grouping occurs in the hospital after the case has been coded. Each discharge is allocated to one group only. The AR-DRG grouping algorithm consists of four steps (see Figure 15.1).[13] In the first step, data on each discharge undergo a series of checks for completeness, validity and consistency. Failing a check may result in a discharge being assigned to an Error AR-DRG. In addition to these checks, HIPE data are subject to rigorous validation checks during the collection process (see subsection 15.3.3).

In the second step, the principal diagnosis determines the allocation to one of 24 major diagnostic categories (MDCs).[14] For certain specialist, high-cost conditions (such as transplants), however, the initial MDC assignment may be altered, with some discharges being reclassified to a Pre-MDC.

The presence of a procedure and its type are used to classify discharges into one of three partitions, which constitutes the third step. A discharge is assigned to the 'surgical' partition if there was at least one operating room (OR) procedure; to the 'other' partition if there was at least one relevant non-OR procedure; or to the 'medical' partition if there were no relevant procedures (that is, a procedure may have been performed, but it was not relevant to the MDC). After the partition is assigned, the discharge is allocated to one of 399 ADRGs, depending

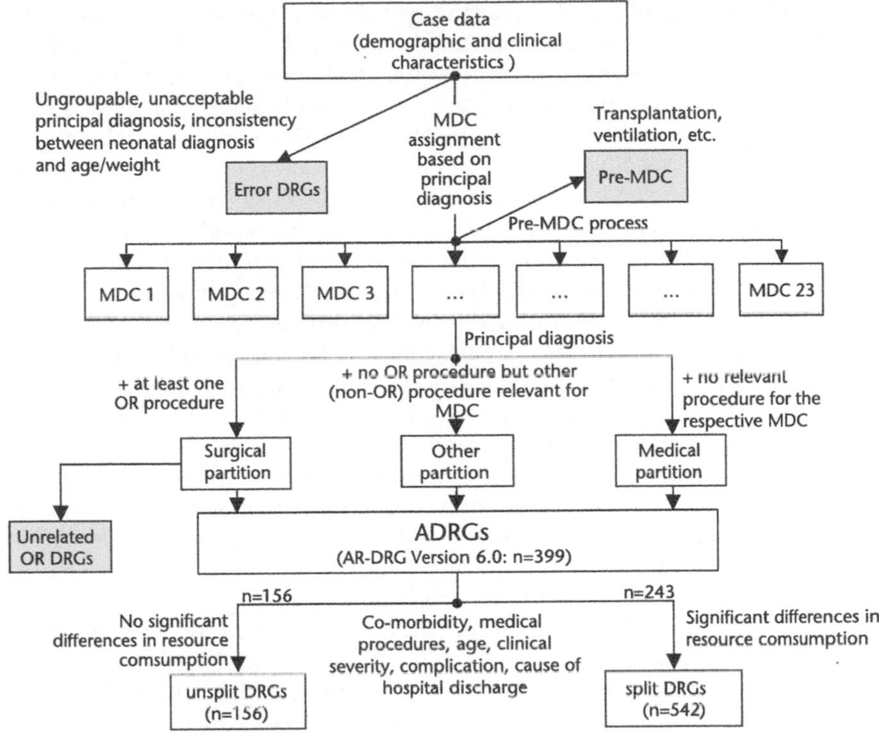

Figure 15.1 Assignment to DRGs using the AR-DRG classification scheme

Source: Adapted from Commonwealth Department of Health and Ageing, 2008.

on diagnoses, procedures and administrative data. The ADRG assignment completes the grouping process for day cases.

Finally, the discharge is allocated to one of 698 AR-DRGs according to severity level, which is determined by characteristics considered to be drivers of resource use (for example, presence of complications and co-morbidities (CCs), age, gender).[15] Usually, CCs are considered in combination to provide a composite score (the Patient Clinical Complexity Level, PCCL) that indicates the patient's overall complexity and determines the final AR-DRG.[16]

Each AR-DRG consists of four alphanumeric characters (Commonwealth Department of Health and Ageing, 2008). The first character is a letter between A and Z indicating the MDC. The second and third characters are numbers, which (together with the MDC letter) define the three-character ADRG. The final character is a letter and indicates whether the ADRG was not split (denoted by 'Z') or the level of severity/resource use (with four categories starting with 'A', indicating the highest resource use).

15.3.3 Data quality and plausibility checks

In addition to the data checks described in subsection 15.3.2, HIPE data are also subjected to several plausibility and validity checks at local (hospital) and national levels. The first set of plausibility checks occurs in hospitals during the data-entry phase and these have been built into the standardized HIPE data-collection software, which has been developed by the Health Research and Information Division (HRID) within the ESRI and is provided free of charge to all participating hospitals. The software has been designed to validate information as it is entered, so that coders can readily reference patient charts if necessary. Such plausibility checks include: validation of diagnosis and procedure codes against patient administrative and demographic details; examining the ordering of diagnoses to ensure that certain diagnosis codes are never used as the principal diagnosis; and notifying coders of certain unusual diagnosis/procedure combinations.

A further set of checks is conducted by the HRID on the national HIPE file. First, year-on-year changes in casemix-adjusted discharges (calculated on the same basis for all years) for a particular hospital are examined. Second, casemix-adjusted discharges are compared to costs in order to identify where activity has increased without a corresponding increase in costs.

Analysis of the national file may highlight specific areas at specialty or AR-DRG level where patient-level audits are required. These audits are carried out by trained coders, external to the hospital. Local audits by hospitals are also supported by the HIPE system and the HRID has developed the HIPE Coding Audit Toolkit (HCAT) to assist in this process.[17]

The National Casemix Programme may revise the number of allocated casemix-adjusted discharges if there is evidence from these checks and external audits that inaccurate data have been submitted (such as the inclusion of outpatient activity in the day-case model). Where costs or activity data are found to be incomplete or inaccurate, this would be expected to result in a lower casemix budgetary adjustment.

15.4 Cost accounting within hospitals

15.4.1 Regulation

Hospitals participating in the National Casemix Programme must submit their cost data to the hospital costing dataset in a standardized format, as outlined in the casemix specialty costing manual. These data are then submitted to the National Casemix Programme, which performs regular data quality audits. In the first step of the audit process, all costs submitted in the costing file are reconciled with the AFS to check for omissions or errors. Hospitals' costs and patient activity data are then linked using the national casemix models. The overall audit process typically involves discussions between the National Casemix Programme and the hospitals. Where issues remain unresolved, the National Casemix Programme can amend the hospital costing file where the costing manual rules have been breached.

15.4.2 Main characteristics of the cost-accounting system

The cost-accounting system for the casemix models starts by adjusting hospitals' AFSs (for example, excluding capital expenditures which are not financed through the national casemix models; National Casemix Programme, 2010b). In line with the HSE's costing manual, the adjusted AFS costs are allocated on a top-down basis to specialty level for inpatients and day cases, as well as to outpatient clinics, primarily using direct allocation.

Once the hospital costing files are submitted and the auditing process by the National Casemix Programme is complete, the national costing file is prepared. For compatibility with the national casemix models, the costing file is arranged into the following 13 cost centres: allied health; critical care; coronary care unit; emergency; imaging; pathology; medical pay; prosthesis; nursing; pharmacy; theatre operating procedures; theatre non-operating procedures; and blood.

When the national casemix models are complete, the combined national patient activity and costing file is used to produce national statistics (for example, average cost per casemix-adjusted discharge).

15.5 DRGs for hospital financing

15.5.1 Range of services and costs included in casemix-adjusted budgets

Public hospitals are invited to participate in the National Casemix Programme by the HSE. The number of participating acute public hospitals increased from 15 in 1993 to 39 in 2009 (HSE, 2010a; National Casemix Programme, 2010a). To ensure comparability, hospitals are assigned to one of four peer groups in the Programme. In the 2009 casemix models, Group I included eight major academic teaching hospitals; Group II contained 26 hospitals; and three maternity and two paediatric hospitals constituted the remaining two groups. Casemix budgetary adjustments are calculated separately for each hospital group.

There are separate national casemix models for day cases and inpatients; non-acute psychiatry, geriatric care and rehabilitation are excluded. All costs are included in the models, apart from those related to capital, depreciation, pensions, bad debts and transfers from other hospitals. Teaching costs are included but research costs are financed separately. Less than 80 per cent of all acute public hospital costs were included in the most recent casemix models (run in 2009; National Casemix Programme, 2010d). As part of the cost-reconciliation process, all participating hospitals can make submissions on a case-by-case basis to the National Casemix Programme for additional funding for unusual and/or high-cost activity.

15.5.2 Service weights and relative values

In Ireland, service weights (locally referred to as cost weights) differ from relative values (RVs).[18] Service weights indicate the share of specialty costs allocated to each AR-DRG and are defined for each of the 13 cost centres listed in subsection 15.4.2. Service weights are based on the patient cost data from

Australia, adapted to the Irish health care system by the inclusion of Irish cost data. In contrast, RVs indicate the relative resource intensity of each AR-DRG.[19] RVs are calculated separately for day cases and inpatients as part of the casemix models using the national cost and activity files. A separate set of RVs is determined for paediatric hospitals, given their specialist nature.

The process for determining the inpatient RVs is described here.

1. Inpatient discharge data are initially trimmed at three standard deviations from the mean length of stay for each AR-DRG to remove cases with extremely short or long lengths of stay from the calculation of the upper and lower length-of-stay thresholds, which are set at 1.96 standard deviations above and below the mean, respectively.[20]
2. The average cost per cost centre and per hospital is determined using the hospital's inpatient cost and activity data, together with inpatient service weights.
3. The inpatient cost and discharge activity data are analysed per AR-DRG to calculate the national average costs per DRG and RVs.

15.5.3 DRG-based budgetary adjustments

The following subsections describe how hospitals' casemix budgetary adjustments are determined.

Calculation of hospital casemix-adjusted activity/casemix units

The casemix unit (CMU) is determined by the RV of the AR-DRG to which the patient is assigned, the patient's length of stay, and the upper and lower length-of-stay thresholds of the AR-DRG. The casemix-adjusted activity of each hospital is the sum of the CMUs across all discharges. Since RVs are calculated using different models and cost data for inpatients and day cases, it is not possible to combine casemix-adjusted inpatient activity with that for day cases.

Figure 15.2 illustrates how the CMU is determined for inpatient discharges. The CMU for a same-day, one-day or inlier case can be determined directly, since same-day, one-day and inlier RVs are calculated separately for each AR-DRG. If the patient is a low outlier, the CMU is determined using the one-day RV with a per diem adjustment. Conversely, the CMU for high outliers is based on the inlier RV of the patient's AR-DRG plus a per diem AR-DRG adjustment for each day in hospital above the upper threshold.

Casemix-adjusted day cases are simply the RV of the applicable ADRG.

Determining hospital casemix budgetary adjustment

Figure 15.3 shows the calculation of a casemix-adjusted budget for inpatients. The casemix-adjusted budget of a hospital depends on the hospital's CMUs and base rate, a peer-group base rate and a blend rate. The hospital base rate is calculated by dividing the total costs of the hospital by the hospital's CMUs.

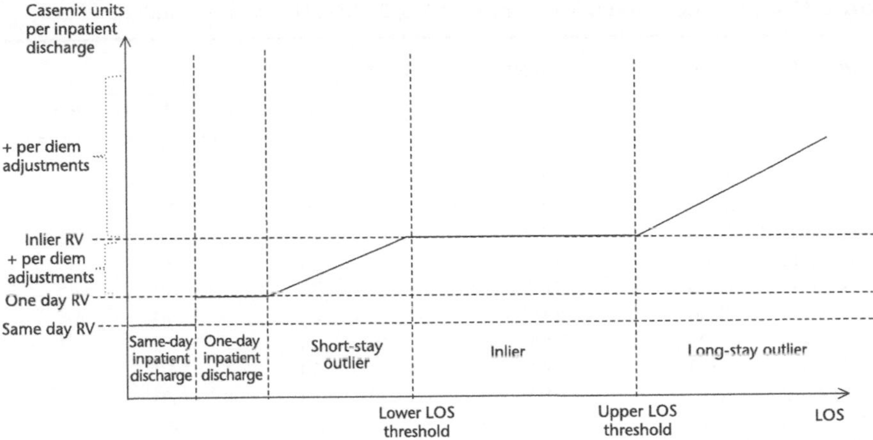

Figure 15.2 Distribution of CMUs for inpatient discharges

Notes: A same-day case is admitted and discharged on the same day. Unlike a day case, which is an elective episode, a same-day case may be admitted as an emergency. A one-day case has admission and discharge dates on consecutive days, thereby spending one night in hospital. An inlier has an LOS between the upper and lower bounds of the AR-DRG. A short-stay outlier is admitted for more than one day and is discharged before their LOS exceeds the lower bound. The RV for this case is a per diem weight. A long-stay outlier case has an LOS which exceeds the upper bound. The RV for this case is a per diem weight.

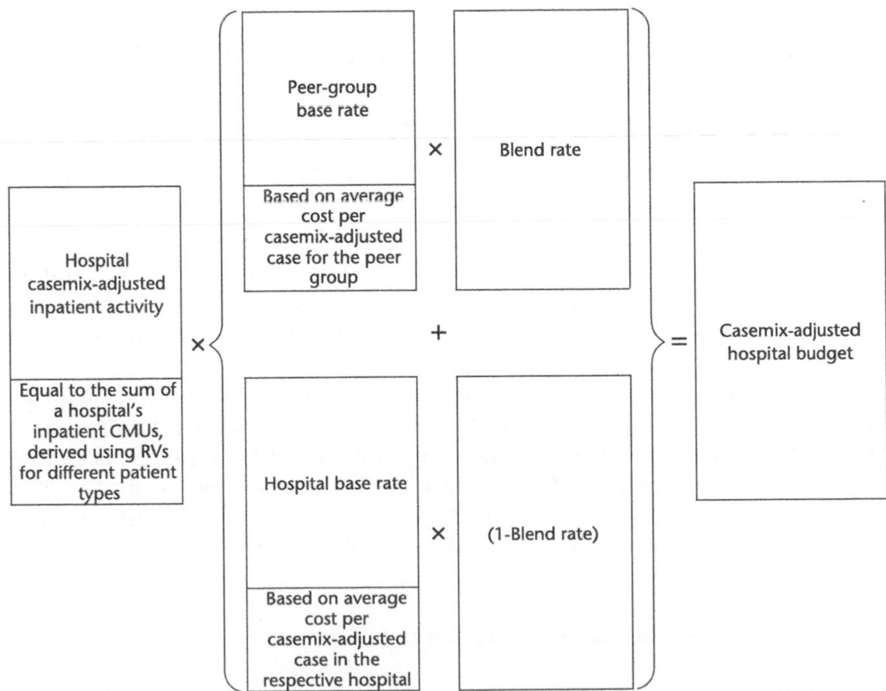

Figure 15.3 Calculation of the hospital inpatient casemix-adjusted budget

Table 15.6 Inpatient and day-case blend rates, 2000–2010 casemix models

Model data[a]	*Model*	*Budgetary adjustment*	*Blend rate*	
			Inpatient (%)	*Day case (%)*
1999/2000	2000	2001	15	5
2000/2001	2001	2002	15	5
2001/2002	2002	2003	20	10
2002/2003	2003	2004	20	10
2003/2004	2004	2005	20	20
2004/2005	2005	2006	30	30
2005/2006	2006	2007	40	40
2006/2007	2007	2008	50	50
2007/2008	2008	2009	60	60
2008/2009	2009	2010	70	70
2009/2010	2010	2011	80	80

Source: National Casemix Programme, 2010a.

Notes: A blend rate of more than 50 per cent implies that hospital budgets are determined more by the costs of treating patients in the hospital's peer group than based on the hospital's own costs. For example, a blend rate of 70 per cent implies that the calculated cost for a casemix-adjusted discharge will be based on 70 per cent of the peer-group costs and 30 per cent of the hospital's own costs. [a]The casemix models include a workload adjustment which is calculated on the basis of activity in the latter half of year *t* and the first half of year *t+1*. Thus, a blend rate of 70 per cent is applied to the inpatient/day-case adjustments (68 per cent) and the workload adjustment (2 per cent).

The peer-group base rate is calculated by dividing total costs of treating patients in a particular hospital group by the total CMUs for that group. The blend rate is used to mitigate any potentially destabilizing effects of the casemix budgetary adjustments on hospitals.[21] Since the early 2000s, the blend rate has progressively increased – a trend which is likely to continue (see Table 15.6). An ADRG-based budget is similarly calculated for day cases.

There is a lag between the time period to which the activity and cost data relate and the application of the casemix budgetary adjustment. For example, the 2009 casemix models used activity and cost data from 2008 and from the first half of 2009 to calculate the casemix budgetary adjustments that applied to hospitals' 2010 budgets.

The difference between the hospital's casemix-adjusted budget and their historic allocation is the casemix budgetary adjustment. A hospital will receive a positive budget adjustment if the calculated casemix-adjusted budget is greater than the historical budgets. The casemix models are revenue-neutral within each peer group, so, where a hospital gains a positive adjustment, another hospital(s) in the same peer group will incur a negative adjustment.

15.5.4 Quality-related adjustments

The national casemix models do not currently incorporate quality-related adjustments.

15.5.5 Main financial incentives for hospitals

The explicit link between activity and cost data under the National Casemix Programme inevitably means that hospitals face a number of potential financial incentives to influence measurement of activity and costs. They may attempt to modify their coding practices to classify patients into AR-DRGs with higher weights (that is, up-coding or 'DRG creep'); submit cases to the incorrect casemix model; or transfer patients as soon as possible to non-participating hospitals or other institutions. However, most of these unintended consequences can be monitored and controlled through regular data audits by the National Casemix Programme and the ESRI.

Participation in the National Casemix Programme may be expected *ex ante* to encourage hospitals to improve their relative efficiency. However, this incentive may be weakened to some extent by the time-lag between when the activity was undertaken and the budgetary adjustment. The inclusion of a workload adjustment in the casemix models reduces this lag to some extent (see subsection 15.5.3).

15.6 New/innovative technologies

Participating hospitals can make submissions on a case-by-case basis to the National Casemix Programme for additional funding for high-cost drugs and innovative treatments. This mechanism is not considered to have a significant impact on the introduction of new technologies. Rather, the availability of capital investment funding would be considered to have a greater influence on the adoption of new technologies.

15.7 Evaluation of the DRG system in Ireland

The application of DRGs in casemix funding has been assessed as part of a number of national reviews within the Irish health sector. The 2001 National Health Strategy considered the National Casemix Programme then in place to be 'the most developed system for assessing comparative efficiency and for creating incentives for good performance' and committed to support it at national and regional level (DoHC, 2001, p. 114). In 2004, the DoHC undertook a 'root and branch' review of the National Casemix Programme, which committed the Department to expanding the number of participating hospitals, increasing the blend rate, and incorporating 'sub-acute' and 'non-acute' care. Progress on each of these commitments is ongoing. The review also confirmed the adoption of ICD-10-AM as the national clinical coding standards in Ireland, thereby confirming the recommendations arising from assessments of the best options available internationally for updating clinical coding and the DRG system (Murphy et al., 2004; Aisbett et al., 2007).[22]

The parameters derived from the national casemix models can provide a useful insight into how the operation of the National Casemix Programme influences hospital behaviour. Figure 15.4 shows the variability in casemix-adjusted average

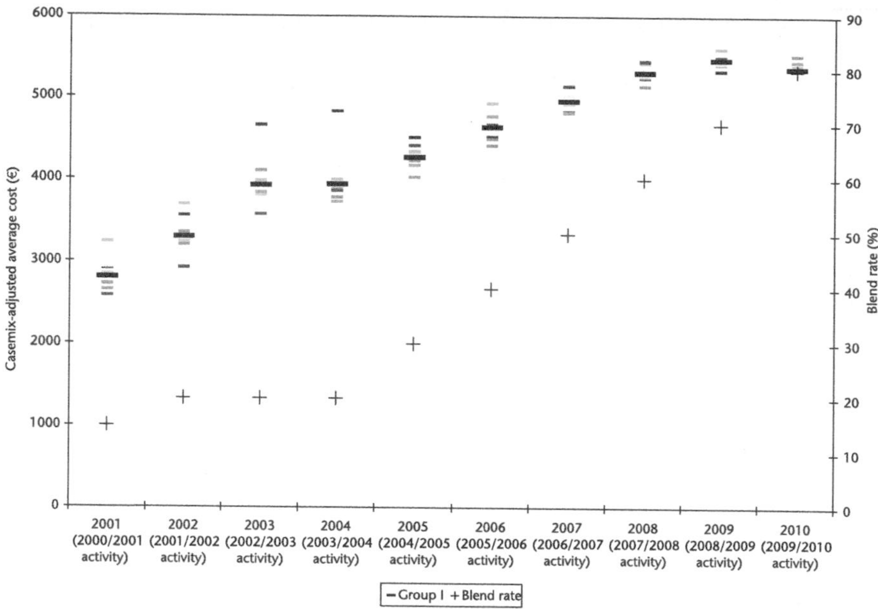

Figure 15.4 Casemix-adjusted inpatient average cost and blend rate for Group I hospitals, 2001–2010

Source: Based on data contained in Circulars prepared by the National Casemix Programme.

Notes: Each horizontal bar represents an observation on a hospital. The larger horizontal bar represents the average for the hospital group. Data for 2001 were converted from Irish pounds to Euros using an exchange rate of €1 = IR£0.787564.

costs for major teaching hospitals from the 2001–2010 inpatient casemix models. Interestingly, there has been convergence in Group I hospitals' average costs over time and across hospitals, towards the mean group cost. This convergence may be associated with the increasing blend rate, which may have encouraged hospitals (particularly those with above-average costs) to change their cost profiles in line with those of their peers.

15.8 Outlook: Future developments and reform

The application of DRGs in the Irish acute public hospital system has travelled an interesting route. The uses of the DRG system have extended beyond hospital reimbursement to informing the planning and reconfiguration of acute public hospital services; facilitating hospital benchmarking; and adjusting and monitoring the hospital consultants' workloads. Most recently, a review of charges associated with private and semi-private treatment in public hospitals has recognized the advantages of a DRG-based case payment system and recommended the piloting of such a system (DoHC, 2010b).

The continued role for DRGs in hospital reimbursement has been recommended in two reports. The first – entitled *Promoting performance-related services* and commissioned by the HSE – suggested implementing cost and volume contracts over a period of ten years. This prompted the HSE to establish a project team, which recognized the advancement of patient-level costing as a key issue. Consequently, the HSE initiated a pilot project in several hospitals in 2009 to assess potential approaches to patient-level costing (National Casemix Programme, 2010c). The second report by an Expert Group established by the Minister for Health and Children in 2009 recommended a mix of hospital payment mechanisms, incorporating DRG-based case payment and lump-sum payments (Ruane, 2010). However, it remains to be seen how this will be translated into policy.

Alongside the continued commitment to the use of DRGs in Ireland has been the simultaneous achievement of improvements in quality, technical factors and the system's scope. As data systems improve and the technical capability to implement increasingly sophisticated measurement systems increases, new and better DRG systems are expected to be developed in the future. However, the core objective of using DRGs in Ireland remains the same: achieving greater transparency in relating resource use to outputs within the acute hospital sector.

15.9 Notes

1 Assistance provided by Brian Donovan and Mark O'Connor is gratefully acknowledged. The authors are also obliged to Wilm Quentin and Conrad Kobel for comments on earlier drafts.

2 Due to profit repatriation by multinational companies located in Ireland, GNP is considered to be a more appropriate indicator of economic performance than GDP (Nolan, 2005; McDaid et al., 2009).

3 A private patient may occupy a public bed only if admitted as an emergency when a designated private bed is not available (Government of Ireland, 1991a, b, c). The Minister for Health and Children approves public/private bed designation (DoHC, 1999).

4 It has been estimated that there are 19 private hospitals operating in Ireland (Brick et al., 2010).

5 Between 2001 and 2008, all those aged 70 years and over, irrespective of income, received a medical card (McDaid et al., 2009; Citizens Information Board, 2011).

6 Some changes in data collection partly account for increased activity reported (see, for example, ESRI-HRID, 2008b).

7 The procedure classification system used in Ireland (namely, ICD-10-AM) is more commonly referred to as the Australian Classification of Health Interventions (ACHI).

8 ADRGs are similar to 'base-DRGs' used in other countries.

9 A hospital's AFSs are subject to audit, typically by the Comptroller and Auditor General (National Casemix Programme, 2010b).

10 Updates to the classification system are covered within a contract between Ireland and Australia.

11 For details of the variables required for grouping, see Commonwealth Department of Health and Ageing (2008).

12 Until 2010, the HIPE scheme collected up to 19 additional diagnoses and up to 20 procedures.

13 Full details and examples of the grouping algorithm are contained in the AR-DRG definitions manual (Commonwealth Department of Health and Ageing, 2008).

14 A discharge may be categorized as 'unassignable to MDC' or to an 'error DRG' where it cannot be directly assigned to one of the 24 MDCs.
15 An ADRG is the first three characters of an AR-DRG (for example, B78 is the ADRG associated with AR-DRG B78B).
16 The PCCL ranges from 0 (lowest complexity level) to 4 (highest). A high PCCL indicates the presence of additional, unrelated CCs that are expected to affect length of stay and cost.
17 For further information on HCAT, see the information leaflet available from the ESRI web site (http://www.esri.ie/health_information/hipe/clinical_coding/data_quality/HCAT_Info_Leaflet_2007.pdf, accessed 10 July 2011).
18 What are termed 'relative values' in Ireland may be referred to as cost weights in other countries.
19 An average AR-DRG has an RV of 1 and more costly AR-DRGs would have an RV greater than 1.
20 For these calculations, length-of-stay values are transformed into natural logarithms.
21 For example, a blend rate of 70 per cent implies that the calculated cost for a casemix-adjusted discharge will be based on 70 per cent of the peer-group costs and 30 per cent of the hospital's own cost.
22 Also, a review of the clinical coder training programme and data quality and audit procedures within the HIPE was commissioned in 2004 by the ESRI and undertaken by Michelle Bramley and Beth Reid, from the University of Sydney.

15.10 References

Aisbett, C., Wiley, M., McCarthy, B., Mulligan, A. (2007). *Measuring Hospital Casemix: Evaluation of Alternative Approaches for the Irish Hospital System*. Dublin: Economic and Social Research Institute (ESRI Working Paper No. 192).

Brennan, N. (2003). *Report of the Commission on Financial Management and Control Systems in the Health Service (The Brennan Report)*. Dublin: The Stationery Office.

Brick, A., Nolan, A., O'Reilly, J., Smith, S. (2010). *Resource Allocation, Financing and Sustainability in Health Care: Evidence for the Expert Group on Resource Allocation and Financing in the Health Sector*. Dublin: Department of Health and Children and Economic and Social Research Institute.

Citizens Information Board (2010). *Charges for Hospital Services*. Dublin: Citizens Information Board (http://www.citizensinformation.ie/en/health/hospital_services/hospital_charges.html, accessed 11 April 2011).

Citizens Information Board (2011). *Medical Cards*. Dublin: Citizens Information Board (http://www.citizensinformation.ie/en/health/entitlement_to_health_services/medical_card.html, accessed 5 April 2011).

Colombo, F., Tapay, N. (2004). *Private Health Insurance in Ireland: A Case Study*. Paris: Organisation for Economic Co-operation and Development (OECD Health Working Paper No. 10).

Commission on Health Funding (1989). *Report of the Commission on Health Funding*. Dublin: The Stationery Office.

Commonwealth Department of Health and Ageing (2002). *Australian Refined Diagnosis Related Groups Version 5.0 Definitions Manual*. Canberra: Commonwealth Department of Health and Ageing.

Commonwealth Department of Health and Ageing (2004). *Australian Refined Diagnosis Related Groups Version 5.1 Definitions Manual*. Canberra: Commonwealth Department of Health and Ageing.

Commonwealth Department of Health and Ageing (2008). *Australian Refined Diagnosis-Related Groups Version 6.0 Definitions Manuals*. Canberra: Commonwealth Department of Health and Ageing.

DoHC (1999). *White Paper – Private Health Insurance*. Dublin: The Stationery Office.

DoHC (2001). *Quality and Fairness: A Health System for You*. Dublin: The Stationery Office.

DoHC (2009a). *Health in Ireland: Key Trends 2009*. Dublin: Department of Health and Children.

DoHC (2009b). *Value for Money and Policy Review of the Economic Cost and Charges Associated with Private and Semi-Private Treatment Services in Public Hospitals – Interim Report*. Dublin: Department of Health and Children (http://www.dohc.ie/publications/pdf/vfm_review_economic_cost_interim_report.pdf?direct=1, accessed 31 May 2010).

DoHC (2010a). *Health in Ireland: Key Trends 2010*. Dublin: Department of Health and Children.

DoHC (2010b). *Value for Money and Policy Review of the Economic Cost and Charges Associated with Private and Semi-Private Treatment Services in Public Hospitals*. Dublin: Department of Health and Children (http://www.dohc.ie/publications/pdf/vfm_review_economic_cost_final_report.pdf, accessed 17 December 2010).

ESRI-HPID (2007). *Activity in Acute Public Hospitals in Ireland: Annual Report 2004*. Dublin: Economic and Social Research Institute, Health Policy and Information Division.

ESRI-HRID (2008a). *Activity in Acute Public Hospitals in Ireland: Annual Report 2005*. Dublin: Economic and Social Research Institute, Health Research and Information Division.

ESRI-HRID (2008b). *Activity in Acute Public Hospitals in Ireland: Annual Report 2006*. Dublin: Economic and Social Research Institute, Health Research and Information Division.

ESRI-HRID (2010). *Activity in Acute Public Hospitals in Ireland: Annual Report 2008*. Dublin: Economic and Social Research Institute, Health Research and Information Division.

Government of Ireland (1991a). *Health (Amendment) Act, 1991*. Dublin: Office of the Attorney General (www.irishstatutebook.ie/1991/en/act/pub/0015/index.html, accessed 26 May 2010).

Government of Ireland (1991b). *Health Services (In-Patient) Regulations, 1991 (S.I. No. 135/1991)*. Dublin: Office of the Attorney General (www.irishstatutebook.ie/1991/en/si/0135.html, accessed 26 May 2010).

Government of Ireland (1991c). *Health Services (Out-Patient) Regulations, 1991 (S.I. No. 136/1991)*. Dublin: Office of the Attorney General (www.irishstatutebook.ie/1991/en/si/0136.html, accessed 26 May 2010).

HCFA (undated). *Diagnosis Related Groups Definitions Manual*, Version 16.0. St. Paul, MN: 3M Health Information Systems.

HSE (2008). *Consultant Contract 2008 – Measurement of Public–Private Mix*. Kildare: Health Service Executive (http://www.hse.ie/eng/staff/HR/tandc/Consultant_Contract_2008__Measurement_of_Public_Private_Mix.pdf, accessed 4 August 2010).

HSE (2010a). *Casemix Budget Outturns for 2009*. Kildare: Health Service Executive (http://www.hse.ie/eng/services/Publications/corporate/2009casemix.html, accessed 12 May 2010).

HSE (2010b). *HealthStat – Supporting High Performance*. Kildare: Health Service Executive (http://www.hse.ie/eng/staff/Healthstat/about/, accessed 4 August 2010).

HSE (2010c). *Hospitals and Cancer Control*. Kildare: Health Service Executive (http://www.hse.ie/eng/services/Find_a_Service/HospsCancer/, accessed 3 August 2010).

HSE (2010d). *Integrated Services*. Kildare: Health Service Executive (http://www.hse.ie/eng/about/Who/is/Integrated_Services.html, accessed 26 April 2010).

McDaid, D., Wiley, M., Maresso, A., Mossialos, E. (2009). Ireland: Health system review. *Health Systems in Transition*, 11(4):1–267.

Murphy, D., Wiley, M.M., Clifton, A., McDonagh, D. (2004). *Updating Clinical Coding in Ireland: Options and Opportunities*. Dublin: Economic and Social Research Institute (ESRI).

National Casemix Programme (2010a). *Casemix Manual: Casemix Annual (Technical) Report 2010 – Part 4*. Dublin: National Casemix Programme.

National Casemix Programme (2010b). *Costing Manual: Casemix Annual (Technical) Report 2010 – Part 5*. Dublin: National Casemix Programme.

National Casemix Programme (2010c). *Technical Aspects of the National Casemix Programme – Part II*. Dublin: National Casemix Programme.

National Casemix Programme (2010d). *C1-10 Casemix Circular Tables*. Dublin: National Casemix Programme.

Nolan, A. (2005). Health: funding, access and efficiency, in J. O'Hagan, C. Newman, eds. *The Economy of Ireland: National and Sectoral Policy Issues*. Dublin: Gill and Macmillan.

Nolan, B., Wiley, M.M. (2000). *Private Practice in Irish Public Hospitals*. Dublin: Oak Tree Press in association with the Economic and Social Research Institute.

OECD (2009). *OECD Health Data 2011. How does Ireland Compare*. Paris: Organisation for Economic Co-operation and Development (http://www.oecd.org/dataoecd/45/53/43216301.pdf, accessed 10 July 2011).

O'Reilly, J., Wiley, M. (2010). Who's that sleeping in my bed? Potential and actual utilization of public and private in-patient beds in Irish acute public hospitals. *Journal of Health Services Research and Policy*, 15:210–14.

Prospectus (2003). *Audit of Structures and Functions in the Health System*. Dublin: The Stationery Office.

Robbins, G., Lapsley, I. (2008). Irish voluntary hospitals: an examination of a theory of voluntary failure. *Accounting, Business & Financial History*, 18:61–80.

Ruane, F. (2010). *Report of the Expert Group on Resource Allocation and Financing in the Health Sector*. Dublin: Department of Health and Children.

Wiley, M.M. (2005). The Irish health system: developments in strategy, structure, funding and delivery since 1980. *Health Economics*, 14:S169–S86.

chapter sixteen

NordDRG: The benefits of coordination

Miika Linna and Martti Virtanen

16.1 Introduction

Since the early 1990s the Nordic countries (Finland, Sweden, Denmark, Norway and Iceland) have been experimenting with patient classification systems. This led to a common Nordic patient classification system known as 'NordDRG' in the mid-1990s. NordDRG is a diagnosis-related group (DRG) grouper which emulates Health Care Financing Administration (HCFA)-DRG Version 12, using definitions based on the WHO International Classification of Diseases 10th revision (ICD-10) and the NOMESCO (Nordic Medico-Statistical Committee) Classification of Surgical Procedures (NCSP). The first grouper was finished in 1996. The grouper is updated yearly, according to the NordDRG maintenance process. This chapter explores the methods the Nordic countries have used to establish a grouping system which is unique on the DRG landscape and functions across the different countries. The implementation of the NordDRGs in Sweden, Finland and Estonia will be examined more closely in the chapters that follow.

During the early 1990s Finland developed a 'FinDRG' grouper based on the HCFA grouping system, which automatically converted Finnish ICD-9 diagnosis and procedure codes into HCFA-DRGs (Salonen et al., 1995; Linnakko, 2001). At the same time, other Nordic countries were also using DRGs, albeit somewhat unsystematically. The groupers used were mainly the 3M™ All Patient (AP)-DRG grouper or the United States HCFA-DRG grouper. DRG application in the Nordic countries was not at this time directly linked to hospital payment, but DRGs were used for benchmarking hospitals, health system evaluation or statistical reporting purposes. However, some of the Swedish county councils used the 3M™ AP-DRGs and the HCFA-DRG grouper in order to reimburse hospitals or inpatient care in some specialties (Håkansson & Gavelin, 2001). In Finland, FinDRGs were mainly used for managerial purposes rather than for hospital reimbursement (Linna, 1997).

Since the beginning of 1996 all Nordic countries decided to start using the ICD-10 classification for clinical diagnoses. However, it was impossible to employ a satisfactory conversion from ICD-9 (used for example, by the HCFA and FinDRG groupers) to ICD-10 and, in addition, the Nordic countries were in the process of implementing the new NCSP. Futhermore, the use of DRGs for hospital reimbursement in Sweden was increasing and several Finnish municipalities had expressed their interest in using hospital service definitions based on DRGs. Thus, the NOMESCO assigned the WHO Collaborating Centre for the Classification of Diseases in the Nordic countries to design a new cross-country DRG system, namely the NordDRG.

The national health authorities and associations in Finland (the Finnish Association of Local and Regional Authorities), Sweden (the National Board of Welfare and Health) and Iceland (the Ministry of Health and Social Insurance) started the NordDRG project, later accompanied by the Danish and Norwegian ministries of health. These organizations established the Nordic Casemix Centre,[1] which is responsible for the distribution, maintenance and development of the NordDRG grouper.

With the introduction of the system in 1996, separate country versions for Sweden and Finland were released, based on common definitions. Later, Denmark (2000), Iceland and Norway (2002) were also included in the set of country versions. In 2002 Denmark decided to leave the joint project in order to build its own system of DRGs (DkDRG), based on different primary classifications (procedures) and major revisions to the NordDRG grouping definitions (Hansen & Nielsen 2001) (Figure 16.1). In 2003 Estonia joined the NordDRG consortium. However, until 2009 they used the 2003 NordDRG grouper, particularly because the Estonian procedure classification (based on the NCSP) was not updated during this period. There is also an agreement with the Ministry of Health of the Republic of Latvia regarding the right to use NordDRGs in Latvia.

Aside from the national NordDRG versions there is also a NordDRG version based on the common Nordic components of ICD-10 and the NCSP. This version is used in Iceland. In 2003 an extended NordDRG version was developed that also includes national modifications to the grouping logic, using national codes that are unique to some of the countries (NCSP+).

16.2 Development and updates of the NordDRG system

The annual maintenance and updating of the NordDRG system is carried out according to a specified protocol and a fixed timetable. This updating process is intended to meet the emerging needs of the main stakeholders of the system within the Nordic countries. Modifications are validated with clinical and cost data to ensure that both economic and medical (clinical) homogeneity are retained or improved. Each country tests and implements these modifications separately, using their own data.

Suggestions for annual system updates are administered through an expert network, which consists of nominated experts from each participating country. The network is the main advisory group and platform for discussions relating to the maintenance, performance evaluation and development of the NordDRG

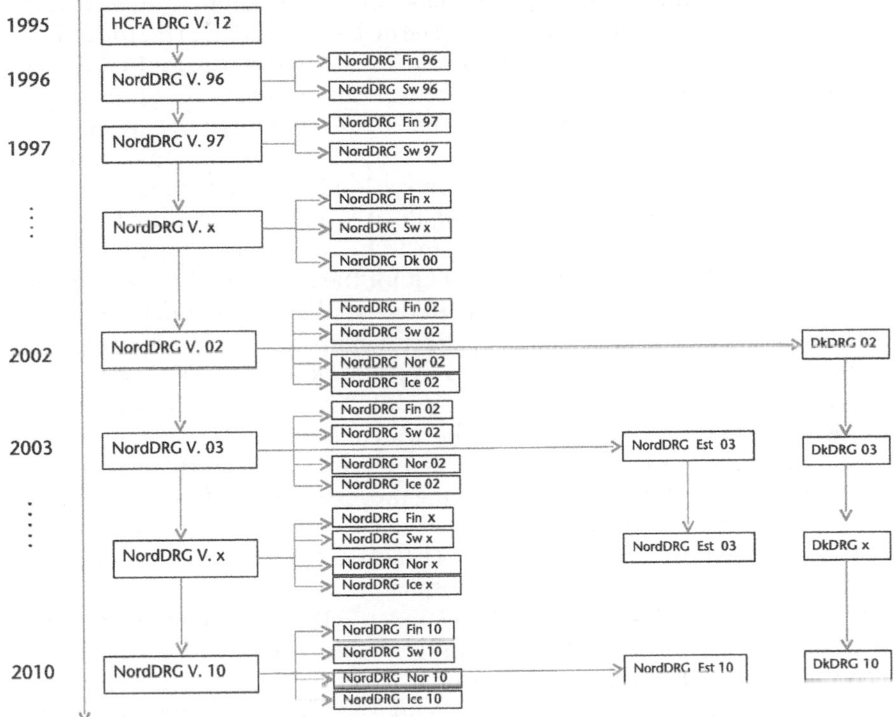

Figure 16.1 The development of the NordDRGs country versions

system. Meetings of the expert network are arranged twice per year. Based on the experts' suggestions, the NordDRG steering group makes the final decision (by consensus) regarding any changes to be made to the system.

The common NordDRG grouper is the reference grouper for inpatient care. Some modifications have been incrementally incorporated to better reflect the Nordic health care system context. Except for Denmark, all of the country-specific modifications represent only minor adaptations in the grouping algorithm for inpatient care. However, the incorporation of outpatient and day care differs markedly. From 2004 to 2007 the grouping of outpatient care was fairly similar in the Finnish and Swedish versions. In 2007 the Swedish version incorporated large revisions to the conservative cases in outpatient care. The operative cases/groups remain quite similar in the Swedish, Finnish and Norwegian versions. Norway integrated DRGs for outpatient care into its NordDRG country version in 2010 and Estonia did so during 2011.

General system information is available through an edited and open NordDRG discussion forum.[2] In addition, the forum is used for proposing updates and answering questions relating to the NordDRG system, and changes made to the NordDRG system each year are also documented.

Each year in which changes are necessary, two evolution versions are produced. The first (planning) version includes changes of the grouping logic of some DRGs for the next year. These changes may include entirely new groups, splitting of DRGs into sub-groups or changes in the assignment rules (patient case being entered into different DRGs). The first version is based on the primary classifications of the concurrent year and can therefore be used to test the effect(s) of the changes. The second (production) version is based on the primary classifications for the next year, but there are no new changes to the assignment logic of the NordDRG. If no errors are revealed, the second version will be accepted as the official production version for the next year.

In Finland all proposed alterations are discussed at the Finnish DRG Centre in cooperation with an expert physician from each medical specialty. They select which of the suggestions are relevant for the system update. If necessary, the suggestions are further discussed with the NordDRG expert network.

In Sweden the National Board of Health and Welfare is responsible for maintaining and developing the Swedish version of the NordDRG system. The National Board works together with the Swedish Association of Local Authorities and Regions (SALAR), representing the 21 county councils and regions in Sweden. There are also a number of expert groups in which the hospitals are represented. The test data for the updating process originate from the National Patient Register. For validating the homogeneity of DRGs, patient-level cost data are supplied by the National Cost Database. This database contains cost-accounting information from several hospitals.

Responsibility for developing and updating the DRG system in Estonia relies on the Estonian Health Insurance Fund (EHIF) and these tasks are carried out according to the DRG development plan.

The calculation of cost weights is accomplished separately in each country, using the NordDRGs and the respective cost data. In Finland the cost weights for the Finnish grouper have been calculated annually, based on patient-level cost data from the hospitals of the largest hospital district in Finland, Helsinki and Uusimaa, covering approximately 30 per cent of the specialized care setting in Finland (Mikkola & Linna, 2002). In Estonia the calculation of cost weights and DRG prices is based on the prices of the health services, not on the actual resource consumption. The main source used to develop the Estonian version is the case costing database of the EHIF. Expertise is also drawn upon from medical professionals' associations and health care providers. In Sweden the Centre for Patient Classification is responsible for the updating process and for calculating the cost weights. It is not mandatory to use the national weight sets in Sweden; there are also local weights in use in some of the counties. National weights are based on the national case costing database (using 'bottom-up' costing approach), which comprises 62 per cent of all inpatients in Sweden. Case costing data are also collected for outpatient care, and weights for day surgery and visits are also based on 'bottom-up' costing data.

The Finnish versions of NordDRGs only included groups for inpatient care until 2004. From then on, the hospital districts have gradually moved away from using the classic (only inpatient and day-care) grouper to using the outpatient DRGs.

Between 2003 and 2009, there were two versions of NordDRGs in effect in Sweden: a full version, which handled both inpatient care and day surgery (including intraluminal endoscopies); and a classic version for inpatient care only. Aside from these, a separate NordDRG grouper that included outpatient care also existed. From 2010, there will be just one version of NordDRGs for handling inpatient care and outpatient care. Estonia has been using the same version of NordDRGs since the year 2000. This is partly because the procedure classification has not been updated during this time. In 2011 DRGs for 'short-term therapy' (day care) were introduced.

16.3 Differences in diagnosis and procedure classification

The responsibility for updating the NCSP lies with the Nordic Centre, which maintains the aforementioned electronic discussion forum for the discussion of changes (see section 16.2). The reference group makes recommendations on changes to the Board of the Nordic Centre, which makes any formal decisions.

To update the NCSP, the reference group requires certain information for taking update proposals into consideration. Proposals should be approved and submitted by a responsible national classification body. The proposal can be prepared by the relevant medical professionals' association. The proposal should include a description of the new method and an account of its indications. In addition, it should include a rough estimate of how many procedures are performed per year in the country submitting the proposal, or the expected annual number in the near future. References should be included to the relevant literature (preferably accessible on the Internet), documenting the fact that proposed new codes represent established procedures and are not purely experimental in nature, giving a broad overview of the indications and techniques of any proposed new code.

However, the classifications of diagnoses and procedures are all slightly different, varying across the countries using NordDRGs. Finland has added a number of 5th-character codes to the ICD-10, but mostly there are no conflicts with the original WHO version. However, the country has made a number of updates to the NCSP (for example, diagnostic radiology, including ultrasound examination, therapeutic radiology and rehabilitation interventions were added). The Finnish Full DRG version (grouping both inpatients and outpatients) has been expanded to outpatient care, with a number of groups for hospital outpatient visits. This is based on the common Nordic model, in which so-called day surgery has its own groups per visit. The national additions refer mostly to the expensive radiology procedures, usually coded in the patient administration systems in Finland. The Finnish model still uses the original concept, from the common Full NordDRGs system, of 'short-term therapy' (in and out during the same calendar day) instead of an outpatient approach. Expensive medication has been another issue for consideration, but – due to the lack of systematic data collection – this has produced only temporary solutions.

The Swedish ICD-10 includes a number of 5th-character additions to the original WHO ICD-10. Similar to the Finnish version, these are mostly compatible with the WHO original. Sweden is the only Nordic country that fully applies the external cause coding of the ICD-10 classification to 5th-character level (~25 000 external cause codes). Sweden uses the NSCP, along with a national classification of conservative interventions that are especially important for

DRGs in outpatient settings. Diagnostic radiology is much less developed in Sweden than its Finnish counterpart but minor (short-stay) procedures and rehabilitation, for example, are more detailed in the procedure classification than in Finland. The Swedish Full NordDRG version is expanded to include all specialized outpatient care (conservative and surgical), along with psychiatry and rehabilitation.

Iceland is using a version of the expanded NCSP called NCSP+ for procedure classification. NCSP+ is based on the different additions to the NCSP in different Nordic countries. NCSP+ was developed for the NordDRG process as a tool that links the different national versions of procedure classifications together, so that the rules for different counties can be defined together and applied through the NCSP+ mapping to all national versions. The ICD-10 in Iceland, similarly to the Estonian version, is a direct translation of the WHO ICD-10.

Norway has modified the NCSP only when the common version has been updated. However, there is a separate classification of 'non-surgical' interventions that can be used together with the NCSP. It covers important areas, even for the classic NordDRG, and thus also includes important features for the outpatient groups. Norway has developed an expanded version of the Full NordDRG system, which is closely related to the Swedish version.

Denmark has revised the ICD-10 coding by replacing the 'dagger-asterisk' system with a large number of predefined combination codes. External cause codes were also replaced by the NOMESCO Classification of External Causes of Injury (NCECI). The procedure classification is mostly taken from the NCSP.

Some countries have added a system of 'nursing interventions' (comprising a number of codes) to the NordDRG system. For example, the Finnish and Swedish Full NordDRG version includes a number of DRG groups for (outpatient-based) nursing procedures.

16.4 Grouping process

The information required by the NordDRG grouper includes the following items: main diagnosis, secondary diagnoses (a list of diagnoses), procedures (a list of procedures), age, gender, mode of discharge and length of stay.

Internally, the grouping algorithm uses various predefined sets and sub-groupings of diagnoses and procedures to determine the properties which affect the grouping of each case (for example, the complication properties for diagnoses and procedures). This information is available in the definition tables for the NordDRG logic. Diagnoses and procedures that have an effect on the grouping are clustered into *intermediate groups* called 'categories' and 'properties'. Each code belongs to only one category, but it may have several properties. Properties relating to co-morbidities and/or complications (CCs) are binary, that is, having only two levels. About 75 per cent of the inpatient DRGs are divided into 'non-complicated' DRGs (without CCs) and 'complicated' DRGs (with CCs). Complicated cases are defined based on secondary diagnoses or in some cases procedures undertaken because of complication(s).

Operating room (OR) properties are binary in the Classic grouper, but in the Full grouper can have three values. Values 1 and 0 indicate whether a surgical procedure has been undertaken or not. According to this information, cases are assigned into 'surgical' and 'medical' DRGs, respectively. Procedures that are important in outpatient setting but do not affect DRG assignment of hospital inpatients have OR-property 2 (OR=2). In the case of hospital inpatients, OR=2 has no impact on the DRG assignment. The grouper algorithm returns three codes: the major diagnostic category (MDC) code, the NordDRG group code and a separate return code which indicates the outcome of the grouping, consistency checks and the reason for unsuccessful grouping.

16.5 Reimbursement via DRGs

The Finnish version of NordDRGs was initially introduced at the Helsinki University Central Hospital at the beginning of 1998. In 2001, five Finnish districts were employing NordDRGs to some extent in their pricing of hospital treatment. Today, 13 out of 21 districts have incorporated DRG-based pricing, but the methodology still varies greatly because regulations or even guidelines for hospital reimbursement are lacking at national level in Finland. Therefore, each district may determine the hospital payment method autonomously (Häkkinen & Linna, 2006).

In Sweden, different DRG systems (but mainly the HCFA-DRGs) have been used since the beginning of the 1990s. Stockholm County Council implemented DRGs as a payment system for inpatient care in 1992. The DRG system was developed as a process of cooperation between the National Board of Health and Welfare and the county councils, and the adoption of the DRGs has mainly been the concern of the county councils. This background – together with a tradition of a high degree of local autonomy – resulted in a situation in which central coordination on DRG-related issues was relatively weak during the 1990s. Since 1999 the National Board of Health and Welfare has coordinated DRG matters. All county councils and regions now use DRGs to some extent.

The DRG system introduced in Estonia in 2003 replaced the previous fee-for-service and per diem payments for hospital reimbursement. In 2011 the update of the current DRG grouping version took place, with the aim of increasing clinical relevance and resource homogeneity in DRGs by introducing them for 'short-term therapy' (day care), taking into account the different costs according to the patient's length of stay.

In Norway the funding of hospital care has largely comprised a mixture of global budgeting and activity-based funding (DRGs) since 1997. The implementation of the 1997 reform changed the format of hospital financing from block grants to a combination of block grants and activity-based reimbursement using NordDRGs.

In Denmark, the Ministry of the Interior and Health introduced casemix rates for the reimbursement of patients who received basic-level treatment outside of their home county ('free-choice patients') in 2000. At the same time, the voluntary 90/10 payment model was introduced in the counties. In the 90/10 model, 90 per cent of the predicted health care delivery/production costs were allocated to hospitals and the remaining 10 per cent of the hospital funding was to be allocated based on health care activities carried out, as measured by DRGs.

16.6 Notes

1 For more details see the Nordic Casemix Centre web site (www.nordcase.org, accessed 10 July 2011).
2 See the Nordic Centre for Classifications in Health Care dedicated forum web site for further details (www.norddrg.net/norddrgforum, accessed 10 July 2011).

16.7 References

Håkansson, S., Gavelin, C. (2001). Casemix in Sweden. Experiences of DRGs 1985–2001, in F. France, I. Mersents, M. Closon, J. Hofdijk. *Casemix: Global Views, Local Actions. Evolution in Twenty Countries*. Amsterdam: IOS Press.

Häkkinen, U., Linna, M. (2006). DRGs in Finnish health care. *Euro Observer*, 7(4):7–8.

Hansen, P., Nielsen, S. (2001). Casemix in Denmark: Status on the development and use of the Nord 'DK' DRG, in F. France, I. Mersents, M. Closon, J. Hofdijk. *Casemix: Global Views, Local Actions. Evolution in Twenty Countries*. Amsterdam: IOS Press.

Linna M. (1997). DRG:n käyttö sairaaloiden tuottavuus- ja tehokkuusvertailuissa [The use of DRGs in hospital productivity comparisons], in M. Neonen. *DRG suomalaisessa terveydenhuollossa [DRGs in Finnish Health Care]*. Helsinki: National Institute for Health and Welfare (STAKES).

Linnakko E. (2001). Casemix in Finland, in F. France, I. Mersents, M. Closon, J. Hofdijk. *Casemix: Global Views, Local Actions. Evolution in Twenty Countries*. Amsterdam: IOS Press.

Mikkola, H., Linna, M. (2002). Utilisation des DRGs dans le système hospitalier finlandais. *Revue Médicale de l'Assurance Maladie*, 33(1):37–43.

Salonen, M., Häkkinen, U., Keskimäki, I., Linna, M. (1995). *DRG-ryhmien kustannuspainot suomalaisella aineistolla [DRG Cost Weights Based on Finnish Cost-Accounting Data]*. Helsinki: National Institute of Health and Welfare (STAKES) (Aiheita 35).

chapter seventeen

Estonia: Developing NordDRGs within social health insurance

Kristiina Kahur, Tõnis Allik, Ain Aaviksoo, Heli Laarmann and Gerli Paat

17.1 Hospital services and the role of DRGs in Estonia

17.1.1 The Estonian health care system

The Estonian health care system is built on a platform of compulsory, solidarity-based insurance and universal access to health services made available by providers that operate under private law (Koppel et al., 2008).

In 2008 Estonia had one of the lowest shares (6.1 per cent) of expenditure on health care relative to gross domestic product (GDP) in Europe (NIHD, 2008). Estonian health expenditure has remained stable over time, with only small variations due to changes in the economic environment. As its main system-level input and output characteristics are comparable with more affluent countries, Estonia is often described as a country with a very cost-efficient health care system (Björnberg et al., 2009).

Since the country's independence in 1991, the Estonian health system has undergone two major shifts: first, from a centralized, state-controlled system to a decentralized one; and second, from a system funded by the state budget to one funded through social health insurance (SHI) contributions (Koppel et al., 2008). In 1992, following the introduction of health insurance and the establishment of autonomous providers, health care professionals ceased to be public employees, lost their civil service status and began to work under private labour regulations. The restructuring of the health system has taken place in several phases. The current organizational and management principles were established between 1999 and 2002 by legislation intended to re-centralize some health system functions.

The Ministry of Social Affairs and its agencies – the State Agency of Medicines (SAM), the Health Board and the National Institute for Health Development (NIHD) – are responsible for the general stewardship and management of the health care system, as well as for health policy development.

The State budget contributes about 11.5 per cent of total health expenditure, mainly for the financing and management of public health services, emergency medical care of uninsured people and emergency ambulance services. Local municipalities have a minor, somewhat voluntary role in organizing and financing health services (Koppel et al., 2008). This means that local municipalities have no defined responsibility to cover health care expenditure and, therefore, financing practices vary widely. Some local governments provide primary care providers with financial support, while some partially reimburse pharmaceutical expenses and nursing care costs for low-income households and for the elderly. In addition, health care providers that treat uninsured people might receive some reimbursement from local municipalities for certain expenditures, to varying degrees depending on the municipality. The majority share of financing for health care services is contributed by the public independent legal body, the Estonian Health Insurance Fund (EHIF), which contributes about 64.8 per cent of total health expenditure (NIHD, 2008). EHIF revenues are pooled from earmarked payroll taxes. Being effectively a single purchaser of care for most providers, the EHIF has gradually become one of the main actors driving developments in the health system. Private spending comprises about 20 per cent of total health expenditure, mostly in the form of co-payments for pharmaceuticals and dental care. Private insurance is almost non-existent in Estonia (0.3 per cent) (NIHD, 2008).

All actors in the Estonian health care market are public or private organizations operating under public or private law, which indicates that direct responsibility for provider performance has been delegated by the Ministry of Social Affairs and the municipalities to the hospital supervisory boards. With regard to purchasers of health care, the main actors are public organizations, such as the EHIF, the Health Board, and the NIHD. The latter two bodies are agencies of the Ministry of Social Affairs. The Health Board acts as a public purchaser of ambulance service providers and ensures sufficient national coverage. The NIHD is the main purchaser of public health services and is responsible for the implementation of all national public health programmes and strategies. However, the planning and coordination of the programmes is carried out by the Ministry of Social Affairs.

The EHIF is the main purchaser of health services. EHIF contracts evolved over a decade of well-established relationships on an equal footing with the service providers. At the beginning of the 1990s the contract content was rather unsophisticated and only the capped total costs were agreed. Currently, the contracts include agreements on rights and obligations of the parties concerned, service quality and access, as well as financial reporting requirements and a detailed cost- and volume-based financial component.

17.1.2 Hospital services in Estonia

An important characteristic of the Estonian hospital system is that since 2001 all hospitals operate under private law in the form of limited liability companies or foundations (Koppel et al., 2008). All hospitals own their capital assets and they are independent in their management decisions. Personnel who work in hospital-based departments have contracts with the hospital and are therefore salaried employees. Between 1991 and 2000 the number of doctors fell by 24 per cent, from 5500 to 4190, and the number of nurses by 14 per cent, from 9900 to 8500 (Jesse et al., 2004). Although the number of doctors and nurses continued to decrease after 1998, the ratio per 1000 inhabitants slightly increased, due to a parallel reduction in the size of the population (Koppel et al., 2008).

However, most hospitals are owned (or founded) by the state, local governments or public legal bodies, and thus effectively act as public hospitals. Estonia has therefore preserved public ownership of the hospital network, but has introduced management concepts specific to the private sector. This has created a framework in which public hospitals are run as networks or integrated providers and as true business entities, with management incentives geared at efficient financial performance.

In many instances, the hospital has multiple owners, for example a number of municipalities, or the state and municipalities jointly owning one hospital. A few hospitals owned by private entities provide specific services (such as gynaecology, obstetrics, rehabilitation, plastic surgery, and so on). The relationship between the EHIF and all hospitals is based on contracts. Owners (including public ones) can influence hospital activity through supervisory bodies or capital investment decisions.

In 2003 the Government approved the Hospital Network Development Plan (HNDP), which drew up a list of hospitals that serve the public interest and are therefore eligible for state aid. The Plan stipulated that hospitals are divided into regional, central, general, local, special, rehabilitation care and nursing care hospitals. Regional, central, general and local hospitals are acute care hospitals providing treatment for acute diseases requiring active medical intervention. Special care hospitals provide inpatient services in orthopaedics, vascular surgery, plastic surgery, psychiatry, obstetrics, gynaecology and otorhinolaryngology.

All hospitals need to be licensed by the Health Board. Differences in requirements according to hospital levels are mainly in the form of a minimum set of medical specialties that certain levels of hospitals must represent.

Each acute care hospital covers a certain area or region. The location has been chosen so that acute care services are available to everyone at a distance of 70 km or 60 minutes' drive; the Government approved the HNDP based on this principle. In order to ensure equal availability of specialist medical services, the HNDP foresees the existence of 19 acute care hospitals, including 11 general, 4 central, 3 regional and 1 local hospital (see Figure 17.1).

In the period 2000–2006 the number of hospital beds decreased by 20 per cent, from 9828 to 7588 beds, and the structure of beds by specialty changed

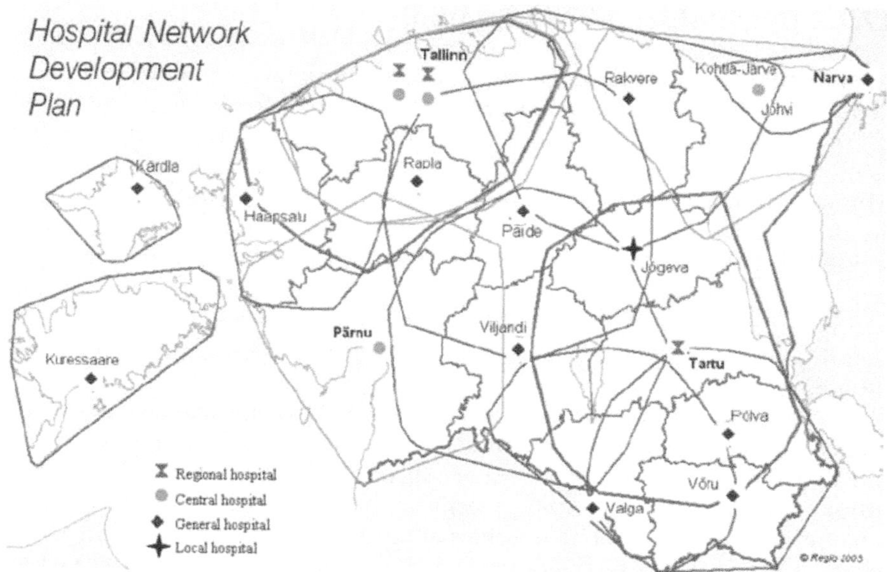

Figure 17.1 Overview of areas served by the Estonian hospital network

Source: Koppel et al., 2008.

significantly; that is, the proportion of nursing care beds increased remarkably, while the proportion of acute care beds decreased (see Table 17.1).

At the end of 2006 there were 55 hospitals in Estonia: 3 regional, 4 central, 12 general, 6 local, 7 special, 3 rehabilitation care and 20 nursing care hospitals, with a total of 7588 beds.

The reduction of acute beds has been related to the establishment of a hospital licensing system. As a result, small hospitals – hitherto predominantly providing long-term care – have lost their licence to provide acute care and have been turned into nursing homes. Other hospitals have been transformed into outpatient care centres providing specialist ambulatory care (Koppel et al., 2008).

In Estonia the range of activities and services in the hospital sector includes specialized outpatient care (including day care and day surgery) and inpatient care (including acute care, follow-up care, nursing care and rehabilitation). The total number of discharges, outpatient contacts, and insured individuals that used specialized medical care services during 2006 and 2009 are shown in Table 17.2.

17.1.3 Purpose of the DRG system

In 2001 the EHIF decided to introduce a DRG-based payment system. Stringent financial constraints exist for Estonian hospitals and the EHIF is not entitled to spend more than its budget (including reserves), since it is not able to raise health insurance contributions to cover the deficit. Therefore, the main motivation

Table 17.1 Hospital indicators, 1998–2008 (selected years)

	1998	*2000*	*2002*	*2004*	*2006*	*2008*
Structure of hospital beds by specialty (%)						
Acute care beds	n/a	77.3	74.2	73.2	69.7	n/a
Psychiatric beds	n/a	11.0	10.7	9.0	9.8	n/a
Beds for TB	n/a	3.2	3.5	3.8	3.6	n/a
Nursing care beds	n/a	8.4	11.6	13.9	17.0	n/a
General indicators of hospital beds						
Number of hospital beds rate per 1000	7.62	n/a	n/a	5.8	5.65	5.7
Acute care beds rate per 1000	5.84	n/a	n/a	4.26	3.94	3.85
Psychiatric beds rate per 1000	0.89	n/a	n/a	0.52	0.55	0.56
Hospital admissions per 1000	204.1	n/a	n/a	n/a	188.3	n/a
ALOS	10.3	9.2	8.4	8.0	7.8	7.9
Bed turnover	26.8	27.7	29.5	33.2	34.6	34.6
Bed occupancy rate (%)	74.6	69.9	67.7	72.6	74.1	74.3
Number of treatment cases						
Ambulatory care per 1000 insured	n/a	n/a	1876	1845	2000	n/a
Day care per 1000 insured	n/a	n/a	n/a	26	35	n/a
Inpatient care per 1000 insured	n/a	n/a	200	197	195	n/a

Source: Koppel et al., 2008.

Note: n/a: not available.

for introducing the DRG system was financial in nature, bearing in mind the particularly strict financial constraints of the EHIF budget. The consequences of these expense limits were particularly serious following the Russian economic crisis that affected the Estonian economy in 1999, driving the EHIF's reserves to zero. During the years that followed, the EHIF's budget revenues slowly increased, while pharmaceutical expenditure also increased rapidly, resulting in serious cost pressure on the EHIF. Thus, the DRG system was mainly seen as a tool to increase productivity and efficiency, rather than to increase the transparency of hospital output.[1] Another motivation for introducing a case-based payment system was

Table 17.2 Overview of discharges, outpatient contacts and insured individuals used specialized medical care services

Indicator	*2006*	*2007*	*2008*	*2009*
Discharges	249 398	248 711	249 784	240 227
Outpatient (excluding family practitioner) contacts	3 481 857	3 624 744	3 722 259	3 573 286
Number of insured individuals that used health care services during one year	796 815	810 834	819 055	800 578

Sources: EHIF, 2008, 2010b.

that the previous fee-for-service and per diem payment systems had led to inflation in the average reimbursement rate per case: inflation reached about 30 per cent between January 2000 and September 2002, while the official price increase was only 13 per cent (Koppel et al., 2008).

The importance of the DRG system has increased gradually with the increase (from 10 per cent up to 70 per cent since July 2009) in the share of the DRG payment system since the introduction of the system. In addition, over time the DRG system has became a tool for benchmarking and analysis. Since 2005, the EHIF provides hospitals with regular information updates regarding average length of stay, casemix index (CMI) (since 2008), use of some DRGs, share of outliers and so on, in order to give them the opportunity to compare with other hospitals, as well as to follow the trend of certain indicators across time.

17.2 Development and updates of the DRG system

17.2.1 The current DRG system at a glance

One DRG system has been in place in Estonia since 2003. No differentiation by region, purpose, or health care provider is applied. The decision to use one DRG system for the whole country was made early in the implementation planning process, and the question of whether to implement more than one system was not under consideration. Before the implementation of the current DRG system, several DRG systems were compared in order to find the best option for Estonia. The final decision was made in favour of the Nordic patient classification system (NordDRG).

The NordDRG system was adopted in 2003, along with the system's DRG grouping logic. In 2011 the grouping logic was updated and the NordDRG 2010 version was implemented. The total number of DRGs in the NordDRG Estonian 2010 version is 786 (496 in the 2003 version), 655 of which (489 in 2003) are used for reimbursement (see Table 17.3). The rest of the DRGs are 'empty'; that is, no cases are assigned to them.

The assignment of cases is based on diagnoses, procedures performed, age, gender, length of stay and status at discharge. DRGs apply only to inpatient care and day surgery, with the exception of long-term care, such as psychiatry, tuberculosis (TB) and nursing care, as well as expensive drugs and inpatient cases which include treatment with cytostatics (see subsection 17.5.1).

17.2.2 Development of the DRG system

The DRG implementation plan in Estonia was prepared in 2001 by the EHIF. It was initially planned for DRG-based reimbursement of hospitals to start in 2002. However, during the preparatory process it became clear that the plan was unrealistic and more time was needed for technical preparation. It was therefore decided that in 2003 the DRG system would be used only as a grouping tool and in 2004 the DRG system would start to be used as a payment tool.

Table 17.3 Summary description of the DRG system

Date of introduction	2003
(Main) purpose	2003 as a grouping tool since April 2004 as a reimbursement tool
DRG system	NordDRG
Data used for development	Database of EHIF
Number of DRGs	496 (until 2010) 786 (since 2011)
Applied to	Health care providers contracted with EHIF, acute inpatient cases and those outpatient cases involving surgical procedure(s)
Proportion of DRG/fee-for-service payments	2004: 10/90 2005: 50/50 2009 July: 70/30
Introduction of NCSP	2003
NCSP update	2010
Introduction of Estonian cost weights	2008
Update of DRG version	2011, NordDRG 2010 Full version

Before the implementation of the DRG system in Estonia, several DRG systems were compared to find the best option. The alternatives under consideration were the Australian Refined (AR)-DRG system, the Nordic NordDRG system and the Estonian case-based system. Various criteria were used to evaluate the available systems, such as other clinical classifications in use, clinical practice, clinical cases, cost of implementation, and technical support. Once the NordDRG system was chosen, work on adaptation began. The Nordic Casemix Centre produced an Estonian NordDRG version that was implemented in 2003.

For DRG weight calculation, two alternatives were considered. First, Estonia would calculate its own DRG weights according to the available historical billing information based on fee-for-service payments. The second alternative was to carry over Health Care Financing Administration (HCFA) weights and the DRG prices would be calculated based on the average reimbursement rate of each case. It was evident that hospitals would not be able to provide DRG-based cost information to use as an input for DRG weights calculation. The fact that Finland had tended to use HCFA weights from the outset without any problems encouraged the EHIF to choose this option. It was thought that starting with the United States HCFA weights system would provide a good basis for further development. In any case, the weight proportions tend to be analogous in different countries (EHIF, 2009). However, health care providers were more supportive of the Estonian national weights idea, as these were seen to better reflect the Estonian context. The decision was therefore made to use a 'home-made' mix of Estonian data and HCFA weights. In 2006 the project of developing Estonian national cost weights began and since 2008 the Estonian cost weights are used in the DRG price calculation. The adjustment of cost weights is in line with the recalculation of the prices of health care services.

Responsibility for developing and updating the DRG system in Estonia lies with the EHIF and it is carried out according to the DRG development plan.

17.2.3 Data used for development and updates of the DRG system

For developing the DRG system (including the grouping logic, cost weights, prices, and so on), the data mainly originate from the EHIF's electronic billing system. The data used for DRG grouping consist of different patient characteristics, such as age, gender, diagnoses, surgical procedures, the way patients arrived at the hospital, their status at discharge, and so on. For the development of the DRG system, other characteristics are used, such as the level of the hospital (regional, central, general hospital), average length of stay, CMI, average cost per case, and so on. Resource-consumption data are used for calculation of cost weights and DRG prices.

According to their contractual obligations with the EHIF, every health care provider must transfer the patient-level data (services provided, length of stay, diagnosis, and so on) to the EHIF database in order to be reimbursed. Thus, the main source used to develop the DRG system is the EHIF database. Expertise from medical professionals' associations and health care providers is also used as an input for system development, but the contribution of these actors to developing the DRG system has remained relatively modest.

17.2.4 Regularity and method of system updates

Since Estonia incorporated the NordDRG system, the regularity and methodology of system updates is steered by the Nordic Casemix Centre (see Chapter 16).

NCSP update

The first NOMESCO (Nordic Medico-Statistical Committee) Classification of Surgical Procedures (NCSP) version in Estonia was the generic classification Version 1.6 that was introduced in 2003. In practice, the NCSP has generic and country-specific versions that can be updated on an annual basis to introduce/change coding. In Estonia, a new updated NCSP version was introduced at the beginning of 2010.

Countries using the NCSP can further develop their own national versions of the classification. However, before proposing updates, local capacities need to be developed at country level and panels convened to facilitate discussions between administrators and medical doctors. Until recently this has not been implemented well in Estonia.

Cost weights and DRG prices update

Updating cost weights and DRG prices is the responsibility of the EHIF. As the calculation of cost weights and DRG prices is based on prices for fee-for-service health services, not on the actual resource need, the updating process is carried out as often as the prices of health services are updated. This update occurs annually (see subsection 17.5.2).

17.3 The current patient classification system

17.3.1 *Information used to classify patients*

Data used to classify patients (cases) are transmitted electronically by health care providers to the EHIF database. The regularity and frequency of data transmission, content of data and so on are regulated by legislation and by contracts. The information needed for grouping consists of the following information: principal diagnoses (in some cases diagnoses of co-morbidities and complications (CCs)), procedures performed, age, gender, length of stay and status at discharge. Resource-consumption data are not used for grouping. The primary classifications used in the NordDRG system are International Classification of Diseases 10th revision (ICD-10) for diagnoses and the NCSP for surgical procedures.

17.3.2 *Classification algorithm*

The overview of the DRG assignment process is depicted in Figure 17.2. It starts from a set of 'Pre-MDC' (major diagnostic category) assignment rules. Pre-MDC definitions refer to the group of DRG assignment rules that ignore the MDC indicated by the principal diagnosis of the patient. This includes DRGs for highly

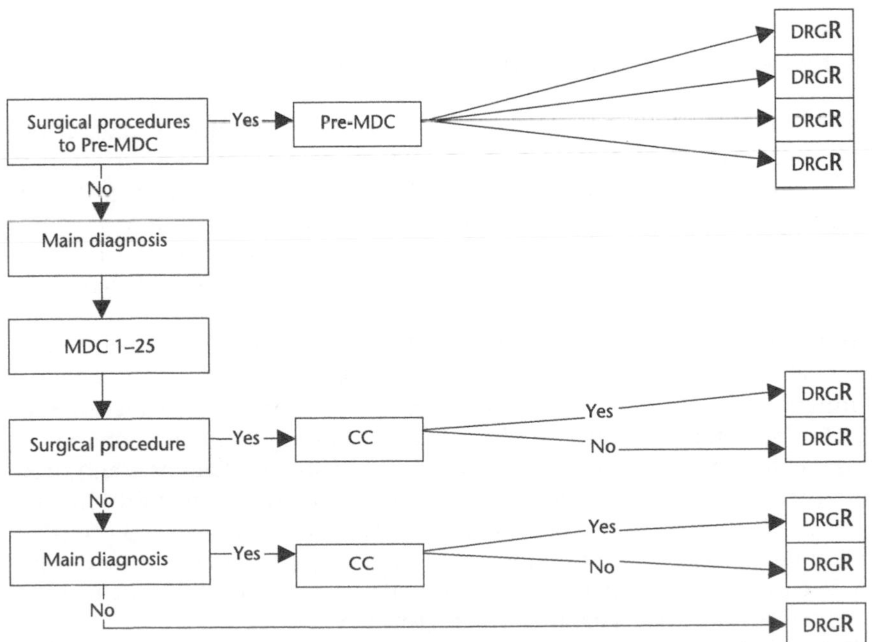

Figure 17.2 Main logic of the NordDRG system

Source: Nordic Casemix Centre, 2003.

specialized and expensive care. Examples of these are lung transplantation and bone marrow transplantation. Second, the Pre-MDC category is needed to avoid misclassification due to some differences between ICD-10 and ICD-9-CM (9th revision, Clinical Modification). Patients with multiple traumas, HIV-related problems, obstetrics and neonatology might entail a principal diagnosis that originally indicates specific MDCs. However, subsequent information may require the cases to be reallocated.

After the Pre-MDC is interpreted, the principal diagnosis of the case indicates the MDC. MDCs are mainly determined by organ systems, such as nervous system, digestive system, ear, nose, mouth and throat, and so on. Some MDCs are related to the etiology of the disease, for example infectious and parasitic diseases, injuries, poisonings and toxic effects of drugs, burns, and so on. There are 26 MDCs in the NordDRG 2010 version used in Estonia (there were 27 in 2003).

For each MDC a decision tree is designed with branching nodes, requiring information relating to the surgical procedure (which needs an operating room (OR)),[2] diagnoses of CCs, age, length of stay, status at discharge, and whether the patient is discharged to home or to another institution, whether the patient died or discharged her/himself against medical advice. At each branching node, the condition at the node is processed by identifying the information needed and comparing it to lists of codes or rules, determining which of the alternative routes to follow. The process is continued until the case ends up in one appropriate DRG.

17.3.3 Data quality and plausibility checks

Different means are used by the EHIF for assessing and improving data quality. All information in the EHIF database is gathered by using the electronic data transmission system. Health care providers complete their medical bills by inputting different patient and provider characteristics, as well as details of services carried out according to the fee-for-service health care service list. Completed bills are gathered together as 'electronic packages' and transmitted to the EHIF.

In the initial stage of data quality checks, format controls are carried out in the electronic system before the electronic packages enter the EHIF database. During format controls, different patient and provider characteristics are checked to determine whether they meet certain requirements, for example those set by legislation or under contract. The format of diagnoses and procedure codes described on medical bills is also checked. All medical bills with mistakes are returned to health care providers, giving them the opportunity to correct the inaccurate information. The health care provider can then transmit the electronic package again. Those bills that contain no mistakes are passed to the provider for final acceptance before payment.

In addition to format controls in the electronic system, some other methods are used for checking data quality. For instance, randomized controls of medical records are carried out by teams of EHIF 'trustee doctors'. These checks aim to compare the ICD-10 and NCSP codes described in the medical records with those on the reimbursement claims and to detect inappropriate use of primary classifications which could lead to the change in assignment of cases into DRGs. On a randomized basis the trustee doctors are sent to the hospitals to check the medical records or the medical records are brought to the EHIF office upon request. The percentage of the medical records checked in order to verify the coding quality amounts to about 4–5 per cent of the total number of records collected.

For most of the cases in which errors are found no financial sanctions are applied, unless fraud or abuse is detected. However, in detecting problems in coding quality, the trustee doctors provide feedback to health care providers, informing them of any inappropriate coding.

17.3.4 Incentives for up- or wrong-coding

There is no clear evidence of up- or wrong-coding. Instead, the results of randomized controls carried out by the EHIF show under-coding by health care providers, mainly due to the lack of accurate reporting of relevant information among medical doctors.

17.4 Cost accounting within hospitals

Cost accounting within hospitals in Estonia can be described as operating on two levels. For reimbursement purposes, hospitals must carry out service volume accounting per patient for all the services listed in the EHIF price list, and they must issue a relevant invoice per patient (volume of services delivered multipled by service prices). In the case of inpatient care and day care, the majority of invoices are recalculated by the EHIF and 70 per cent of the value is replaced by the relevant DRG price (see subsection 17.5.1).

This chapter deals with another level of cost accounting in hospitals, relating to the cost of providing services. This information is an input for fee-for-service pricing, and billing information relating to fee-for-service pricing is an input for DRG pricing (on an annual basis) (see subsection 17.5.2).

Cost accounting in hospitals in Estonia is not regulated in a specific way, as there is no requirement to report costs to health care authorities. Hospital steering and financial control is carried out by hospital supervisory board, and the Ministry of Social Affairs receives hospitals' annual reports (including financial reports). The only cost item monitored by the Ministry of Social Affairs is the average salaries of medical professionals, such as doctors, nurses and assistant nurses. That said, in the case of approving new health care services or updating prices of existing services, there is a regulated process for presenting relevant information to the EHIF (see subsection 17.4.1).

17.4.1 Regulation

The service costing process is regulated by ministerial decree and is an integral part of the benefits package (service list) update process, which is regulated by law (Health Insurance Act) and by governmental decree. According to the content of the regulation, the Government approves services and the DRG pricelist, the EHIF is responsible for expertise relating to cost-efficiency analyses of services within the benefits package and all applications for new services. Updating of existing services or elimination of services is processed in collaboration with the EHIF and professional associations or providers' associations (see subsection 17.6.1).

According to regulation, applications for new or updating existing services must include relevant cost information. In order to process applications, the EHIF needs to receive actual cost data from at least one hospital from each category of hospitals (regional, central and general). The regulation of costing (and pricing) of hospital services in Estonia can therefore be described as centralized and 'top-down' in approach.

17.4.2 Main characteristics of the cost-accounting system(s)

For the costing process of services in specialized medical care, the EHIF has set up a standard costing model which – according to regulations – comprises an activity-based costing methodology, whereby each service is described through certain activities and those activities are related to the costs of resources.

Recourses are allocated to direct and indirect resource categories , including, for example, drugs; single-use medical devices; multi-use medical devices; labour, including training and administration,; infrastructure-related costs, including investment (loan interest not included); and auxiliary services. From July 2003, infrastructure costs have been included in the prices paid to providers by the EHIF, in order to ensure geographical consistency and fairness in infrastructure development. The infrastructure costs in health service prices include the facilities' depreciation costs based on the market price of buildings, and a 36-year depreciation period. The mark-up has been calculated according to providers' optimal capacity per bed (which includes a standard number of square meters per bed that will produce an optimal occupancy rate). Since 2008, infrastructure cost expenditures were covered by the state budget as an earmarked allocation to the EHIF's budget, and will still be allocated to providers through the service prices. In 2009 the state stopped allocating infrastructure costs to the EHIF due to the economic downturn and therefore the EHIF must cover these from the regular health insurance budget.

Within all resource categories (except drugs and single-use medical devices), annual costs and effective utilization of resource units (in minutes or usage frequency) are determined, along with unit costs per utilization unit. Annual costs of resources are established by regulating degree (for doctors', nurses' and assistant nurses' salaries), expert opinion (for infrastructure investment costs) and all other resources are determined based on actual cost data presented by hospitals. The level of effective utilization is determined by the EHIF; usually 8 hours per working day (minimum one shift effective utilization).

Utilization of resource units by activity and by service is based on the expert opinion of professional associations, but this is checked by the EHIF against actual unit data from hospitals and often negotiated in the event of discrepancies.

Cost and resource-utilization data presented by hospitals should represent the total cost of the previous year's audited financial statements. As costs in hospitals are recorded mostly at the department or hospital level, and not at the service level (top-down approach), cost data presented by hospitals are aggregated only by medical specialty or at hospital level. This creates some uncertainty and results in an averaging approach within the EHIF cost model (costs defined at service level) in terms of checking pre-calculated costs against actual data presented.

Although there are several hospitals where costs are recorded at the level of service(s) delivered to the patient, the generated information is not comparable due to a lack of standardization of hospital information systems.

17.5 DRGs for hospital payment

17.5.1 Range of services and costs included in DRG-based hospital payments

How applicable the DRG system is to health care providers depends on the existence of a contract with the EHIF, regardless of the ownership, geographical location, teaching status, size, and so on, of health care providers. It means that the DRG system is applied to all specialized medical care providers contracting with the EHIF. The health care providers working without an EHIF contract are mainly financed on the basis of fee-for-service payments paid out of pocket.

The DRG system is used in combination with the fee-for-service payment method. To minimize any financial risk in the new system, the share of DRG payment applied upon submitting a reimbursement bill was initially (in 2004) set as low as 10 per cent. In 2005 the share of DRG payment was raised to 50 per cent and since July 2007 it amounts to 70 per cent. The share of fee-for-service payment applied upon submitting a reimbursement bill has decreased accordingly, from 90 per cent in 2004 to 30 per cent in 2009.

In practice, every bill lists the health care services delivered to the patient during their hospital stay. The bill is calculated by adding together the fee-for-service prices of each of the services. In addition, every bill is assigned to one DRG with its respective price. The combination of DRG and fee-for-service reimbursement means that the total sum of the medical bill is calculated as follows: (1) the fee-for-service element of the bill is multiplied by 0.3 (since July 2009); (2) the corresponding DRG price is multiplied by 0.7; (3) the latter is added to the fee-for-service sum.

DRGs are used for reimbursement in acute inpatient cases and for those outpatient cases involving surgical procedure(s). However, the DRG payment system does not apply to all assigned cases. A system of DRG outliers (rules to detect cases that do not come under the DRG-based reimbursement system) exists in Estonia. The outliers can be divided into two groups, as detailed here.

1. Cases with certain characteristics (types of care), such as psychiatry, rehabilitation, TB and follow-up cases. This same group of outliers also contains cases determined according to their principal diagnosis (for example, Z51.1 and Z51.2 – chemotherapy; and Z76.3 – healthy person accompanying ill person), as well as some referred cases (for example, while referring the patient from a higher level hospital to a lower level one, the patient is considered an outlier).
2. Cost-outliers; that is, cases that are too low cost or too high cost.

All above-mentioned cases are treated as DRG outliers and are reimbursed fully through fee-for-service payment(s). Pricing of DRGs is based on prices and casemix (according to reimbursement information) of the health services provided, rather than on the explicit cost information (see subsection 17.5.2). DRG prices – along with health service prices – are equal for all providers and there are no higher rates for teaching hospitals or for other higher level or specialized hospitals. Health service prices cover all costs related to providing services, except those related to scientific and teaching activities, which are funded separately. All prices approved are maximum prices and providers and the EHIF can agree on lower prices for specific contracts.

17.5.2 Calculation of DRG prices/cost weights

DRG price calculation is conducted by the EHIF and alongside updating the prices of health services; that is, when the prices of health services are going to change, current DRG prices need to be recalculated and the cost weights adjusted accordingly. The DRG price calculation is carried out at patient level and is based on fee-for-service billing information, taking into account the latest available data from all health care providers. DRG prices are equal for all health care providers.

The calculation of DRG prices can be divided into separate steps, as detailed here.

- The process starts with data quality analysis, in order to detect and eliminate data of poor quality.
- Second, the coefficient of volume inflation is calculated, in order to take into account the changes in the structure of health services by comparing specified periods of time.
- Third, the impact of change of health service prices is calculated by comparing current DRG prices with the new average price *per* DRG, calculated on the basis of new fee-for-service prices. For calculation of the average price *per* DRG, two-phase trimming is used in order to eliminate the impact of outliers (see Figure 17.3). In the 1st phase of trimming, the outlier cases with costs outside 3 standard deviation are excluded and in the 2nd phase, outlier cases with costs outside 2 standard deviation are excluded.
- The correction of the average price per DRG is carried out by applying to the current DRG price the above-mentioned coefficients of volume inflation and impact of change of health service prices.

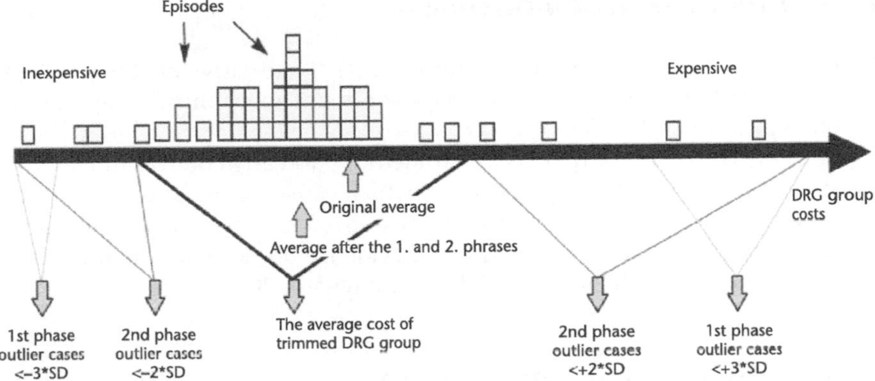

Figure 17.3 Trimming method used in the calculation of the DRG price

Source: Compiled by Jorma Lauharanta.

- For calculation of the base rate, all bills remaining after two phases of trimming are taken into account. The base rate is calculated by dividing the total sum of fee-for-service prices by the total number of bills.
- Cost weights *per* DRG are calculated by dividing the corrected DRG price by the base rate. Cost weights are compared with current ones and adjusted if necessary;
- The limits of each DRG are set up – the upper and lower limits are identified according to the last trimming points (see Figure 17.3). In many cases the lower limit is a negative value and therefore the lower limit is set equal to the lowest per diem rate.
- Finally, the calculation of the price for each DRG is carried out by multiplying the base rate by the cost weight of the corresponding DRG.

17.5.3 Use of DRGs in hospital payment

As already mentioned, three different payment methods are used for inpatient care – DRGs, fee-for-service payments and per diem payments. As the share of DRG payments has increased throughout the years (see subsection 17.5.1), the utilization of the DRG-based payment method has increased accordingly and in 2009 it accounted for 39 per cent of total hospital expenditure for inpatient care (see Table 17.4).

Table 17.4 Proportion of different payment mechanisms for inpatient care in acute care hospitals, 2006–2009

Payment method	*2006*	*2007*	*2008*	*2009*
Fee-for-service (%)	35	36	37	33
DRG (%)	36	34	33	39
Per diem (%)	29	30	30	28

Source: EHIF, 2010a.

17.5.4 Quality-related adjustments

Although introducing the pay for performance (P4P) initiative has been considered, no quality-related adjustment reimbursement mechanism is applied to hospitals in Estonia thus far.

The implementation of new payment methods and any changes in payment methods – together with the processes by which care is commissioned – should be undertaken carefully and with emphasis on making the most of available evidence and contributing to the body of evidence on how trading incentives affect the efficiency of health care delivery (Maynard, 2008).

17.5.5 Main incentives for hospitals

Not many incentives exist to set up DRG systems for hospitals. The main argument of the EHIF in favour of setting up such a system was that hospitals could control the increase of services in the casemix. However, in the current approach to DRG pricing, the change in the average reimbursement rate for the casemix is taken into account. The only incentive for hospitals is to maximize outpatient and day-care services, for which DRGs are not applicable.

17.6 New/innovative technologies

17.6.1 Steps required prior to the introduction of new/innovative technologies in hospitals

Estonia has no systematic programme for health technology assessment (HTA), mainly due to a lack of interest on the part of policy-makers and a lack of trained human resources. The main activities in this field include assessing new services to be added to the benefits package and prescription drugs to the positive list; evaluating the need for high-cost technologies; and ensuring the safety of medical equipment. These activities are carried out at national level and there is no evidence on the use of HTA at the organizational level. However, hospitals conduct some cost-analysis studies when high-cost technologies are purchased (such as magnetic resonance imaging (MRI) or computerized tomography (CT) scanners) (Koppel et al., 2008).

During the 1990s, the inclusion and exclusion of services from the benefits package was decided by the Ministry of Social Affairs, following evaluation by a ministry committee made up of provider and sickness fund representatives. Evaluations were based on treatment effectiveness criteria and, where possible, proposals for adding new treatments were weighed against existing treatments.

Since 2002, there have been clearer and more explicit rules for adding new services to the benefits package and establishing the appropriate level of cost-sharing. In 2002, when the EHIF was established as an independent public body, it was tasked with the responsibility for defining the benefits package in collaboration with other stakeholders. The benefits package is agreed by the EHIF and the Ministry of Social Affairs, and a final decision is made by the

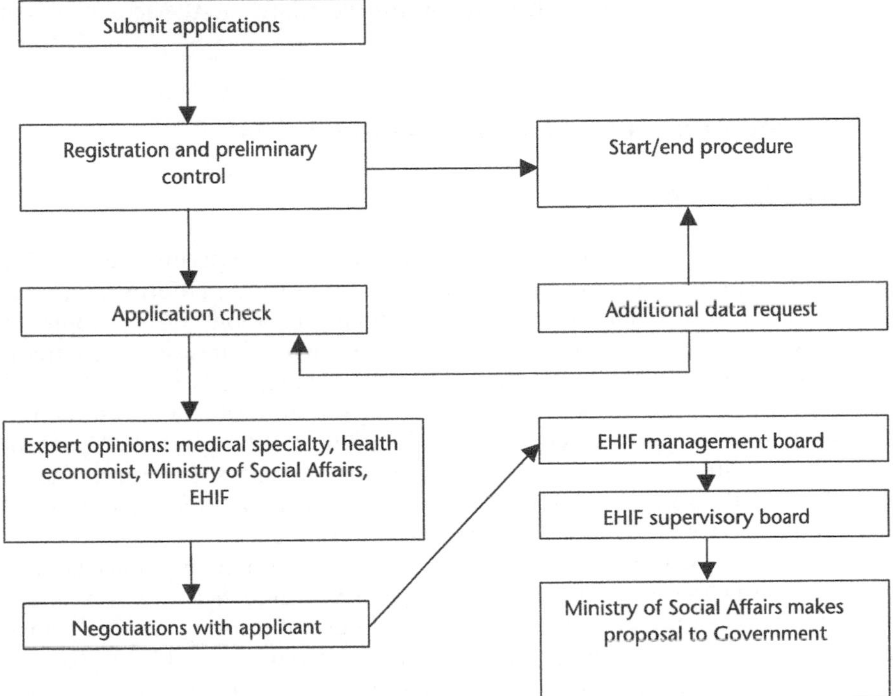

Figure 17.4 Procedure for amending the benefits package

Source: EHIF, 2008, 2010b.

Government, which endorses the price list. The procedure for amending the benefits package is presented in Figure 17.4.

17.6.2 Payment mechanisms

The funding of new technologies included in the benefits package does not differ from the funding of any other services within the package and there is no specific or separate funding for innovative technologies before they are included.

17.6.3 (Dis-)incentives for hospitals to use new/innovative technologies

No straightforward system of incentives exists for the utilization of new or innovative technologies in Estonia. The driving force is the interest and initiative of clinicians and leadership of medical groups in certain hospitals or at country level. However, due to some historical decisions, utilization of some technologies (high-end radiology, interventional radiology and cardiac surgery, for example) is increasing, as these are overpriced relative to the actual costs of providing the service(s).

17.7 Evaluation of the DRG system in Estonia

17.7.1 Official evaluation

Evaluation of the NordDRG system relies on the Nordic Casemix Centre. The NordDRG expert network is the main advisory group and platform for discussions relating to the maintenance, performance evaluation and development of the NordDRG system. The suggestions for annual updates of the common NordDRG are based on expert network recommendations.

In addition, the Nordic Casemix Centre carries out evaluation, testing and certification of DRG groupers to ensure compatibility with the NordDRG definitions. The Centre also cooperates with the main NordDRG software provider(s) in delivering the common NordDRG version (as well as national versions based on national codes) to the NordDRG users, as appropriate.

In terms of evaluation at national level, there has not been any official evaluation of the DRG system. However, the EHIF has conducted various analyses in order to assess the data quality (mainly the use of primary classifications), DRG pricing methodology, preparedness for and impact of shifting to new NCSP and DRG grouper versions, as well as the impact of increasing the share of DRG-based payment in reimbursement, and so on. The results of the analyses have been used to further develop and fine-tune the DRG system in Estonia.

17.7.2 Authors' assessment of successes and problems

One of the central arguments for the introduction of the DRG system was to increase efficiency and contain the health insurance expenditure. From the purchaser point of view, during the initial years of the adoption of the DRG payment system in Estonia the set objective was met; namely, the DRG system has contained the average cost per case compared to the situation that would have arisen if only a fee-for-service and per diem-based payment system had been used (as it was before the implementation of the DRG system).[3] However, the results show the differences between various hospitals. Therefore, bearing in mind the strategic goal of the DRG system, the further development and fine-tuning of the system is carried out according to the four-year DRG development plan.

The use of the DRG system as a benchmarking tool began in 2005 and has developed over time. Since 2009 the range of indicators has broadened and hospitals listed in the HNDP are provided the data via a web page of EHIF. This provides the opportunity to compare and assess different performance indicators. Until recently, hospitals in Estonia were benchmarked (length of stay, use of some DRGs, percentage of outliers, and so on) mostly at the specialty level, without standardizing for case structure and severity. The introduction of the

CMI since 2008 affords hospitals (and other authorities) additional dimensions for more objective comparison of performance results.

Comparisons are a powerful way of driving performance improvement. However, there is a great deal of potential in Estonia to use this information in order to locate and pinpoint the strengths and weaknesses of hospital performance and to use the data to support decision-making processes.

17.8 Outlook: Future developments and reform

17.8.1 Trends in hospital service (or general health care) delivery

The most fundamental changes for building a functioning health system in Estonia were made in the early stages of reform, during the early 1990s. The incremental arrangements that followed were implemented to support the public health, primary health care and hospital sector reforms and to strengthen the EHIF's purchasing function. Therefore, the attention has shifted to improving and monitoring performance of the system as a whole.

In terms of service delivery, the main challenge is presented in the need to optimize the system. The strength of the current delivery system is in family medicine-centred primary health care. This system covers a wide range of services, without co-payments and with minimal waiting times. It is complemented by the ambulance (emergency) services for care outside normal working hours. The challenge lies in making the delivery system more patient-centred and coordinating care at the primary care level, with the development of additional nursing and rehabilitation services.

17.8.2 Trends in DRG application/coverage

The EHIF is responsible for the development of the DRG system in Estonia. This is carried out in line with the four-year DRG development plan approved by the management board of the EHIF.

The strategic goal of the DRG system is to contribute to increased efficiency in the use of health insurance resources. In order to achieve this goal, the EHIF will implement the following measures:

- improve the quality of coding
- develop DRG-based analysis and feedback
- develop transparent pricing and funding principles.

Improving coding quality involves, *inter alia*, the correct and unified use of primary classifications (ICD and NCSP) by health care providers, and the improvement of coding quality assessment. The development of methods of analysis and benchmarking is related to improvement in technical resources, together with the respective competences of the staff of the EHIF. Actions to develop transparent methodology of DRG pricing and funding principles include, *inter alia*, the regular updating of the current DRG grouping version.

17.9 Notes

1 Due to the former fee-for-service payment structure and well-developed electronic data transmission systems, Estonia already had a relatively transparent overview of hospital output.
2 Cases with an OR procedure are assigned to the 'surgical' DRGs and those without an OR procedure are assigned to the 'medical' DRGs.
3 More details are available at the EHIF web site (www.haigekassa.ee, accessed 1 August 2011).

17.10 References

Björnberg, A., Garrofé, B.C., Lindblad, S. (2009). *Euro Health Consumer Index 2009 Report.* Brussels: Health Consumer Powerhouse.

EHIF (2008). *Estonian Health Insurance Fund Annual Report 2008.* Tallinn: Estonian Health Insurance Fund.

EHIF (2009). *Overview of Estonian Experiences with DRG System.* Tallinn: Estonian Health Insurance Fund (http://www.haigekassa.ee/uploads/userfiles/Implementation_DRG_EST_291209_cover(1).pdf, accessed 21 June 2010).

EHIF (2010a). *DRG tagasiside aruanne [DRG Feedback Report].* Tallinn: Estonian Health Insurance Fund (http://www.haigekassa.ee/uploads/userfiles/DRG_tagasiside_aruanne_2009.pdf, accessed 21 June 2010).

EHIF (2010b). *Estonian Health Insurance Fund Annual Report 2010.* Tallinn: Estonian Health Insurance Fund.

EHIF (2011). *Estonian Health Insurance Fund.* Tallinn: Estonian Health Insurance Fund (www.haigekassa.ee, accessed 1 August 2011).

Jesse, M., Habicht, J., Aaviksoo, A. et al. (2004). *Health Care Systems in Transition: Estonia.* Copenhagen: WHO Regional Office for Europe on behalf of the European Observatory on Health Systems and Policies.

Koppel, A., Kahur, K., Habicht, T. et al. (2008). Estonia: health system review. *Health Systems in Transition,* 10(1):1–230.

Maynard, A. (2008). *Payment for Performance (P4P): International Experience and a Cautionary Proposal for Estonia.* Copenhagen: WHO Regional Office for Europe (Health Financing Policy Paper, Division of Country Health Systems).

NIHD (2008). *Department of Health Statistics, Health Statistics and Health Research Database* [online database]. Tallinn: National Institute for Health Development (http://pxweb.tai.ee/esf/pxweb2008/dialog/statfile2.asp, accessed 20 January 2010).

Nordic Casemix Centre (2003). *NordDRG System.* Helsinki: Nordic Casemix Centre (http://www.nordcase.org, accessed 10 July 2011).

chapter eighteen

Finland: DRGs in a decentralized health care system

Kirsi Kautiainen, Unto Häkkinen and Jorma Lauharanta

18.1 Hospital services and the role of DRGs in Finland

18.1.1 The Finnish health system

In its institutional structure, financing and goals, the Finnish health care system is closest to those of other Nordic countries and the United Kingdom, to the extent that it covers the whole population and its services are mainly delivered by the public sector and financed through general taxation (for more details, see Häkkinen, 2005, 2009; Häkkinen & Lehto, 2005; OECD, 2005; Vuorenkoski, 2008). However, compared to the other Nordic countries, the Finnish system is more decentralized (Magnussen et al., 2009); in fact it can be described as one of the most decentralized in the world. Even the smallest of the 342 municipalities (local government authorities) are responsible for arranging and taking financial responsibility for a whole range of 'municipal health and social services'. From an international perspective, another unique characteristic of the system is the existence of a secondary public financing scheme (the National Health Insurance scheme) also covering the whole population, which partly reimburses the same services as the tax-based system, but only services which are provided by the private sector. The National Health Insurance also partly reimburses the use of private hospital care.

Municipally provided services include primary and specialized health care. In addition, municipalities are responsible for other basic services, such as nursing homes and other social services for the elderly, child day-care, social assistance and basic education. Municipal health services are financed through municipal taxes, state subsidies and user charges. Primary health care is mainly provided at health centres, which are owned by municipalities or federations of municipalities. Preventive care for communicable and non-communicable diseases, ambulatory, medical and dental care, an increasing number of outpatient specialized services, and various public health programmes (such as maternity and school health care) are provided by the health centres. They also provide occupational health services and services for specific patient groups (for example, clinics for diabetes and hypertension patients). Health centres include also inpatient departments. The majority of patients in these departments are elderly and chronically ill people, but in some municipalities, health centres also provide acute short-term curative inpatient services. In addition to the inpatient departments of the health centres, long-term care is provided at homes for the elderly that in administrative terms come under municipal social services.

Specialized care (psychiatric and acute non-psychiatric) is provided by hospital districts, which correspond to the federations of municipalities. Each municipality is obligated to be a member of a hospital district. In addition to services provided through health centres and hospital districts, municipalities may purchase services from a private provider.

18.1.2. Hospital services in Finland

Acute somatic hospital care is mostly publicly provided by hospital districts and, to a lesser extent, some health centres are supplemented by care provided in private hospitals. In 2007, specialized care comprised in total 33 per cent of the total health care expenditure, of which the share of private service provision was only 1 per cent (THL, 2010).

There are 21 hospital districts in the country. Most hospital districts have a central hospital and in some districts, care is supplemented by small regional hospitals. There are 14 regional hospitals in the country. Tertiary care is provided in five university hospitals, which also act as central hospitals for their hospital district. All of the 34 hospitals owned by hospital districts provide both inpatient and outpatient services; in 2007, on average 59 per cent of resources were allocated to inpatient care, 7 per cent to day-case surgical care, and 34 per cent to ambulatory care. In addition, some acute somatic care is provided in health centres owned by municipalities or federations of municipalities, as well as in private hospitals (Table 18.1).

Hospital districts are managed and funded by the member municipalities. Funding is mainly based on municipalities' payments to hospital districts, according to the services used (see Figure 18.1). In 2008, the share of municipal payments of all costs of somatic care was 89 per cent. A total of 2 per cent of the total funding of hospitals comes from state subsidies for research and teaching, and 4 per cent from user charges. The Government defines the maximum fees that hospitals can charge. In practice, every hospital applies the maximum fees. In 2010 these were €32.50 for an inpatient day, €27.40 for outpatient visits and €89.90 for day surgery. User charges within public sector health care have an annual ceiling (€633), after which patients receive services free of charge.

Table 18.1 Acute hospital key figures by type and ownership, 2009

Type and ownership	*Number of hospitals*		*Patients (inpatient and day-case surgical care)*		*Discharges (inpatient and day-case surgical care)*		*Bed days (inpatient and day-case surgical care)*		*Average length of stay, days*	*Emergency discharges*		*Day-case surgery discharges*	
	Number	*Share*	*Number*	*Share*	*Number*	*Share*	*Number*	*Share*		*Number*	*Share*	*Number*	*Share*
University hospitals	5	5.4	271 104	39.7	394 975	41.0	1 396 570	40.76	3.5	162 968	39.4	58 892	32.4
Central hospitals	15	16.1	245 278	35.9	355 703	36.9	1 240 606	36.20	3.5	180 566	43.6	59 078	32.5
Regional hospitals	14	15.1	79 094	11.6	103 520	10.8	353 804	10.33	3.4	48 359	11.7	21 103	11.6
Health centres (specialised)	15	16.1	37 868	5.5	51 186	5.3	281 331	8.21	5.5	20 866	5.0	9 317	5.1
Public hospitals	49	52.7	633 344	92.7	905 384	94.0	3 272 311	95.50	3.6	412 759	99.8	148 390	81.5
Private hospitals	44	47.3	49 954	7.3	57 579	6.0	154 321	4.50	2.7	984	0.2	33 605	18.5
Total	**93**	100.0	**683 298**	100.0	**962 963**	100.0	**3 426 632**	100.00	3.6	**413 743**	100.0	**181 995**	100.0

Source: Authors' own compilation based on the national hospital discharge data.

Note: Finland no longer compiles data on hospital bed numbers since this is recognized as an inaccurate measure of hospital capacity.

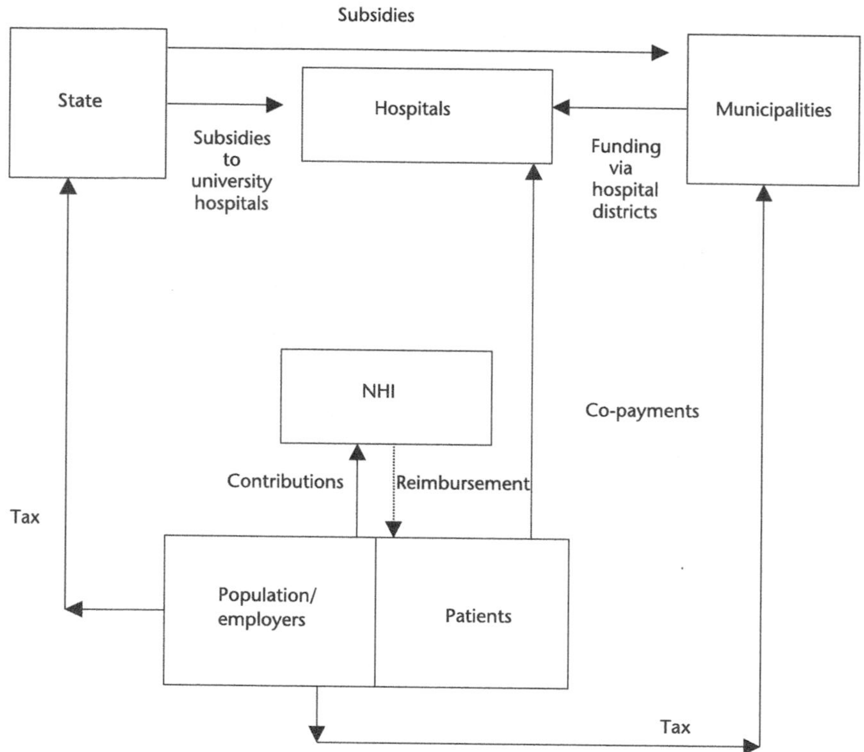

Figure 18.1 Funding of hospital care in Finland

Note: NHI: National Health Insurance

As purchasers, municipalities negotiate annually the provision of services with their hospital district. There are different contractual or negotiation mechanisms between hospital districts and municipalities for agreeing target volumes and payments. Both the volumes and costs are planned based on the previous year. In many cases, the municipalities and the hospital districts differ in opinion regarding the correct size of the resource allocations. There is a tendency for budgets to be set too low, which means that agreements sometimes need to be revised during the year, according to the actual amount and type of hospital services delivered. Usually, no explicit sanctions are applied if agreed plans and targets are deviated from, and municipalities cover any deficits and retain any savings in their accounts. The negotiation mechanisms have been under continuous change and development.

The budget of each hospital district is formally decided by a council, the members of which are appointed by each municipality. The council also approves the financial statements (such as payment methods and levels of payments (prices)) and makes decisions regarding major investments. The hospital payments from municipalities are based on the total budget and the predicted use of services. If the hospital budget is exceeded, the municipalities must cover the deficit from their own revenues, usually by paying higher prices for services. In the case of budgetary surplus, the prices per service can be lowered. Thus, the major purpose of hospital pricing systems has been to cover the costs of production and to allocate hospital costs fairly between the municipalities that finance the provision of services within a hospital district.

In the absence of nationally set regulations or even guidelines, each hospital district determines the payment methods used to reimburse its hospitals. Payment methods are organized according to district and as such they vary from district to district. The trend of pricing has been consistently moving away from a price-per-bed-day approach towards case-based pricing. Currently, 13 out of 21 districts are using DRG-based payment methods. The principles and rules for DRG usage vary greatly between hospital districts.

In order to diminish municipalities' financial risk from expensive patients, a compensation system has been created. With this system, treatment costs per patient above a particular limit are shared between all the member municipalities of a hospital district. In most hospital districts this limit is between €50 000 and €60 000. Variation exists, and in some districts the limit is even higher than €80 000. The payment share for each municipality is defined based on the number of citizens living in the municipality.

18.1.3 Purpose of the DRG system

Within the hospital districts, the DRG system (as well as other prevailing payment systems) is not used for resource allocation but mainly as a method of collecting payments from municipalities; that is, as a billing instrument. Hospital districts use DRG-based prices to charge municipalities for the services they have delivered. The Finnish payment system does not create similar incentives to the prospective payment system used in many countries. This is because hospitals do not bear any responsibility for financial loss, as municipalities cover their deficits.

In addition to the collection of payments, DRGs are used for patient classification in the planning, evaluation and management of hospital services. The motivation behind using DRGs was to simplify the hospital product definitions, in order to assess hospital performance, develop hospital operating processes, monitor the quality of care and develop performance-based budgets.

At national level, DRGs are used for hospital benchmarking. In 1996 the then National Research and Development Centre for Health and Welfare (STAKES, now the National Institute for Health and Welfare) launched a project, called the Hospital Benchmarking Project, in cooperation with the hospital districts (Linna & Häkkinen, 2008). Its main purpose was to provide hospital managers with benchmarking data for improving and directing activities in hospitals. The project designed and implemented an Internet-based information system supporting continuous data gathering and processing, as well as displaying benchmark measures at the desired level of aggregation. The project has taken advantage of the existing information systems in hospitals (the patient administration systems, cost-accounting and pricing/reimbursement data, and cost-administration processes) to collect patient-level data on delivered services and their costs. Now, annual data are collected routinely. Productivity and efficiency calculations are made with traditional activity measures, such as DRG admissions and outpatient visits, with a more advanced DRG-weighted measure for episodes of care.

The quality as well as efficiency of specialized care has been evaluated since 2004 in the PERFECT project (PERFormance, Effectiveness and Cost of Treatment episodes).[1] Within the framework of this project, protocols have been developed for eight diseases/health problems (acute myocardial infarction; revascular procedures (percutanous transluminal coronary angioplasty, coronary artery bypass grafting); hip fracture; breast cancer; hip and knee joint replacements; very low birth weight infants; schizophrenia; and stroke) (Häkkinen, 2011). The development has been undertaken in seven separate expert groups, the members of which are leading clinical experts on the aforementioned diseases. DRGs are used for calculating the costs of diseases. At present, register-based indicators (at both the regional and hospital levels) relating to the content of care, as well as costs and outcomes between 1998 and 2008 are available for seven health problems. The indicators are freely available on the Internet, and they are to be routinely updated using more recent information. They have been widely used in local decision-making and have also been discussed in the media. The Ministry of Social Affairs and Health uses the information in strategic planning: the indicators developed in the project will be used to evaluate the development of regional differences in the effectiveness of specialized care. The Ministry has also used the information in its recommendation concerning the centralization of certain services (such as care of low-birth-weight infants) to university hospitals with adequate resources.

18.2 Development and updates of the DRG system

18.2.1 The current DRG systems at a glance

Currently, two different DRG systems are in use: the NordDRG Classic and the NordDRG Full systems (see Chapter 16). The main difference between these two groupers is that the Classic system covers only hospital inpatient and day-case surgical activities, whereas the Full system extends the coverage to hospital outpatient activities, that is, to scheduled and emergency visits. Because of the lack of outpatient groups, the Classic DRGs were supplemented in productivity analysis with a separate outpatient grouping based on visit types by specialty. This grouping has been developed as part of the Finnish Hospital Benchmarking Project and is not used as a pricing method.

In the Classic DRG system, inpatient and surgical day cases with the same diagnosis and procedures are grouped to the same DRG. The Full DRG system takes lengths of stay into account and classifies one-day cases into so-called O-groups. As such, the O-groups contain both surgical and medical day cases. The O-groups are equivalent to inpatient groups, except that they have a lower cost weight indicating the lower cost structure of day cases.

18.2.2 Development of the DRG systems

The development of the NordDRG system is described in the NordDRG chapter of this volume (see Chapter 16). In Finland the growing significance of hospital outpatient services during the late 1990s created demand for a more advanced grouping structure for these services. In 2004 the Nordic Centre for Classifications in Health Care implemented a NordDRG Full version for both hospital in- and outpatients. The first Full grouper comprised 831 groups, of which 91 were ambulatory care groups. The ambulatory care groups consist of series of groups for endoscopies (so-called '700-series'), non-extensive procedures ('800-series'), and 'short therapies' (short-stay treatment) without significant procedures ('900-series'). Since the first version, the ambulatory care grouping has been developed markedly; the 2010 Full grouper comprises 370 ambulatory care groups and in total 1020 groups. The Full grouper applies the same rules that are used in inpatient settings in assigning patients to specific outpatient groups. The Finnish Full DRG version has been in use in the Helsinki and Uusimaa hospital district (HUS) since 2004. At the beginning of 2008 the system was also introduced in one central hospital. Since 2008, the Finnish Hospital Benchmarking Project has used the Full grouper.

A summary of all the DRG systems that have been used in Finland is presented in Table 18.2. The information represents the official national DRG groupers, which are not used in every hospital district. In the absence of national guidelines for DRG usage, hospital districts are free to change the national groupers; for example, splitting groups further if they find it necessary for their own purposes. The actual number of DRG groups used in different hospitals may therefore vary.

Table 18.2 Main facts relating to the different DRG versions

	FinDRG	*NordDRG Classic version**	*NordDRG Classic version*	*NordDRG Full version**	*NordDRG Full version*
Year of introduction	1995	1996	2010 (current)	2004	2010 (current)
(Main) Purpose	Research	Billing		Billing	
DRG system	HCFA Version 3 modified	HCFA Version 12 modified		HCFA Version 12 modified	
Data used for development	Cost data from 3 university hospitals	Cost data from Helsinki and Uusimaa hospital district		Cost data from Helsinki and Uusimaa hospital district	
Number of DRGs	470	495	650	831	1020
- *of which scheduled and emergency visits*	–	–	–	91	370
Applied to	Some public hospitals, inpatients	Some public hospitals, inpatients		Some public hospitals, in- and outpatients	

*Updated annually.

18.2.3 Data used for development and update of the DRG systems

The Finnish version of NordDRGs is based on patient-level data from the HUS district hospitals. These hospitals provide about 30 per cent of specialized care in the country. In HUS hospitals a patient information system is used, which collects all relevant information needed in the DRG grouping. In 2010, about 2 million cases were used to calculate DRG cost weights for the NordDRG Full grouper. Data are now available from all university hospitals (about 370 000 cases) for calculating cost weights for the NordDRG Classic version.

18.3 The current patient classification system

18.3.1 Information used to classify patients

In the Classic DRG system, the grouping algorithm used to assign a patient to a DRG is based on the inpatient hospital discharge dataset, which consist of: major diagnosis, secondary diagnoses, procedures, patient characteristics (gender, age, weight of neonates) and discharge status (death, transferred to other institution, left against medical advice). In the Full DRG system the grouping algorithm is similar to the Classic one, except that it uses both in- and outpatient data to assign patients to a specific DRG. Moreover, it uses the length of stay as a grouping criterion alongside the aforementioned criteria.

18.3.2 Classification algorithm

In the grouping process, patient discharge data are fed into a special software tool, the so-called 'grouper'. The process is described in detail in the NordDRG Users' Manual (Nordic Centre for Classification of Health Care, 2009). In NordDRGs the grouping rules are presented as a series of ten tables.

Diagnoses and procedures that have an effect on the grouping are clustered into larger subsets called 'categories' and 'properties'. Each code belongs to only one category, but it may have several properties. A CC property (co-morbidities and complications) is binary; that is, it has only two levels. An OR property (operating room procedure) is binary in the Classic DRG grouper, but in the Full grouper it can have three values. Values 1 and 0 indicate whether a surgical procedure has been carried out or not. According to this information, cases are assigned into 'surgical' and 'medical' DRGs, respectively. Procedures that are important in the outpatient setting but do not affect the DRG assignment of hospital inpatients have OR property 2 (OR=2). In the case of hospital inpatients OR=2 has no impact on the DRG assignment (see Figure 18.2).

Because of the complexity of the decision process, as well as for logistical reasons, one specific DRG can be represented by several rows in the DRG logic table. The complexity of the table is a reflection of the detailed nature of the original assignment rules. The rows in the table follow the hierarchy of the original assignment rules. Therefore, when allocating patient cases, each row

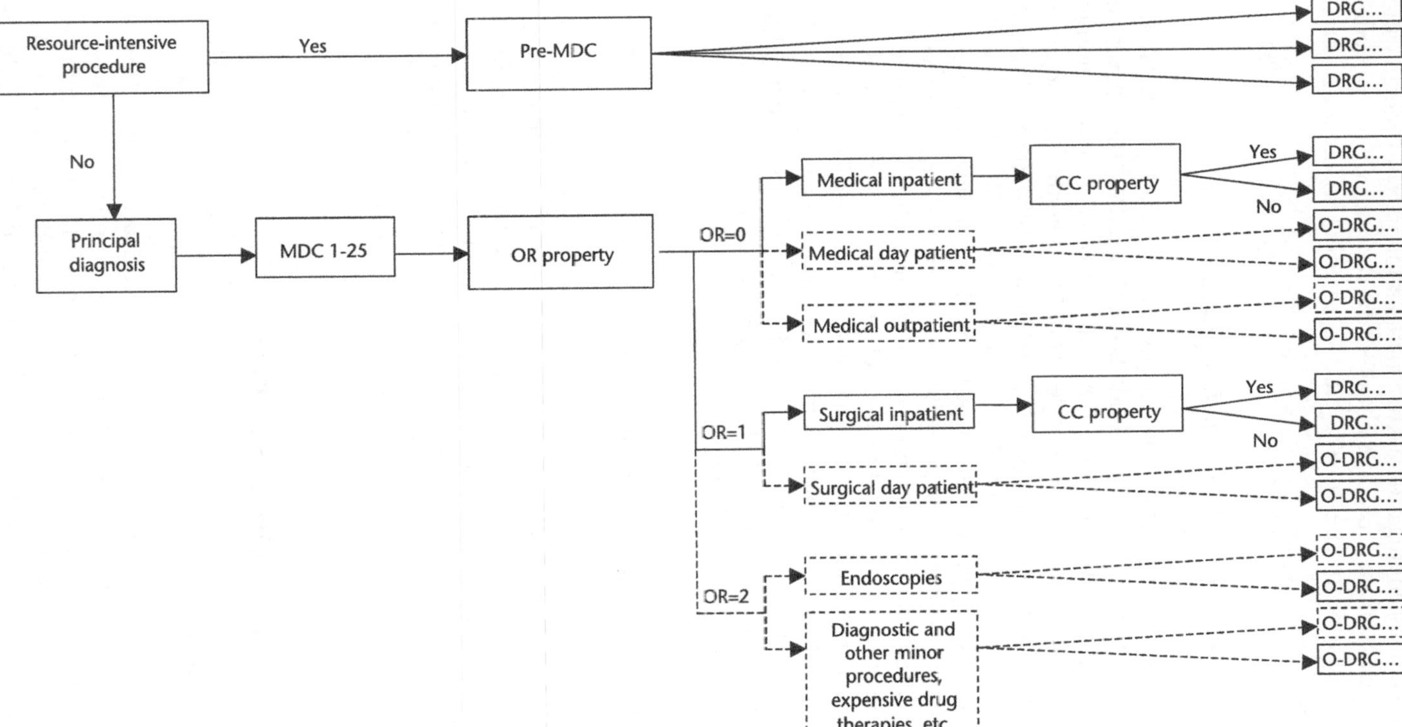

Figure 18.2 Grouping process in the NordDRG system

Source: Nordic Centre for Classifications in Health Care, 2009.

Note: The Classic system is depicted by continuous lines, the Full system also includes the parts presented with dashed lines.

has to be checked in ascending order until a match is found. The order in which variables are checked on each row does not affect the allocation, while preceding through the logic rows in the correct order is essential to obtain a correct grouping result.

18.3.3 Data quality and plausibility checks

Due to the lack of national guidelines for the use of DRGs, no official data quality and plausibility checks are undertaken. Hospitals themselves are responsible for data quality assurance. Hospitals use DRGs in billing municipalities for the services they have provided and it is therefore important for the hospitals that patient cases are correctly assigned to DRG groups. Incorrect DRG assignment leads to a failure in the billing process. After the patient is discharged, the DRG grouping system performs the grouping automatically, using information on diagnoses; procedures; and patients' age, gender and discharge status. Special attention has been paid to the coding of diagnoses and procedures. One problem has been the insufficient coding of secondary diagnoses and additional procedure codes – so-called 'Z-codes' which indicate, for example, long lengths of stay, bilateral operation and emergency status. The lack of these codes leads to a 'down-coding' and therefore a lower billing price. To enable correct billing, a manual check is performed to ensure that each patient is assigned to a correct DRG group.

18.3.4 Incentives for up- or wrong-coding

Since DRGs are not used as a prospective payment system, there are no strong incentives for up- or wrong-coding. Hospitals only need to cover their operating costs and therefore they do not have any profit-based incentives for upcoding. The use of DRGs as a payment system has increased the accuracy of coding secondary diagnoses and procedure codes. Information from the STAKES hospital benchmarking database[2] shows that the coding quality is much higher in those hospital districts that use DRGs as a payment method, compared to the hospitals without DRG payment.

18.4 Cost accounting within hospitals

18.4.1 Regulation

In Finland there are no national guidelines for cost accounting. Hospital districts or individual hospitals are therefore allowed to choose their own level of cost accounting and the cost-accounting system used. For DRG purposes, however, a particular standard is required. Advanced patient-level cost-accounting systems were originally only used in the HUS hospitals. Today, some other large hospitals have also developed patent-level cost-accounting data systems that fulfil the requirements for calculating cost weights. In 2010, national weights for the Classic DRG version were calculated using data from all five university hospitals.

18.4.2 *Main characteristics of the cost-accounting system(s)*

In the HUS hospitals, an advanced cost-accounting system (Ecomed IC) is in use.[3] Cost accounting starts with the calculation of the overhead costs, which are then allocated to lower organizational levels, using a top-down approach. All overhead costs (such as administrative costs) are allocated to the organizational level relevant for hospitalization days, outpatient visits, operations or ambulatory procedures. After this stage, the 'bottom-up' cost-analysis phase begins. For each treated patient the following costs are defined: nursing (basic care – 'price of the hospital day'), procedures undertaken in OR and ambulatory care settings, radiology, laboratory tests, expensive drugs, blood products, and pathological services (see Table 18.3). These costs include both staffing and devices. The bottom-up cost accounting is undertaken in each of the five hospitals, at department level. 'Controllers' bear the main responsibility for cost accounting, and nurses and doctors are used as experts in the process.

18.5 DRGs for reimbursement

18.5.1 *Range of DRGs used for reimbursement*

In Finland, DRGs are not used as a prospective payment system, as in many other countries, but rather as a financing instrument in hospital districts,

Table 18.3 Distribution of cost by categories used in cost accounting in the HUS, 2009

Cost category	*Inpatient and day surgery DRGs (Classic)*	*Scheduled and emergency visit DRGs (O-groups) (%)*	*Classic and O-groups total (%)*
Basic (inpatient) care	50.5	14.1	45.8
Basic (outpatient) care	0.2	14.2	2.0
Inpatient consultations	0.4	0.0	0.3
Laboratory tests	4.2	1.4	3.9
Blood products	1.9	0.2	1.7
Pathological services	1.1	1.4	1.2
Physiological services	0.1	0.0	0.1
Radiology	3.7	2.7	3.6
OR procedures	26.9	49.8	29.8
Procedures in outpatient departments	9.1	15.4	9.9
Expensive drugs	1.6	0.4	1.4
Expensive products	0.3	0.5	0.4
Total	**100.0**	**100.0**	**100.0**
Share of total cost	**87.1**	**12.9**	**100.0**

Source: Compiled by the authors on the basis of information provided in a personal communication from Virpi Alander (HUS).

used to collect payments related to services use by municipalities. As explained in section 18.1.1 the total budget (including capital, administration) for hospital districts is decided first and prices are then set in such a way that they fit the budget.

Not all hospitals use the system, and those that do use it do so in different ways. For example, some hospitals have split the DRGs further where necessary for their own purposes, which is acceptable due to the lack of national guidelines relating to the use of DRGs.

There are no national guidelines that obligate hospitals to use DRG. The Finnish National DRG Centre – which is a part of the private FCG Finnish Consulting Group OY – maintains and develops the groupers, as well as providing recommendations for their use. Currently 13 out of 21 hospital districts use DRG billing, but the extent to which it is used varies a lot between the hospital districts. Moreover, the type of services covered by DRG billing varies; in all hospitals, psychiatric patients and patients requiring long-term intensive treatment (such as patients with respiratory arrest) are excluded and in some hospitals dermatological and cancer patients, for example, are also excluded. DRG billing covers outpatient visits (completely or partially) in four hospital districts. The pricing and billing of services excluded from the DRG system is based on bed days or treatment packages in inpatient settings and on visit types by specialty in outpatient settings.

18.5.2 Calculation of DRG prices/cost weights

The national cost weights calculated by the National DRG Centre are based on patient-level costing data from the HUS and (since 2010) university hospitals (the costing data are described in more detail in subsection 18.4.2). The National DRG Centre also calculates cost weights for individual hospitals based on their patient-level cost data. Trimming is used in defining the average cost of a DRG group, and because of skewed distribution (SD) of cost. The trimming process is depicted in Figure 18.3. The trimming is undertaken in two phases: in the 1st phase, patient cases for which treatment costs are ± 3 SD from the mean cost of all patient cases are excluded; in the 2nd phase, patient cases for which the treatment costs are ± 2 SD from the mean cost of the 1st phase patient population are excluded. In 2010 the centre also calculated the outliers using a method based on variation coefficients. The National DRG Centre recommends that university hospitals should use outlier methods in their pricing, since a considerable proportion of the high-cost patients come from municipalities not belonging to their own hospital districts. The centre does not recommend applying an outlier approach in central and regional hospitals, in which almost all patients came from municipalities within their own districts.

18.5.3 DRGs in actual hospital payment

Five out of thirteen hospital districts (using DRG as payment method) have calculated cost weights based on their own patient-level costing data. Other hospital districts use the national relative cost weights calculated by the National

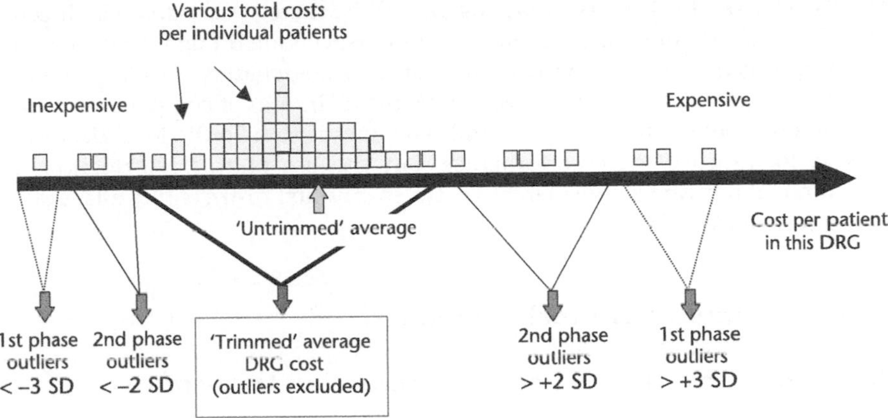

Figure 18.3 Definition process of the average cost of a DRG group

Source: Compiled by Jorma Lauharanta.

DRG Centre, but have calculated the price for a DRG point (that is, base rate), based on their own cost accounting. The price of a DRG point represents the costs of an average DRG group in the whole system; the billing price of each individual DRG group is obtained by multiplying the price of a DRG point by the respective cost weight. In most hospital districts, irrespective of whether they use their own or national cost weights, the price for a DRG point is defined separately for each hospital, and in many hospitals, separately for each department. This is because the casemix complexity – and hence the average treatment cost – varies between hospital and department types; this variation is not captured perfectly by the cost weights. For example, large university hospitals treat on average more complex and expensive patients than small local hospitals, and the current DRG system is too rudimentary to take this into account.

Many hospitals have a defined upper outlier limit based on the number of bed days above which DRG billing is not used, but the billing is based instead on bed days. The outlier limit varies markedly between hospital districts and this creates great variation in terms of the billing prices for the outlier patients. For these patients the billing price consists of the DRG price and the sum of outlier bed-day prices.

As already explained, the use of DRGs varies considerably between hospital districts. In the HUS, where DRGs have been in use since 1998, about 65 per cent of service charges paid by the municipalities were based on NordDRGs in 2008; the rest of the billing was based on bed days and outpatient visits (HUS, 2009). Similar data are not available from other hospitals.

18.5.4 Quality-related adjustments

As explained in subsection 18.1.2, the budgetary and payment system used in Finland does not create similar incentives for hospitals to use DRGs to those that a prospective payment system is known to create. There are no quality-related adjustments in pricing and, thus, there are no financial incentives for efficiency or quality. In Finland these aspects are thought to have been taken into account by involving municipalities as purchasers as well as owners in decision-making within the hospital districts. The aim of comparative information on productivity, efficiency and outcomes is to help the local decision-makers to improve their performance, but the use of this information in decision-making varies considerably between hospital districts (Junnila, 2004; Linna & Häkkinen, 2008).

18.6 New/innovative technologies

18.6.1 Steps required prior to introduction in hospitals

Funding decisions are made at hospital district or department/clinic level, based on the total budget approved by the hospital district. There is no national regulation. It is assumed that the introduction of new technologies is based on health technology assessment. It is generally accepted that before the introduction of new equipment, treatment practices or drugs can take place, evidence relating to cost–effectiveness is required. University hospitals and some large central hospitals carry out these kinds of research activities on their own. The Finnish Office for Health Technology Assessment (Finohta) – in cooperation with hospital districts – provides information on the effectiveness and safety of new technologies for national use. Systematic literature reviews are undertaken in order to gather all relevant information. Finohta does not issue any guidelines, but it provides hospitals with information needed for decision-making. However, there is no exact information available as to how decisions are made in each hospital district and to what extent they are based on scientific evidence.

18.6.2 Payment mechanisms

Hospital districts have different practices for funding new technologies. The funding can be based on surpluses from previous years, internal financing or loans. The costs of new technologies are at least partly transferred to DRG prices via depreciation and interest on loans. Exact information is not available regarding the principles of funding new technologies in hospital districts.

18.6.3 (Dis-)incentives for hospitals to use new technologies

No direct financial incentives or disincentives exist for the use of new technologies. The system is based on the idea that municipalities – as providers of specialized care for their citizens and as financiers of hospital districts – are interested on the one hand in receiving the best possible care for their populations and on the other hand in controlling for the how the money they have paid to hospital districts has been used. With this dual role in mind, municipalities are likely to be interested in making sure that the money is used for effective technologies, rather than it being wasted on something less effective.

18.7 Evaluation of the DRG system(s) in Finland

18.7.1 Official evaluation

In Finland the right to make decisions regarding specialized care is afforded to hospital districts, which can decide independently their own method of charging municipalities for the services that their citizens use. It has therefore not – so far – been of interest to the central Government to evaluate how the DRG system (or other prevailing payment systems) works in practice.

18.7.2 Authors' assessment

In Finland the main problem concerning DRGs is that there are no national guidelines on how to use the system. Not every hospital uses the system and those that do are free to use it in different ways. The main purpose of the DRG system in Finland is to make hospital billing transparent by encouraging hospitals to introduce the same billing system. However, as long as hospital districts keep modifying the system in order to make it perfectly suitable for each individual hospital, using different rules (for example, differing outlier limits and department-level DRG point prices), comparison of billing prices between hospitals is impossible. Each municipality is obligated to be a member of one hospital district and without being able to compare the prices, municipalities are not able to make rational choices. This prevents competition, which, in turn, does not incentivize hospitals to improve their operating efficiency. In order to make the DRG billing system function properly and to enhance efficiency, the Ministry of Social Affairs and Health should introduce national rules and obligate all hospital districts to use the DRG billing, as has been implemented in many other countries. This is also important because private and non-profit-making – and even multinational – firms are now entering the health care market. In addition, a new Health Care Act (accepted by the Finnish Parliament in December 2010) introduces patient choice of hospital. However, so far, it has not been decided (or indeed proposed) how municipalities would pay hospitals within the new framework. If the central Government is to take a more active role in developing the pricing rules, the development of the DRG system should also be carried out by a public authority, not by a private firm (National DRG Centre) as is currently the case in Finland.

In individual hospitals the introduction of DRG billing has brought about improvements. In these hospitals it has been necessary to pay more attention to the coding of diagnoses and procedures, and indeed the coding has been improved compared to hospitals not using the DRG billing system. This has made hospital billing more accurate, but also improved hospital management. It is therefore possible that the introduction of a DRG-based pricing system could lead to much improvement in the management and provision of hospital services, such as greater transparency and more accurate cost information (Häkkinen & Linna, 2005). However, if the system moves in the direction of a general prospective payment system, the potential for incentives/bias should be considered (see Chapter 6 of this volume). Given the current structure of the Finnish health care system, the choice of pricing method is not the most crucial one to be made. Efforts should be directed towards more important questions, such as the development of contracts between municipalities and hospitals, the management and control of care chains (total episodes of care), quality of services, or (even more generally) the governance role of central Government, as well as the issue of centralization – that is, increasing the size/impact of the purchasing and providing functions. All these elements are currently under considerable scrutiny in Finland.

18.8 Outlook: Future developments and reform

18.8.1 Trends in hospital service (or general health care) delivery

Finland places a strong emphasis on the public provision of health services. However, the importance of private service provision has been growing rapidly in recent years. Simultaneously, the boundary between public and private service provision has become blurred. Public hospitals order services from private producers if they are not able to produce the services themselves within the required time scale. Municipalities can also order private services directly. This trend is expected to continue.

Finnish public hospitals have not traditionally been highly specialized. Hospital districts have tried to be as self-sufficient as possible in treating their patients. In recent years it has been realized that it is not efficient, or even conducive to delivering high-quality health care, to provide all services in each hospital district. A trend has been developing towards more specialized units. At the same time, an increasing number of patients are treated as outpatients, in day-care and ambulatory care settings. This has led to the reduction of inpatient capacity.

Since the early 2000s, several local reforms have been implemented to integrate municipal service provision into a single organization. The purpose of these reforms is to enhance cooperation between primary and secondary health care and social welfare services (Vuorenkoski, 2008). The reforms include merging health centres and local hospitals into one organization, creating new regional self-regulating administrative bodies for all municipal services (including health and social services, upper secondary schools, and vocational services) with their own regional councils, and hospital districts also taking responsibility for primary health care. In 2008 about 10 per cent of the Finnish population lived in areas in which most primary and secondary care is provided by the same organization. The most recent initiative from the Ministry of Social Affairs and Health is to create 40–60 health and social regions (federations of municipalities or large municipalities) that are responsible for social services as well as primary and (most) specialist care services, along with five districts with special responsibility, which would be responsible for the most expensive tertiary care. If the trend continues and the proposal is to be implemented, the contract and payment systems for hospital care should also be reconsidered.

18.8.2 Trends in DRG application/coverage

In 2005–2007 the National DRG Centre organized a project related to the usage of DRGs in Finnish hospitals, in cooperation with Finnish DRG experts and hospital districts. In the final report (Kuntaliitto, 2007) the project team offers suggestions and a schedule relating to how to proceed in the implementation and development of a DRG system in hospitals in the near future. The main targets are as follows.

- The DRG billing would be implemented in all Finnish public hospitals by 2010, covering at least inpatient and day-care activities.
- The coverage of DRG billing would be extended to outpatient services by 2011 and at the same time the grouping would be developed to correspond better to outpatient and psychiatric services.
- By 2011 all the hospitals would have advanced patient-level cost-accounting systems in place, in order to calculate their own DRG cost weights.
- Hospitals would stop using the department-level pricing and use the same DRG prices across departments within a hospital.
- Hospitals would use a national handbook in order to ensure that all hospitals apply the same principles for cost accounting and coding for diagnoses and procedures; the coding handbook should be available on the Internet and it should be updated constantly.
- A certification system should be created for hospitals, which would obligate them to maintain their own system of internal quality standards in terms of coding, and to submit to regular external auditing.

Most hospitals that do not currently use the DRG billing system have already launched a DRG implementation project and are planning to introduce the system as soon as possible. For some hospitals, however, the target time frame for introducing the system by 2010 was too tight. Similarly, many hospitals currently using the Classic DRG system are preparing to implement the Full DRG system. Currently, four of the thirteen hospital districts (using DRGs) use the Full DRG system, at least in part.

There has been a trend towards outpatient production in Finnish hospitals since the early 2000s and the importance of developing a grouper which is able to take into account treatment episodes in ambulatory care is therefore growing. The Full DRG grouper contains outpatient groups, but it still functions mostly on a fee-for-service basis. The challenge will be to develop the Full DRG system so that it will be able to capture the whole treatment pathway, instead of separate visits. This will not be straightforward, as patient treatment in an ambulatory care setting is not as homogeneous as in an inpatient setting. Further development of inpatient groups is also needed, in order to ensure that they better take into account patient casemix. Currently, the DRG system underestimates the complexity level of patients treated in university hospitals.

18.9 Notes

1 More information available on the National Institute for Health and Welfare web site (http://www.thl.fi/fi-FI/web/fi/tutkimus/hankkeet/perfect, accessed 10 July 2011).
2 Outdated database available at the STAKES web site (http://info.stakes.fi/benchmarking/EN/benchmarking.htm, accessed 1 August 2011).
3 The system was developed by a private firm, Datawell. It was first introduced in the HUS but is now used in many other hospitals.

18.10 References

Häkkinen, U. (2005). The impact of changes in Finland's health care system. *Health Economics*, 1(September):101–18.

Häkkinen, U. (2009). Finland, in E. Jonsson. *Cost Containments in National Health Systems*. Weinheim: Wiley International Science.

Häkkinen, U. (2011). The PERFECT project: measuring performance of health care episodes. *Annals of Medicine*, 43(S1):1–3.

Häkkinen, U., Lehto, J. (2005). Reform, change and continuity in Finnish health care. *Journal of Health Politics, Policy and Law*, 30(1–2):76–96.

Häkkinen, U., Linna, M. (2005). DRGs in Finnish health care. *Euro Observer*, 7(4):7–8 (http://www2.lse.ac.uk/LSEHealthAndSocialCare/LSEHealth/pdf/euroObserver.Obsval7n04.pdf, accessed 10 July 2011).

HUS (2009). *Tilinpäätös ja toimintakertomus 2008 [Financial Statement and Annual Report 2008]*. Helsinki: Hospital District of Helsinki and Uusimaa.

Junnila, M. (2004). *Sairaaloiden tuottavuus: Benchmarking-tietojen käyttö erikoissairaanhoidon toiminnan suunnittelussa, seurannassa ja arvioinnissa [Productivity of Hospitals: the Use of Benchmarking Information on the Planning, Follow-up and Evaluation of Specialized Care]*. Helsinki: National Institute for Health and Welfare (STAKES) (Reports 280).

Kuntaliitto (2007). *Erikoissairaanhoidon palvelujen tuotteistus Suomessa [Product Definition in Specialized Care in Finland]*. Helsinki: Kuntaliitto.

Linna, M., Häkkinen, U. (1998). A comparative application of econometric and DEA methods for assessing cost-efficiency of Finnish hospitals, in P. Zweifel, ed. *Health, the Medical Profession and Regulation*. Boston: Kluwer Academic Publishers.

Linna, M., Häkkinen, U. (2008). Benchmarking Finnish hospitals, in J. Blank, V. Valdmanis, eds. *Evaluating Hospital Policy and Performance: Contributions from Hospital Policy and Productivity Research*. Oxford: JAI Press.

Magnussen, J., Vrangbæk, K., Saltman, R.B. (2009). *Nordic Health Care Systems: Recent Reforms and Current Policy Challenges*. Maidenhead: Open University Press.

Nordic Centre for Classifications in Health Care (2009). *NordDRG Users' Manual* (Version 2009). Oslo: Nordic Centre for Classifications in Health Care (http://www.norddrg.net/norddrgmanual/NordDRG_2009_NC/index.htm, accessed 23 October 2009).

OECD (2005). *OECD Reviews of Health Systems – Finland*. Paris: Organisation for Economic Co-operation and Development.

THL (2010). *Terveydenhuollon menot ja rahoitus vuonna 2008 [Health Expenditure and Financing 2008]. Statistical Report 12/2010*. Helsinki: National Institute for Health and Welfare (STAKES).

Vuorenkoski, L. (2008). Finland: Health system review. *Health Systems in Transition*, 10(4):1–170.

chapter nineteen

Sweden: The history, development and current use of DRGs

Lisbeth Serdén and Mona Heurgren

19.1 Hospital services and the role of DRGs in Sweden

19.1.1 The Swedish health care system

Sweden has a decentralized health care system. There are three political and administrative levels; central Government, county councils and local municipalities. All are involved in financing, providing and evaluating health care activities. The central Government has a legislative supervisory role and partially finances health care, while the county councils and municipalities are responsible for both financing and providing health services. The municipalities and county councils are also politically accountable through their directly elected assemblies. The 21 county councils/regions are responsible for most health care services, except long-term care of the elderly and disabled people (including mentally ill people), for whom the 290 municipalities are responsible.

The Swedish health care system is mainly financed by taxes. The county councils and municipalities are entitled to collect direct income tax revenues as their major financial source; council tax amounts to about 10 per cent of the residents' income. There is also a grant from the Government, which amounts to about 9 per cent of the counties' revenue. The individual patient's co-payment is low – fees account for about 2.5 per cent of the total county revenues. In total, Sweden spent about 9 per cent of its gross domestic product (GDP) on health care in 2009.

19.1.2 Hospital services in Sweden

In total there are 81 hospitals in Sweden (as of 2009). Of these hospitals, seven are university hospitals (with 7300 disposable beds) (for more details relating

Table 19.1 Hospital beds in acute care, psychiatric and long-term care, and beds per 1000 people, 2009

	2009
Acute care hospital beds	18 944
per 1000 people	2.0
Psychiatric hospital beds	4 449
per 1000 people	0.5
Long-term care beds	2 167
per 1000 people	0.2

Source: SALAR, 2010.

specifically to acute care hospitals, see Table 19.1). The vast majority of Swedish hospitals are publicly funded. There are only three private profit-making hospitals and some smaller private non-profit-making hospitals (SALAR, 2010).

Annually, there are about 1.5 million inpatient care cases and 10 million visits by physicians for specialized outpatient care carried out at Swedish hospitals. In addition, there are 3 million private specialist visits, outside of the hospitals. Acute cases account for 75 per cent of inpatient care and elective care for 25 per cent. Outpatient care is distributed as 25 per cent acute care and 75 per cent elective care (Forsberg et al., 2009).

The hospital services encompass inpatient care, day surgery, day medicine and specialized outpatient care. Inpatient care is divided into specialized care, psychiatry, rehabilitation and geriatrics. Rehabilitation care is mostly carried out as a hospital treatment, but there are also units that offer rehabilitation services as care delivered outside of hospitals. GPs in ambulatory care refer patients to specialists at hospitals. All elective patients at hospitals are referred from GPs in their role as gatekeepers.

Each of the 21 counties/regions decides independently how their health care should be organized and reimbursed.

19.1.3 Purpose of the DRG system

In the early 1990s, the Swedish health care system needed save money. There was also a strong movement towards a more patient-oriented system. This signalled the emergence of incentives to start using diagnosis-related groups (DRGs); the main motive for introducing DRG-based payment schemes was to increase productivity and thereby to save (or make better use of) the money used for health care. Long waiting lists for elective surgery were another reason for this change. A third important reason for introducing DRG-based payment systems was to allow the patient freedom of choice to select a hospital for treatment. The idea was that, by giving freedom of choice to the patients – and if the money follows the patient – a degree of competition could be introduced among the hospitals. By providing good services and thereby attracting patients, the hospitals would secure higher revenues. There was also a need for higher quality information and greater transparency in health care. The global budget encouraged neither productivity nor patient-oriented care, so the move to a DRG-based funding system was initiated. However, the need for cost control was also important, and budget ceilings were introduced to prevent oversupply and overuse.

In accordance with the counties' right to self-determination in health care activities, use of the Nordic patient classification system (NordDRG) in Sweden is voluntary. The counties decide for themselves independently how to use DRGs within their own payment systems and what complementary rules should be applied (such as reimbursement of outliers, cost ceilings, and so on). The counties are also responsible for the follow-up of fraudulent activity and any other misuse of the system. The availability of health care represents another issue for the county councils. The most common method used for controlling the supply of health care activities has been to limit availability.

Today, aside from their application as a payment mechanism, DRGs are used for managerial purposes, benchmarking, health statistics, measuring hospital performance and calculating productivity (and efficiency) at all levels of health care. The National Board of Health and Welfare has started working to find a method for calculating efficiency in Swedish health care. In order to do so, DRGs were used to describe performance, as well as process costs.

19.2 Development and updates of the DRG system

19.2.1 The current DRG system at a glance

The NordDRG system is currently the only DRG system in Sweden. Thus far there are only two different licensed software suppliers for NordDRGs. Each of them provides groupers, either available as interactive single cases, or as a 'batch' grouper.

The Full version of NordDRG 2009 embraces a total of 983 DRGs (see Table 19.2). Of these groups there are 216 outpatient groups designed for day surgery, day medicine and endoscopies. There are also 190 groups for specialized

Table 19.2 Number of NordDRG codes in different settings in 2009

Setting	*Number*
Inpatient care	577
– Specialized care	514
– Psychiatry	30
– Rehabilitation	33
Day surgery	162
Day medicine	34
Endoscopy	20
Outpatient specialized care	190
Total	**983**

Source: Nordic Centre for Classifications in Health Care, 2009.

outpatient care visits. The groups for other day-treatment visits and outpatient care carry an 'O' or a 'P' at the end of the DRG code. Day surgery is allocated the same number as the corresponding inpatient group, but with an 'O' in the DRG-code (Nordic Casemix Centre, 2011).

The counties in Sweden can be divided into three categories with regard to their usage of DRGs. The first category uses DRGs for reimbursement to hospitals for a large range of care (both in- and outpatient care, to some extent). The eight counties/regions in this category represent more than half of the Swedish health care system (calculated by health care expenditure). Psychiatry is included in the payment system of one of the counties. The second category of counties use DRGs only as a tool for analysis, to calculate casemix, for hospital budgeting or for reimbursement of patients across county borders. The third category of counties uses DRGs as a component in the reimbursement system for a smaller component of health care; for example, for patients across county borders, or for a single hospital.

In total, about 90 per cent of inpatients are grouped into DRGs, and 65 per cent are financed by DRGs. In outpatient care, 80 per cent are grouped into DRGs, and 30 per cent are financed by them.

19.2.2 Development of the DRG system

The National Board of Health and Welfare is responsible for developing and maintaining the Swedish version of the NordDRG system. In validating the resource homogeneity process in DRGs, the Board cooperates with the Swedish Association of Local Authorities and Regions (*Sveriges Kommuner och Landsting*, SALAR) which is responsible for the Swedish National Case Costing Database. All cost data in use with respect to DRG maintenance are calculated using a 'bottom-up' approach.

The Swedish NordDRG version has been developed to comprise both in- and outpatient care, as well as psychiatry and rehabilitation (see Table 19.3). The NordDRG system can be implemented in any type of hospital. In 2011, the 15th version of NordDRG was introduced.

Between 2003 and 2009, two versions of NordDRG were operating in Sweden; a Full version, which handled both inpatient care and day surgery (including intraluminal endoscopies), along with outpatient specialized care, and a Classic version for inpatient care only. Since 2010, just one version of NordDRG is in effect for handling all in- and outpatient care using the same logic.

19.2.3 Data used for development and updates of the DRG system

Test data from the National Patient Register (NPR) (except the personal identification number) are used to inform the update process. The National Case Costing Database is used to validate the resource homogeneity in the DRGs.

Table 19.3 Various NordDRG versions in Sweden, 1995–2008 (selected years)

	1st DRG version	*6th DRG version*	*8th DRG version*	*10th DRG version*	*11th DRG version*	*12th DRG version*
Date of introduction	*1995*	*2001*	*2003*	*2005*	*2006*	*2008*
(Main) Purpose	Reimbursement, and to describe performance	Reimbursement, and to describe performance	Reimbursement, and to describe performance	Reimbursement, and to describe performance	Reimbursement, and to describe performance Benchmarking Productivity Measurement	Reimbursement, and to describe performance Benchmarking Productivity Measurement
DRG system	NordDRG	NordDRG	NordDRG	NordDRG	NordDRG	NordDRG
Data used for development	Cost weights, USA	National Cost Database, NPR	National Cost Database, NPR	National Cost database, NPR	National Cost Database, NPR	National Cost Database, NPR
Number of DRGs	500	498	722	740	929	976
Applied to	All hospitals, only inpatients	All hospitals, only inpatients including children/ neonatology	All hospitals, inpatients and day surgery	All hospitals, inpatients, plus psychiatry and day surgery	All hospitals, inpatients and all outpatients	All hospitals, in- and outpatients, including rehabilitation

Source: Designed for this report by Lisbeth Serdén at the National Board of Health and Welfare[2] in 2011.

This database contains bottom-up cost data collected directly from hospitals. The hospitals join the database on a voluntary basis. National cost data have been available since 1997 and the quality of the data has improved significantly over time (see section 19.4) (Ludvigsson et al., 2011).

The tradition of collecting data at the individual patient level is strong in Sweden; the NPR has been in use since the 1960s and contains all individual inpatient records in Sweden. All data can be linked to the individual patient by the personal identification number that is given to all citizens at birth. The register has traditionally been used mainly for research purposes. The use of the register for measuring productivity and various types of follow-ups in health care is gradually increasing over time.

19.2.4 Regularity and method of system updates

The NordDRG system is updated yearly. The original development work carried out in advance of major changes is normally conducted in each country that uses the system. Some major changes can be implemented as joint projects between the countries concerned.

Changes in DRGs may be initiated by problems with either cost heterogeneity or clinical relevance, according to the basic concept that applies to all DRG systems: patient cases are to be assigned to clinically relevant groups with the least possible variance in cost.

For all types of changes (splitting DRGs, merging DRGs, partial or total reassignment), there are specified statistical criteria that must be evaluated with cost-per-case data from at least one of the Nordic countries. Changes can sometimes be made even if not all criteria are met, but in those cases a clear rationale must be put forward (Lindqvist, 2008).

19.3 The current patient classification system

19.3.1 Information used to classify patients

The Nordic countries have a long tradition of collaborating on classification systems – as manifested in the Nordic Centre for Classifications in Health Care (which is a WHO collaborating centre). The Nordic countries collaborate concerning the basic classifications, but are also obligated to maintain national versions of the classifications in their national languages.

For coding diagnosis, the Nordic countries use a national version of the International Classification of Diseases 10th revision (ICD-10) and, for surgery procedures, the common Nordic classification of surgery is used (NOMESCO Classification of Surgical Procedures, NCSP). In Sweden, a new national classification system for non-surgical procedures was introduced in 2006 (KMÅ). Combined, the classification of surgery and non-surgical procedures is called KVÅ. The surgical procedures in KVÅ are in general the same as the procedures in the NCSP, but the medical procedures are national in scope.

19.3.2 Grouping algorithm

NordDRG is a system for classifying inpatient cases and outpatient visits into categories with similar resource use (see Figure 19.1). The grouping is based on diagnoses, procedures performed, age, birth weight, gender and status at discharge. The history, design and classification rules of the DRG system – as well as its application in terms of patient discharge data and updating procedures – are presented in the *DRG Definitions Manual* (Nordic Casemix Centre, 2011).

19.3.3 Data quality and plausibility checks

The NPR – managed by the National Board of Health and Welfare – is quality checked on an annual basis. For each record reported to the NPR, a data control is performed to check that compulsory variables are reported, such as the patient's personal identification number, the hospital and the main diagnosis. Codes for different variables and dates are also checked. Some obviously incorrect data are corrected in the quality controls, while other data are sent back to the hospital for correction. In the same way, the cost data in the National Case Costing Database are checked annually by the SALAR.

Many performance indicators can be deducted from Swedish national health data registers; for example, registers have been used for analysing the differences in case fatality within 28 days after acute myocardial infarction or stroke. Significant efforts are now being made, at both the national and local levels, to find valid and accepted quality indicators for following up health care performance, and also for productivity/efficiency measurements. Some counties already have models in use for the follow-up of performance indicators. Since 2006, Sweden has used national performance indicators to measure performance at county level on an annual basis. (National Board of Health and Welfare, 2010). For the year 2010, 134 quality indicators were published. The National Board of Health and Welfare also publishes reports on coding activity and quality on a yearly basis.

The county councils are responsible for checking the quality of DRG-grouped data by means case record audits. Some of the county councils carry out audits of case records on a regular basis in order to identify incorrect coding. The process in place in the event that fraud is identified in the records differs from county to county. In most cases the hospital or private clinic will be obligated to pay back the discrepancy. Coding quality has improved and continues to improve in Sweden. As such, there are attempts to introduce more time for coding issues in physicians' education programmes, and many county councils are educating their medical secretaries in coding and encouraging them to play a larger role in this field.

19.3.4 Incentives for up- or wrong-coding

Very few cases of up-coding occur because of the small number of private hospitals in Sweden. However, a problem still exists in terms of 'down-coding'

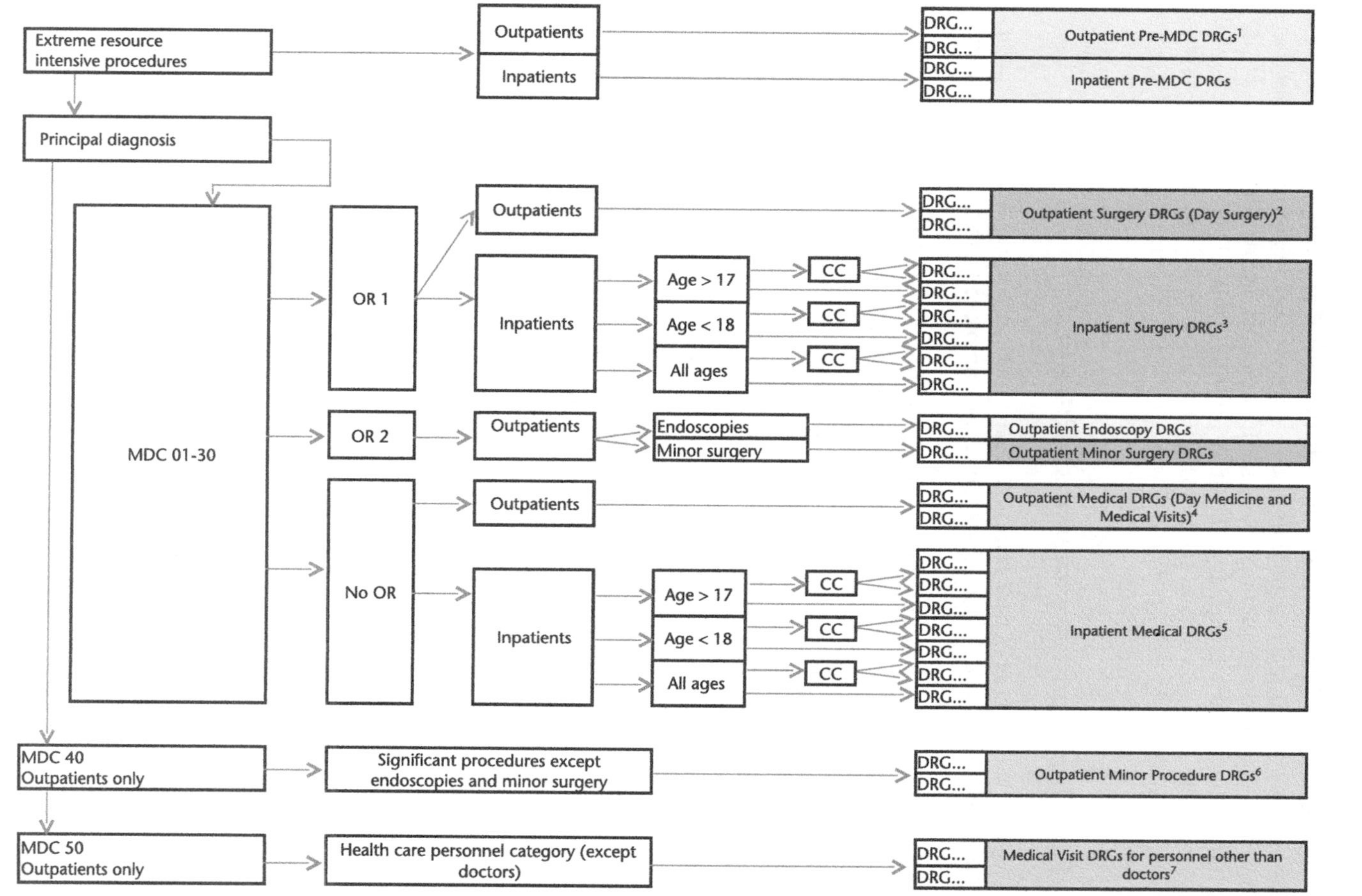

Extreme resource intensive procedures
Outpatients
Inpatients
Outpatient Pre-MDC DRGs[1]
Inpatient Pre-MDC DRGs
Principal diagnosis
MDC 01-30
OR 1
OR 2
No OR
Outpatients
Inpatients
Age > 17
Age < 18
All ages
CC
Endoscopies
Minor surgery
DRG...
Outpatient Surgery DRGs (Day Surgery)[2]
Inpatient Surgery DRGs[3]
Outpatient Endoscopy DRGs
Outpatient Minor Surgery DRGs
Outpatient Medical DRGs (Day Medicine and Medical Visits)[4]
Inpatient Medical DRGs[5]
MDC 40
Outpatients only
Significant procedures except endoscopies and minor surgery
Outpatient Minor Procedure DRGs[6]
MDC 50
Outpatients only
Health care personnel category (except doctors)
Medical Visit DRGs for personnel other than doctors[7]

Figure 19.1 Grouping algorithm in the Swedish version of NordDRG system

Source: Designed for this publication by Mats Fernström at the National Board of Health and Welfare in 2011.

Notes:

1 **Outpatient Pre-MDC DRGs**: extremely resource-intensive procedures are seldom performed on outpatients, so there are few cases in these DRGs.

2 **Outpatient Surgery DRGs (Day Surgery)**: these DRGs are also called Day Surgery and they have a grouping logic very similar to the Inpatient Surgery DRGs, but there is no age split or CC split.

3 **Inpatient Surgery DRGs**: about 50 per cent of these DRGs are split based on age and/or CC. The age split is less than 18 years, but for MDC 15 the patient must be less than 1 year old.

4 **Outpatient Medical DRGs**: some of these DRGs are for longer visits (for example for some hours of observation) and are called Day Medicine.

5 **Inpatient Medical DRGs**: like the Inpatient Surgery DRGs, about 50 per cent of the groups are split based on age and/or CC. The common age split is identical to the split for Inpatient Surgery DRGs but the DRGs for Diabetes are divided into > 35 or < 35 years of age.

6 **Outpatient Minor Procedure DRGs**: these DRGs are for minor procedures, except endoscopies and minor surgery. These procedures are often performed by personnel other than doctors and therefore a principal diagnosis is not mandatory.

7 **Medical Visit DRGs for personnel other than doctors**: according to Swedish law, only doctors are obliged to report diagnoses, so the grouping logic for these DRGs is based on profession and the type of visit (single, team or group).

(due not to failings of the financial system, but rather the tradition of entering only few codes into the system). At national level, the authorities encourage hospitals to operate better coding practices, which has often led to a greater number of registered secondary diagnoses per case. Systematic selection of patients for financial reasons (cherry-picking or cream-skimming) has not occurred in public hospitals, but has occurred to some degree among private providers in Stockholm.

Several record audits in Sweden (2300 medical records altogether) show that abuse of secondary diagnosis coding can create an increase, but also (at the same time) a decrease in DRG weights compared with accurate coding. Audits can lead to adjustments in reimbursement to hospitals and other providers of health care (National Board of Health and Welfare, 2006). Most wrong-coding is not in fact a sign of abuse of the system, but rather a matter of ignorance.

19.4 Cost accounting within hospitals

19.4.1 Regulation

It is not mandatory to implement case-costing databases within a hospital. The incentive for the hospitals to do so is that they will achieve not only a greater degree of cost control within the hospital management, but also an influence over the national DRG weights. National guidelines have been developed for cost-per-case calculations. About 65 per cent of inpatient cases and 36 per cent of outpatient visits were individually calculated in 2009.

Case costing is a costing method that uses a bottom-up approach. All costs, including indirect costs, should be incorporated. There are some exceptions, such as costs for research and teaching, external projects, ambulances, and the counties' politicians and their staff (SALAR, 2011).

19.4.2 Main characteristics of the cost-accounting system

Case costing data have been collected from hospitals with case costing systems since the mid-1990s and added to the National Case Costing Database (Heurgren, et al., 2003; SALAR, 2011). The data are held in a common database for the calculation of Swedish DRG weights, managed by the SALAR. The information in the National Case Costing Database is almost the same as in the NPR, except that the cost data are added and the personal identification numbers are missing.

Case costing model

The case costing model comprises four steps: (1) accurately identifying the total cost of the hospital; (2) allocating indirect costs to the cost centres (that are absorbing the cost); (3) identifying intermediate products and calculating their costs; (4) distributing products and costs to the patients. Figure 19.2 provides more details.

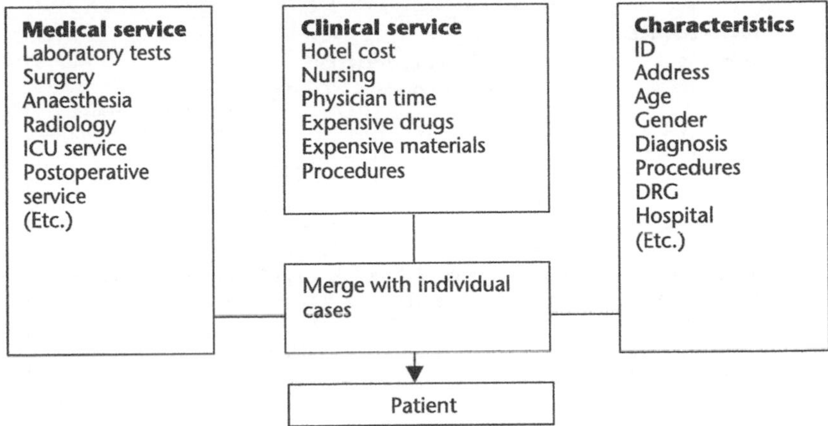

Figure 19.2 The Swedish case costing model

Source: SALAR 2009.

In the case costing process, all costs are distributed to the individual cases by the unique personal identification number. A patient-specific service mix is tied together with patient characteristics. The case costing system provides information about activities such as surgery, laboratory tests, intensive care, and nursing care. Their costs are calculated uniquely for each patient. The system also holds information on diagnoses, procedures, DRG, and so on, for each patient. National guidelines have been implemented to ensure data quality and comparability (SALAR, 2009).

The most common IT-structure for case costing is the integration model, in which data are collected from various databases in the hospital into a 'data warehouse'. The case costing system uses these data to link the relevant case and patient by means of the personal identification number for each patient and the date of their stay or visit (see Figure 19.3). It is also possible to collect data for a case costing system directly from medical records, but in general this does not take place in Sweden (except for a few hospital departments), since current medical records are not designed for this purpose.

The IT structure is important when implementing case costing systems. Access to information must be highly automated, and an important principle to apply is to use existing data as much as possible in order to minimize manual work and obtain higher data quality.

The use of case costing is important from many perspectives. In Sweden, case costing data are used in the following areas:

- management support for hospital departments and hospitals – process management;
- support for buyers of health care;
- benchmarking studies of costs and medical praxis;
- development of the DRG system and calculating prices in health care;
- calculating relative cost weights in the NordDRG system;
- calculating productivity and efficiency.

Intermediate products	Costs	Characteristics		
Nursing care	11 950	Length of stay	5 days	
Physician (ward)	3 540	DRG	211	(Hip and femur procedures except major joint, age > 17, without CC)
Hotel costs	5 700	Clinic	311	
Surgery	6 522	Age	72	
Intensive care	2 911	Gender	Female	
Anaesthesia	10 957	Acute	Yes	
Laboratory tests	1 846	Principal diagnosis	S7240	Fracture on lower part of femur
Imaging exams	2 629	Procedures	NFJ59	Fracture surgery, femur
Other products	4 333		NFJ09	"
			NFJ99	"
Total cost	**SEK 50 388**			

Figure 19.3 An example of a patient in the Swedish National Case Costing Database: femur fracture

Source: SALAR, 2009.

19.5 DRGs for hospital payment

19.5.1 Range of services and costs included in DRG-based hospital payments

In the public health care sector, the decision to use a DRG for reimbursement is made at the county council level.

Swedish hospitals are traditionally financed via global budgeting. This is due to the fact that Sweden has a tradition of publicly owned hospitals, and therefore cost control has always been an important issue. Moreover, before the introduction of DRGs, there was no general, accepted system in use for describing performance. The counties' knowledge of hospital activity and productivity was poor, and therefore a great need existed to find ways to measure productivity.

The main reasons for introducing the DRG system as a financing tool for hospitals included to improve productivity and efficiency, to increase transparency in the hospital sector, and to create a 'market', with purchaser and providers sharing the financial risk.

In Sweden there are differences in the way DRGs are used for financing in different types of hospitals (regional, teaching hospitals, acute care, psychiatric, rehabilitation, and so on). Until recently, DRGs were used only for somatic care (inpatient and outpatient) in Sweden. In 2010, one county used DRGs for financing psychiatry. Rehabilitation is another new field for DRG use in Sweden, introduced in 2008, but only a few counties have adopted DRGs for financing purposes. Others simply use this part of the DRG system to describe performance.

On the other hand, the use of DRGs has been quite similar within hospitals, regardless of whether they are teaching hospitals or rural hospitals. Both acute and planned care have been included, but the teaching hospitals have incorporated more exceptions from the DRG list, such as fee-for-service prices for unusual and costly treatments. There are no differences in the way DRGs are used in terms of the legal status of the hospital (that is, whether it is public, private profit-making or non-profit-making).

In Sweden, the cost all health professionals' (for example doctors', nurses') fees are included in the DRG weights and prices. The vast majority of health care professionals are employed by the hospitals/counties. The costs of infrastructure, important medical equipment and installations, communication systems or informatics are also included.

Costs for outliers are not included in the DRG weights. Burn injuries are also not included. In some counties, specific regional care and rehabilitation are excluded. Some unusual and expensive drugs/materials might also be excluded. All these exceptions are reimbursed separately, and the exclusion list varies widely between counties.

The cost of education, and of research and development (R&D) are not covered by DRGs. The majority of R&D costs are covered by grants from the Government. Most counties also offer local grants to their hospitals for R&D activities. Other activities of general interest (such as accreditation, incentives to hospital personnel, participation in social or other projects, and so on) are covered by specially designated project budgets.

The most used model for reimbursement of all areas of the health care sector is a mixed model, with global budgets, prospective payment systems, retrospective payment systems and payment for performance (P4P) in use within the same system.

19.5.2 Calculation of DRG prices/cost weights

There is no 'national price' per DRG in Sweden, but there are reference cost weights. Sums vary by county and by hospital, resulting in different prices per DRG. The county councils are the payers and purchasers of hospital services and the DRG prices are set according to the budget and regulation of the council.

The National Board of Health and Welfare develops and publishes national prospective weights for NordDRGs (both in- and outpatients) on an annual basis. It is not mandatory to use the national weight sets; local weights are also in use in two counties/regions. A goal for the future is that all counties will use the same weights.

The average real cost in the cost database from last year is used to calculate the national weights. The average cost is adjusted by the budgeted cost increases and decreases for the next year and sometimes also by an estimated increase in productivity (about 1 per cent). The most common method variant is that hospitals use the same weight set within and between counties, but that the prices per DRG are different for each hospital/council.

Items that are reimbursed on a 'fee-for-service' basis (rather than by cost weights) represent very unusual and expensive treatments that cannot be properly described in the DRG system, such as burns or special treatments delivered at teaching hospitals.

The national DRG weights are based on individual patient costs, as are the outlier limits. In addition, also outlier limits are also calculated based on length of stay by those hospitals that do not yet calculate individual patient-related costs. Outliers are reimbursed outside the DRG system, with money from the global budget of the county councils.

The cost trim-point is calculated using the quartile (Q) method, given 5 per cent outliers by the following formula: Q3 + cost constant x (Q3 – Q1). The cost constant is chosen to give 5 per cent outliers.

19.5.3 DRGs in actual hospital payment

The councils decide independently how to pay for health care. The reimbursement model is set up in negotiation between purchaser and provider, within the councils. The councils are free to use the DRGs or part of the DRG system, or other models such as capitation or fixed reimbursement.

Over 65 per cent of all discharges from Swedish acute somatic care are reimbursed by NordDRGs to some extent. Outpatient care is reimbursed by the NordDRG system to a more modest degree, and psychiatry and rehabilitation even less so.

Various methods are used in different counties for keeping within the budget. The county's purchases and their volume are set, in negotiation with the hospitals. In some counties a ceiling is in place for expenditures and the hospital faces making a loss if it treats too many patients. In other counties, this could be a gradual shift of responsibility, with a shared risk for when the negotiated volume is exceeded.

19.5.4 Quality-related adjustments

The counties use quality indicators to describe performance and to some extent for reimbursement purposes, in addition to the use of DRGs. Most hospitals contribute to the national quality registers and also report to the national waiting-time database.[1] Sanctions are decided upon in each individual county.

There is no quality assurance tool attached to the DRG-based health care production in Sweden. Every county must decide themselves how to monitor quality. Most counties use the national quality indicators, among other tools.

19.5.5 Main incentives for hospitals

Following the introduction of DRGs in Swedish health care, there has been a significant increase in coding diagnoses; in 1998, there were 1.8 diagnoses per case and in 2009 there were 2.7 diagnoses coded per case in inpatient care (Serdén at al., 2003). Quality has been improved to some extent in the national registers, by educating the medical secretaries who input diagnosis and procedure codes into the administrated systems.

19.6 New/innovative technologies

19.6.1 Steps required prior to introduction in hospitals

County councils and hospitals should take the initiative to develop health care by introducing new technologies. The adoption of innovations into the DRG system is decided in the updating process, which itself is published in reports. At national level, the DRG system is administrated and developed by the National Board of Health and Welfare. Within the updating process, innovations are discussed at Nordic level in the NordDRG expert group(s) and finally in a steering group in which decisions are made.

19.6.2 Payment mechanisms

During the first two years, new and innovative technologies are funded either separately, outside of the DRG system, or via the DRG system (through additional payments for high-cost outliers), depending on the regulations in each county council. Most hospitals negotiate with the county regarding separate prices for new technologies. When the innovations are adopted into the DRG system, their funding is embraced within the DRGs.

19.6.3 Incentives for hospitals to use new/innovative technologies

There is a delay in the process, from the decision to use new technologies until those technologies are incorporated into the reimbursement system. The whole process usually takes about two years.

19.7 Evaluation of the DRG system in Sweden

19.7.1 Official evaluation(s)

County councils are responsible for the primary coding of and registration of DRGs at the hospital. The councils are also responsible for evaluating the DRG results. Unfortunately, only a few counties carry out audits to check the DRG results. As already mentioned, Sweden does not have a significant problem in terms of up-coding, but a problem does exist relating to too few diagnoses and procedures being coded (in some counties). In counties in which this is a problem, it is characteristic for them to only use DRGs to a minor extent.

19.7.2 Authors' assessment

The original goals that were set out before the introduction of the DRG system have been reached: a rise in productivity and transparency in hospital activities, creating a common 'language' between professionals and administrators, resulting in a financing system focused on hospital activities instead of organization, along with better describing performance, and a tool for benchmarking and productivity calculation.

In the early 1990s, many physicians were opposed to DRGs. To start with there was very little knowledge relating to DRGs, in terms of how they worked and how the system could be utilized. This lack of knowledge was a problem. Many actors had also unrealistic expectations of the benefits of the system; for example, that it would save a lot of money and solve the issue of quality monitoring. In addition, many politicians disliked activity-based funding. This has now changed, and most are in favour of activity-based funding to some degree.

As time passed, users learnt more and the expectations became more realistic, along with the ability to see the good and bad aspects of the system. In addition, the introduction and use of cost-outliers achieved better acceptance levels – today, most professionals accept the system. Extending the system to encompass both outpatient care and psychiatry has also been a positive development. In psychiatry, DRGs were not accepted until 2005, when 26 new groups for psychiatry were incorporated. There is just one county using DRGs for financing in psychiatric care; predominantly, it is used as a tool to describe performance (in eight counties).

There were not many technical problems in implementing the grouper system. The period of time needed for technical implementation of the system was different in each hospital. The cost of developing and implementing DRGs (for the Government, hospitals, taxpayers, and so on) remained fairly low and did not exceed expected levels.

The DRG impact

After introducing DRGs in Sweden, there was an increase in productivity and service delivery increased. At the start, the Stockholm County Council had a problem with the use of DRGs to control total costs; when the system was introduced, the increase in volume resulted in the costs exceeding the global budget. Within a few years, this could be controlled. In general, the hospitals that are using DRGs have better control (with some exceptions) over their activities and have a lower cost per DRG point than hospitals that do not use the system.

In terms of the impact on the patient, the introduction of the DRG system has shortened waiting times, due to the increase in productivity (more services carried out) (Charpentier & Samuelson, 1998).

Sweden has had a major reduction in length of stay since the early 2000s – for a number of reasons, but partly because of the use of DRGs. Counties that use DRGs tend to have shorter lengths of stay than others. Whether the present length of stay is too short or not is a matter for debate, but most will agree that it is good for the patients if the length of stay is short. A short length of stay shows that the process works and that the patient is well informed. The argument against short lengths of stay is mainly that elderly people are sent back to their homes too early in the health care process, but there is no evidence of an increased level of readmission when introducing DRG-based reimbursement systems.

The introduction of the DRG system has not had a direct impact on the way inpatient and outpatient care is organized on a daily basis, although it may have had an indirect effect. The DRG system has exerted no influence on hospital organization as a whole.

DRGs are not a 'miracle cure'

The most important experience gained from working with DRGs for reimbursement is that the introduction of payment systems does not solve all the problems that health care systems are facing (Lindqvist, 2008). When DRGs for reimbursement were introduced in some counties in the early 1990s, there was a strong notion that this was a 'miracle cure'. The few that were opposed to the transformation, on the other hand, saw the change as the end of the Swedish health care model as we know it. Both of these expectations have been proven wrong. Other political decisions and changes, economic conditions and the general public's expectations have had more of an impact on health care than the introduction of DRG-based payment systems.

One of the most significant problems with using DRGs for reimbursement, at least from a Swedish perspective, has been the mechanisms of cost control. In the case of Stockholm County, productivity rose quite dramatically during the years following its introduction, but the increased production also led to higher total expenditures. To secure cost control, budget ceilings were introduced – which led to a reduction in the increased rate of productivity. Finding a balance between the desire to increase productivity and the need to control cost (given limited resources) has been the biggest challenge in the introduction of payment systems.

A casemix reimbursement system improves productivity

It is quite simple – when a funding system based on recorded activity is introduced, the activity increases – or, to be more precise, the recorded activity increases (Lindqvist, 2008). The first problem is to determine whether the increase is an effect of better or changed recording, or of an actual increase in volume. The experience in Sweden, especially in the outpatient care setting (where there was no tradition of good recording), is that the initial increase seen following the introduction of DRG-based payment systems was to a great extent due to changes in recording. However, the number of inpatient admissions also increased, and this effect is better documented, since the medical recording of admissions was of good quality in Sweden.

Good information systems and good data are crucial

When shifting to a system in which clinical data are the basis for reimbursement, the increasing need for data and information system is of great importance (Lindqvist, 2008). In Sweden, the tradition of collecting clinical data and the use of a personal identification number have been beneficial, but a new information system for follow-up and analysis needed to be developed. This development was regrettably slow in terms of tools for analysing production at hospital and department levels. This was quite ironic, considering that the responsibility for the hospitals' economy was to a large extent moved to the department heads.

The data quality must also be considered. In spite of a long tradition of data collection, the quality of data was poorly analysed in Sweden. This necessitated efforts to improve the quality of basic clinical data. There is a trend towards 'going back to the basic data quality'. More efforts are being directed towards correct registration and regular revisions of coding. One key question concerns access to and quality of data. Working with prospective payment systems based on DRGs means dealing with core health care data, and the performance of the systems is heavily dependent on the quality of the basic data. To implement the systems, access to individual patient data is required – to both reimburse and assess performance more accurately.

19.8 Outlook: Future developments and reform

19.8.1 Trends in hospital service (or general health care) delivery

The National Board of Health and Welfare has received a government commission to improve the reimbursement system in primary care; specifically, a system promoting health care activities and results. Uniform classification of diagnoses and procedures in primary care is necessary when creating high-quality squared systems to describe performance, which form the basis of reimbursement and high-quality follow-up in primary care. Uniform classification systems are also necessary to compare health care within primary care. It is beneficial if the classification is comparable to other settings.

A Swedish classification system for *diagnoses* exists for Swedish primary care, but it is not generally used and, when it is, it is not used properly. Since there is no classification system for *procedures* in primary care, the need exists to develop such a system or to improve existing classification relating to procedures. There is much to be done before a new secondary patient classification system in primary care can be established.

19.8.2 Trends in DRG application/coverage

An extensive amount of work in exchanging and improving the system has taken place during the 2000s. Sweden has just finished the development of a new grouper, which will be available in Sweden from 2012. The purpose of this grouping system is to divide DRGs into three severity sub-group levels. The role model is the grouper of the Centers for Medicare & Medicaid Services (CMS) in the United States (3M, 2011).

19.9 Notes

1 More information is available at the relevant web site of the Swedish Association of Local Authorities and Regions (www.vantetider.se, accessed 1 August 2011).
2 More details available at the National Board of Health and Welfare web site (http://www.socialstyrelsen.se/klassificeringochkoder/norddrg/logikenidrg, accessed 1 August 2011).

19.10 References

3M (2011). *Definitions Manuals*. St Paul, MN: 3M Health Information Systems (http://solutions.3m.com/wps/portal/3M/en_US/3M_Health_Information_Systems/HIS/Products/Definition_Manuals/, accessed 1 August 2011),

Charpentier, C., Samuelson, L.A. (1998). *Effekter av en sjukvårdsreform – En analys av Stockholmsmodellen [The Effects of the Stockholm Model]*. Stockholm: Nerenius & Santérus Förlag.

Forsberg, L., Rydh, H., Jacobson, A., Nygvist, K., Heurgren, M. (2009). *Kvalitet och innehåll i patientregistret. Discharge from inpatient treatment 1964–2007 and visits to specialist outpatient care (excluding primary care visits) 1997–2007 [Quality and Content of the Patient Register]*. Stockholm: National Board of Health and Welfare.

Heurgren, M., Nilsson, H., Erlö, C., Sjöli, P. (2003). What does the individual patient cost? CPP – the Cost Per Patient method – is the answer. *Lakartidningen*, 100(42):3312–15.

Lindqvist, R. (2008). From naïve hope to realistic conviction: DRGs in Sweden, in J.R. Kimberly, G. de Pouvourville, T. D'Aunno, eds. *The Globalization of Managerial Innovation in Health Care*. Cambridge: Cambridge University Press.

Ludvigsson, J.F., Andersson, E., Ekbom, E. et al. (2011). External review and validation of the Swedish national inpatient register. *BMC Public Health*, 11(450):1–16.

National Board of Health and Welfare (2006). *Diagnosgranskningar utförda i Sverige 1997–2005 samt råd inför granskning [Audits Performed in Swedish Health Care 1997–2005]*. Stockholm: National Board of Health and Welfare (http://www.socialstyrelsen.se/publikationer2006/2006-131-30, accessed 10 July 2011).

National Board of Health and Welfare (2010). *Quality and Efficiency in Swedish Health Care – Regional Comparisons 2009* [English version]. Stockholm: Swedish Association of Local Authorities and Regions (SALAR) (http://www.socialstyrelsen.se/Lists/Artikelkatalog/Attachments/18023/2010-4-37.pdf, accessed 10 July 2011).

Nordic Casemix Centre (2011). *Swedish Version*. Helsinki: Nordic Casemix Centre (http://www.nordcase.org/eng/norddrg_manuals/versions/swedish, accessed 1 August 2011).

SALAR (2009). *Nationella KPP-principer, version 2. [National Case Costing Principles, Version 2]*. Stockholm: Swedish Association of Local Authorities and Regions.

SALAR (2010). *Statistik om hälso- och sjukvård samt regional utveckling 2009 [Health Care Statistics and Regional Development in 2009]*. Stockholm: Swedish Association of Local Authorities and Regions.

SALAR (2011). *Swedish National Case Costing Database*. Stockholm: Swedish Association of Local Authorities and Regions (www.skl.se/vi_arbetar _med/statistik/sjukvård/KPP, accessed 1 August 2011).

Serdén, L., Lindqvist, R., Rosén, M. (2003). Have DRG-based prospective payment systems influenced the number of secondary diagnoses in health care administrative data? *Health Policy*, 65(2):101–7.

chapter twenty

Poland: The Jednorodne Grupy Pacjentów – Polish experiences with DRGs

Katarzyna Czach,
Katarzyna Klonowska,
Maria Świderek and
Katarzyna Wiktorzak

20.1 Hospital services and the role of DRGs in Poland

20.1.1 The Polish health care system

Poland has a mixed system of public and private health care financing. Total health expenditure amounts to about €667 per capita per year, which corresponds to 6.6 per cent of gross domestic product (GDP) (European Commission, 2009). Public expenditure accounts for roughly 72 per cent of total health expenditure and is mostly based on mandatory social health insurance contributions. Private expenditure accounted for about 24 per cent of total health expenditure in 2008, and predominantly took the form of out-of-pocket payments and co-payments from members of social health insurance schemes, for example for food and accommodation at rehabilitative care facilities, or for a certain percentage of the costs of medicines and diagnostic examinations (Kuszewski & Gericke, 2005; European Commission, 2009).

The three most important actors in the system are: (1) the Ministry of Health, (2) the territorial governments, and (3) the National Health Fund (NFZ) (Kuszewski & Gericke, 2005). The Ministry of Health is responsible for policy-making and regulation. As such, it designs national health policies, finances major capital investments and oversees medical science and medical education. The territorial governments (local, county and municipality levels) manage the majority of public hospitals; they develop strategies and health plans for their populations, as well as engaging in health promotion activities. The NFZ, which was established in 2003 is the purchaser of health care services for all members of the social health insurance system.

About 98 per cent of the population are members of a social health insurance scheme and contributions currently amount to 9 per cent of most individuals' taxable income. Contributions are paid either to the Social Insurance Institution (ZUS) or to the Agricultural Social Insurance Fund (KRUS), which forward collected contributions to the NFZ. Health care benefits for uninsured people, the unemployed population and individuals requiring complex and expensive medical care are financed directly from tax-funded state budgets or the budgets of local governments. State budgets also contribute to capital expenditures of health care providers, while recurrent costs are paid from health insurance contributions managed by the NFZ (Ministry of Health, 2008).

The NFZ is composed of 16 regional branch offices, plus one central office. It is supervised by the NFZ Council, consisting of nine members appointed by the Prime Minister for a five-year term. The NFZ pools and manages all revenue received through contributions from social health insurance members. As the purchaser of health care, the NFZ operates within a budget that is fixed for a given year. A 'Universal Catalogue of Services' is defined at the national level and the regional branches of the NFZ negotiate contracts with providers competing for contracts in the form of a competitive bid. There are strict regulations prohibiting the NFZ from engaging in the direct provision of health care services and from undertaking income-generating activities.

20.1.2 Hospital services in Poland

Historically, there has been a relatively strict separation between outpatient care and inpatient care in Poland (Kuszewski & Gericke, 2005). Outpatient care (both delivered by general practitioners (GPs) and specialists) is mostly provided in private medical practices or in independent health care institutions. Hospital care is provided either in general (county) hospitals, specialized (province (*voivodship*))-level hospitals, or highly specialized university hospitals.

Throughout most of the 1990s, hospitals in Poland had the status of budgetary units that received funds from the Ministry of Health or from territorial governments. This changed fundamentally with the Law on Universal Health Insurance that came into effect in 1999. The law introduced a split between the purchasers and providers of health care and all public hospitals were obligated to change their status into independent institutions that must generate revenue through health service delivery. As a result of the reform, hospitals can incur deficits and make profits. However, most hospitals are still public and are owned by territorial governments (Kozierkiewicz, 2008).

At the end of 2007, there were 578 public hospitals and 170 non-public hospitals in Poland (Table 20.1). The share of non-public hospitals increased from 4 per cent in the year 2000 to almost 23 per cent in 2007. Changes in the total number of hospitals have been difficult to identify. However, the number of hospital beds has continued to decrease since the year 2000. In absolute numbers, there were 8 per cent fewer hospital beds in 2007 than in 2000, a decrease that is even more pronounced when looking at the number of hospital

Table 20.1 Number of hospitals, hospital beds and patients in Poland, 2000, 2005 and 2007

Year	*2000*	*2005*	*2007*	*Change in %*
	Number (%)	*Number (%)*	*Number (%)*	*2000 to 2007*
Hospitals by ownership				
Total	716	781	748	4
Public	686 (96)	611 (78)	578 (77)	–16
Non-public	30 (4)	170 (22)	170 (23)	467
Number of hospital beds				
Total	190 952	179 493	175 023	–8
Beds per 100 000 inhabitants	515	469	459	–11
Number of patients treated in hospitals				
Number of inpatients (in thousands)	6 007	6 739	6 850	14
Number of day cases in hospital wards (in thousands)[a]	–	895	1 014	–

Sources: Central Statistical Office, 2009b; [a]Central Statistical Office, 2007 (p. 124), 2008 (p. 135), 2009a (p. 145).

beds per 100 000 inhabitants. That said, some departments have seen increases in the number of beds over the same period of time (for example, the number of beds in cardiology, oncology, psychiatry, and intensive care units (ICUs) increased by more than 10 per cent (Świderek, 2009)). Although the number of hospital beds decreased from 2000 to 2007, the total number of patients treated in hospitals increased by 14 per cent.

In recent years, the number of day-care patients in hospitals has increased dramatically, and during the course of 2007, hospitals treated more than 1 million patients as day cases.

A typical treatment episode starts when a patient visits a primary health care physician who issues a referral to a specialist physician or a hospital. There is a group of specialist physicians (dermatologists, oculists, gynaecologists, oncologists, psychiatrists), for which no referral is required. In an emergency, a patient is admitted directly to a hospital. Treatment is completed when the patient is discharged from the hospital. If further treatment is required, the patient is referred to another hospital, a primary health care physician or a specialist physician (see Figure 20.1).

Since the introduction of social health insurance in 1999, hospitals must raise the majority of their revenues through the provision of health services to social health insurance members. In 2007, this is thought to have accounted for more than 60 per cent of total revenues for hospitals. In order to improve purchasing for social health insurance members, the NFZ introduced a

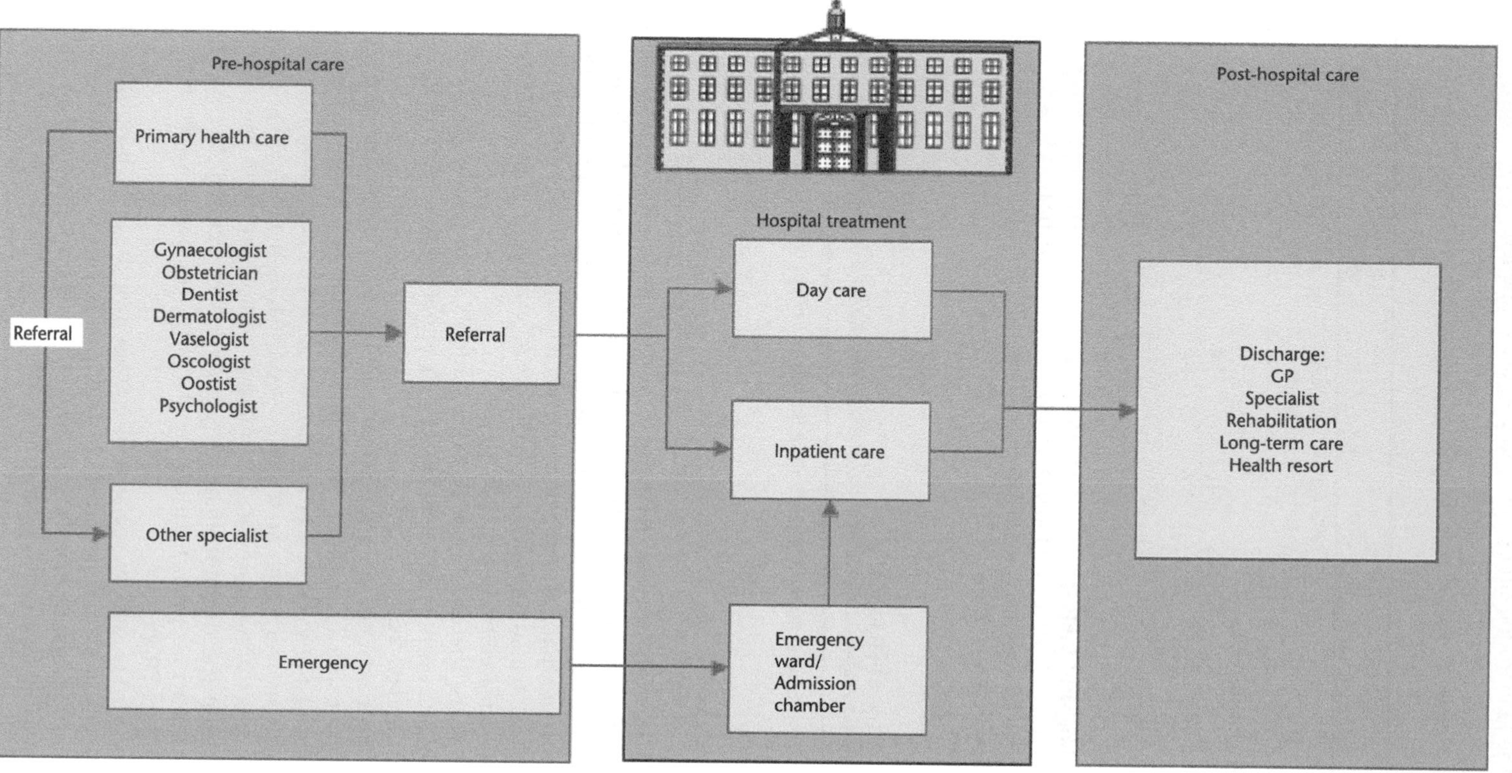

Figure 20.1 Typical episode of care across sectoral borders

Source: NFZ, 2010.

diagnosis-related group (DRG)-based hospital payment system in 2009, which means that the majority of hospital revenues are now related to DRG-based hospital payment. However, in addition to these revenues, hospitals still receive financial contributions from national and territorial governments for capital investments, for teaching and research, and for highly specialized services. In addition, hospitals also receive funds from private sources (benefactors).

20.1.3 Purpose of the DRG system

Prior to the introduction of DRG-based hospital payment in Poland, hospital payment was based on a 'Catalogue of Health Care Products' that was annually updated by the NFZ (Kozierkiewicz et al., 2006). Similar to DRGs, health care products were defined through specific diagnoses or procedures, and hospitals received a flat payment per admission based on the point value of a given product. However, in contrast to DRGs, the system was not based on systematic coding of all the diagnoses and procedures of the patients. Consequently, information was available only for the specific services defined by the Catalogue of Health Care Products. Since the definitions of products changed every year and the number of items in the catalogue continued to increase, the system lacked transparency. In addition, because of the constantly changing product definitions, hospital performance could not be assessed across time. Furthermore, the NFZ used its position of power to negotiate hospital payment rates that were often below the costs of service provision (Kozierkiewicz et al., 2006). This led to a deterioration of service quality and compromised access to hospital care through the emergence of waiting lists.

The main goals of introducing DRG-based hospital payment in Poland were: (1) to improve resource allocation to hospitals, and (2) to increase transparency of service provision.

DRG-based hospital payment was considered to be better able to provide adequate (fair) reimbursement to hospitals for delivered services, which was thought to increase the availability of services and to improve quality. Furthermore, DRG-based hospital payment was assumed to promote cost-accounting practices within hospitals, which would enable effective auditing of provider accounts, and would – ultimately – restrict unjustified increases in health care costs.

Transparency of hospital services was expected to improve because DRG-based hospital payment requires the collection of detailed data on every patient admitted to hospital (including primary diagnosis, secondary diagnoses, procedures, length of stay, gender and age). Given the need for data collection, hospitals would be encouraged to develop information technology (IT) systems that could facilitate the flow of information between the regional NFZ branch offices and service providers. Consequently, the NFZ would have better data regarding patients treated by contracted providers, and provider performance.

Last but not least, the international success of DRG-based hospital payment systems influenced the decision to introduce a similar system in Poland.

20.2 Development and updates of the DRG system in Poland

20.2.1 The current DRG system at a glance: the Jednorodne Grupy Pacjentów

In July 2008, a national DRG system was introduced in Poland, entitled *Jednorodne Grupy Pacjentów* (JGP), which can be translated as 'homogeneous groups of patients'. The British Healthcare Resource Groups (HRGs) (Version 3.5) served as the starting point for the JGP system, resulting in similarities between the two systems. Each JGP represents a distinct group of patients with similar characteristics (for example, diagnoses, procedures, patient age) and similar resource-consumption patterns or costs. Table 20.2 summarizes some of the main facts regarding the first national DRG system in Poland (Schreyögg et al., 2006).

Since July 2008, all hospitals (public and private) that have contracts with the NFZ must classify their patients using JGPs in order to receive DRG-based hospital payment for services they deliver. The system covers only hospital inpatient services and (similar to the British system of HRGs) differentiates between emergency admissions, planned admissions and day-care treatment episodes. Rehabilitation is only partly included, and psychiatry is not included in the JGP system. Rehabilitative care is mostly financed using fee-for-service payments; psychiatric services are paid for by means of per diem payments. However, plans are being developed to extend DRG-based hospital payment to include these areas of care (see section 20.8).

The NFZ enters into contracts with hospitals, specifying which JGPs hospitals are permitted to provide. In order to receive payments under the JGP system, hospitals must group each patient into a specific JGP and report such data to the regional branch of the NFZ. Each JGP has a predetermined score between 5 points (for example, 'minor procedure on eye's protective apparatus') and

Table 20.2 Main facts relating to the first national DRG version in Poland: the JGP system

Date of introduction	Patient classification: July 2008 Hospital payment: January 2009 (voluntarily since July 2008)
(Main) purpose	DRG-based hospital payment
DRG system	Homogeneous Groups of Patients (JGP) (based on British Healthcare Resource Groups (HRGs) Version 3.5)
Data used for development	Expert consultations, data on length of stay
Number of DRGs (as of 2010)	518
Applied to	All hospitals (public and private) that have contracts with the NFZ
Range of included services	All hospital inpatients and day cases except psychiatric and rehabilitative care. Since October 2010, also including neurological and cardiological rehabilitation
Range of included cost categories	Capital and recurrent costs, excluding major investments
Update of JGP	Scheduled for 2011

Source: Compiled by the authors based on grey literature from the NFZ.

4706 points (for example, 'transplantation of hematopoietic cells'), specified in the JGP catalogue. Depending on the score, hospitals receive a fixed sum of money, which is the same for all hospitals contracted by the NFZ.

Four documents are essential for the JGP system: (1) the JGP catalogue, which contains a full list of all JGPs, their scores and some further specifications; (2) the JGP characteristics file, which specifies the variables that define each JGP; (3) the grouper algorithm, which describes how to develop a grouper software tool by outlining all steps necessary in order to select the correct JGP; and (4) a parameterization file that is a functional form of the grouper algorithm (Gilewski, 2010).

The JGP catalogue is divided into 16 sections (or major diagnostic categories, MDCs) that correspond to anatomic or physiological systems of the body or to a specific clinical specialty (see Table 20.3). The 16 sections contain a total of 518 JGPs. Within each section, JGPs are arranged from highest to lowest scores. There are a total of 283 procedural JGPs and 235 medical JGPs.

20.2.2 Development of the JGP system

When the first national JGP system was introduced in July 2008, it was the result of several years of preparation and experimentation with different DRG systems in Poland: at the end of the 1990s, regional sickness funds had used DRGs for hospital payment in the Łódzkie, Dolnośląskie and Podkarpackie *voivodships* for several years (see Figure 20.2). After 2003, when sickness funds had been replaced by the NFZ, interest in DRGs remained strong.

Table 20.3 Sections of the JGP system

Section	*Section name*	*Number of DRG groups*
A	Diseases of the nervous system	36
B	Eye diseases	31
C	Diseases of the face, oral cavity, throat, larynx, nose and ears	27
D	Diseases of the respiratory system	29
E	Heart diseases	57
F	Diseases of the digestive system	39
G	Diseases of the liver, bile ducts, pancreas and spleen	24
H	Diseases of the musculoskeletal system	47
J	Diseases of breasts and skin, and burns	30
K	Diseases of the hormonal system	27
L	Diseases of the genitourinary system	45
M	Female genital diseases	22
N	Obstetrics and care of neonates	22
P	Paediatrics	27
Q	Vascular diseases	30
S	Diseases of blood-forming organs, poisoning and infectious diseases	25
Total		**518**

Source: Regulation of the President of the NFZ No. 69/2009.[5]

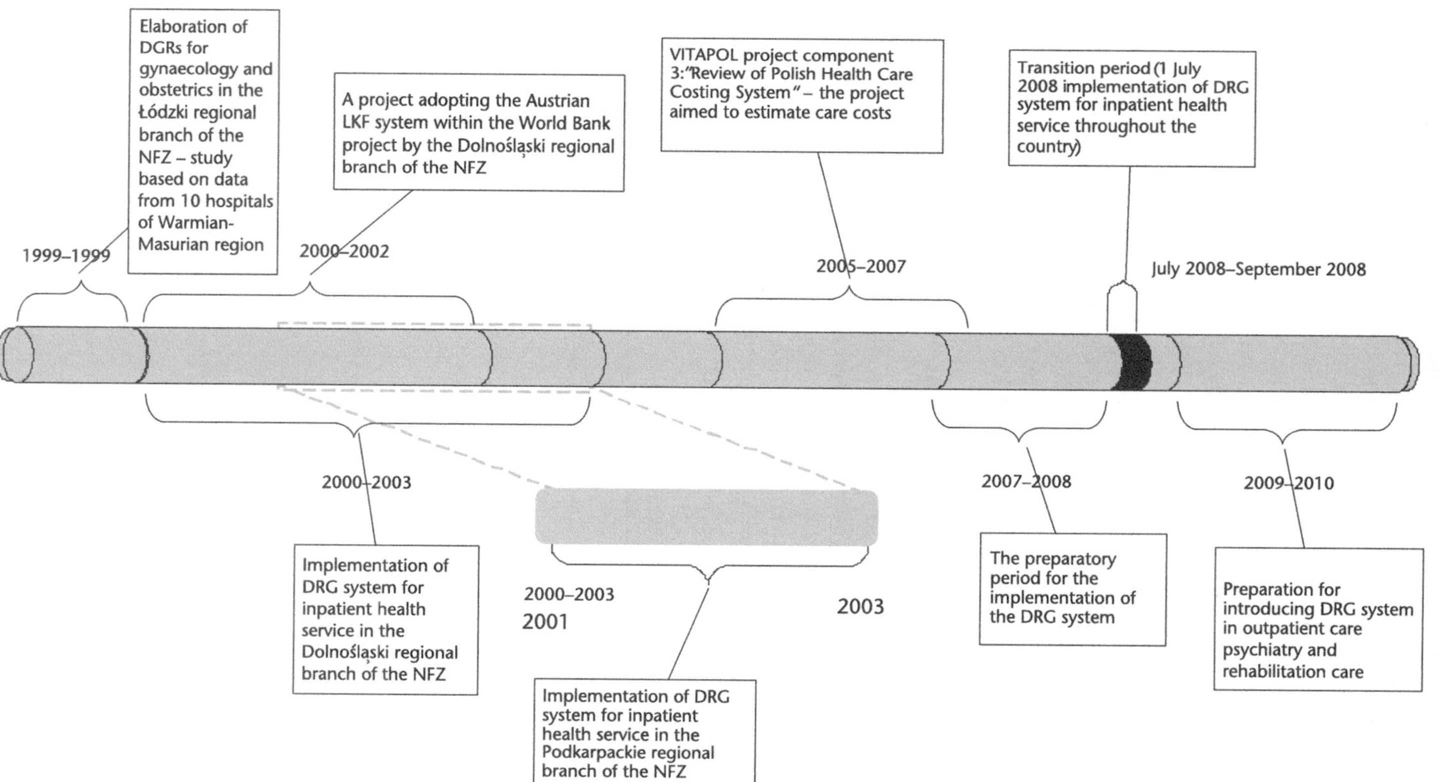

Figure 20.2 Timeline: introduction of the national JGP system in Poland and prior sub-national uses of DRGs

Source: NFZ, 2010.

Between 2004 and 2006, a European Union (EU)-funded research project on hospital costs in Poland (VITAPOL) contributed to the establishment of a close working relationship between British experts and Polish NFZ managers. The project generated interest in British HRGs and, in early 2007, the final decision was made by the President of the NFZ to introduce DRG-based hospital payment in Poland on the basis of British HRGs.

The process of developing the Polish JGP hospital payment system stretched over a period of about two years. In a first step, the NFZ adapted British HRGs to the Polish context. In order to do so, the British Classification of Interventions and Procedures (OPCS) was mapped to ICD-9-PL codes (WHO International Classification of Diseases 9th revision, Polish Clinical Modification). In a second step, hospital services from the previously existing Catalogue of Health Care Products were matched to HRGs. Since the number of hospital products in the old system was greater than the number of 'homogeneous groups of patients' (there were 1500 hospital products in 2005 but only 518 JGPs), the new groups of patients sometimes contained different types of hospital services. Therefore, in a third step, the (old) prices for the different types of services within one JGP were assessed, and – if possible – homogeneity of prices was increased by reassigning cases to different JGPs.

Once the draft version of the patient classification system had been prepared, a score (or price) per JGP was calculated by the NFZ: the price of each of the old hospital products within a JGP was weighted by the relative frequency of the service within the JGP, in order to calculate a (weighted) average price for the services grouped into one JGP. This calculated score per JGP was then compared with price ratios in the British HRG system. Furthermore, length-of-stay thresholds were determined for certain JGPs in order to define outlier cases, for which hospitals would receive supplementary payments.

Finally, the financial impact of the new DRG-based hospital payment system was estimated, based on data relating to the payment rate per JGP and the anticipated number of patients per JGP. The estimated expenditures (for the NFZ and regional branches of the NFZ) and estimated revenues (for selected providers) were compared to expenditures and revenues under the old system, in order to assess the financial impact of the hospital payment reform.

A draft version of the JGP system was published in August 2007 and discussed in a process of broad consultations with medical professionals and hospital managers. During numerous meetings between the NFZ and national consultants (recognized experts in a specific medical specialty, appointed by the Minister of Health), a number of modifications were agreed upon that were introduced into the President of the NFZ's draft ordinance. In March 2008, an early JGP version was tested as a pilot project in 44 selected hospitals. On the basis of the information gathered, the NFZ further modified the ICD-9-PL classification of procedures and the definitions and payment rates of JGPs (Kozierkiewicz, 2009).

As part of a broader process of extending the JGP system to other areas of care (see section 20.8), the NFZ started to introduce JPGs for neurological and cardiological rehabilitation patients treated at hospitals in October 2010. Rehabilitation patients are grouped on the basis of their primary diagnosis, medical procedures, secondary diagnoses and the assessment of each patient's health status according to the Barthel Activity of Daily Living scale, the American Spinal Injury Association scale and the Gross Motor Function Classification System. A total of 14 DRGs were created within neurological rehabilitation and three within cardiological rehabilitation.

During most of the process of introducing JGPs, Poland experienced a period of sustained high economic growth, which resulted in increased revenue for the NFZ. As a result, the NFZ had sufficient funds to increase total expenditure for hospital care and to raise payment rates for previously underfunded services. These additional revenues were an important positive influence in the process of introducing DRG-based hospital payment in Poland, since they helped to assure support from providers for the new payment system.

20.2.3 Sources of information used for developing and updating the JGP system

As already described, the JGP system is mostly based on imported British HRGs. However, Polish data were used to assess the adequacy of HRGs in the Polish context and to calculate JGP scores: first, information about the prices of hospital products under the previous payment system was used to assess the homogeneity of JGPs in Poland. Second, national hospital statistics from 2006/2007 were used to estimate the relative frequency of services bundled within each JGP, in order in turn to estimate payment rates. Third, data on hospital patients' lengths of stay were used to determine length-of-stay thresholds that delimit the number of days for which hospital payments are calculated on the basis of JGPs. Furthermore, information about innovative medical technologies is used to update the system. Unfortunately, data on costs of hospital services are not systematically collected by the NFZ and are not used to develop the JGP system. However, cost data from specific hospitals were used (albeit in a non-systematic way) to inform decisions during the process of setting the payment rate(s) under the old hospital payment system (Kozierkiewicz et al., 2006), and such data are still being used under the new system.

20.2.4 Regularity and methods of system updates

The JGP system was introduced by the NFZ in mid-2008. Since then, a number of minor updates have been introduced into the system (mostly in the second half of 2008). In most cases, these were motivated by suggestions from medical consultants or health care providers, but also by economic analyses conducted by the NFZ. In some cases, these suggestions have resulted in the creation of new JGPs. However, in order to introduce new JGPs, it must be demonstrated that the proposed group would comprise more than 300 cases, or that total payments for patients in the JGP would amount to more than PLN (Polish Złoty) 1.5 million per year (about €370 000).

At present, JGP scores are updated annually and are the same for all health care providers in Poland. In the years to follow, the principle of universal applicability of scores may be subject to change. The point value, used to convert scores per JGP into PLN depends on the resources available in the NFZ's annual financial plan.

Decisions relating to the introduction of new medical technologies into the Polish hospital sector are made by the Ministry of Health on the basis of recommendations from the Health Technology Assessment Agency (*Agencja Oceny Technologii Medycznych*, AOTM) (see section 20.6).

Major updates to the JGP system are planned for the year 2011. Among other things, the NFZ plans to introduce a new process of regular updates to the patient classification system and to the payment rates (see section 20.8).

20.3 The current patient classification system

20.3.1 Information used to classify patients

Each JGP is defined on the basis of data available from the common hospital discharge dataset. This contains information about the diagnoses of patients (primary diagnosis and secondary diagnoses coded using ICD-10; procedures coded using ICD-9-PL; demographic variables (age and gender); reason for hospital admission/discharge; and length of stay). After hospital discharge, one JGP is selected for the entire hospital stay by a specialized software program called a 'grouper', which uses information about diagnoses, procedures, age, type of admission, type of discharge and length of stay to classify patients into the appropriate group of patients.

20.3.2 Classification algorithm

The grouping algorithm is illustrated in Figure 20.3. In a first step, the grouper checks whether any services were provided that are reimbursed without being assigned to a specific JGP. For example, very costly procedures such as transplantations, treatment of drug-resistant epilepsy, and chemotherapy are excluded from the further grouping process (see Figure 20.4 for reimbursement components besides those for JGPs). The next step of the grouping algorithm is to check whether any significant procedures were performed. If this is the case, the grouper determines for each procedure a rank between 0 and 6. The highest ranked procedure is then indicated as the dominant procedure for the hospital stay. However, unlike in the British HRG system, the grouper does not automatically select the dominant procedure. Instead, health care providers can manually select the procedure that was the most important during the hospital stay in question.

Subsequently, this procedure determines the section of the JGP system. If the rank of the procedure is > 2, which is the case for most operating room (OR) procedures, the JGP is determined directly (94 basic 'surgical' procedural JGPs). If the procedure rank is ≤2, the grouper checks whether additional conditions concerning secondary diagnoses, secondary procedures, age, gender, and so on are met, in order to determine the JGP (191 procedural JGPs).

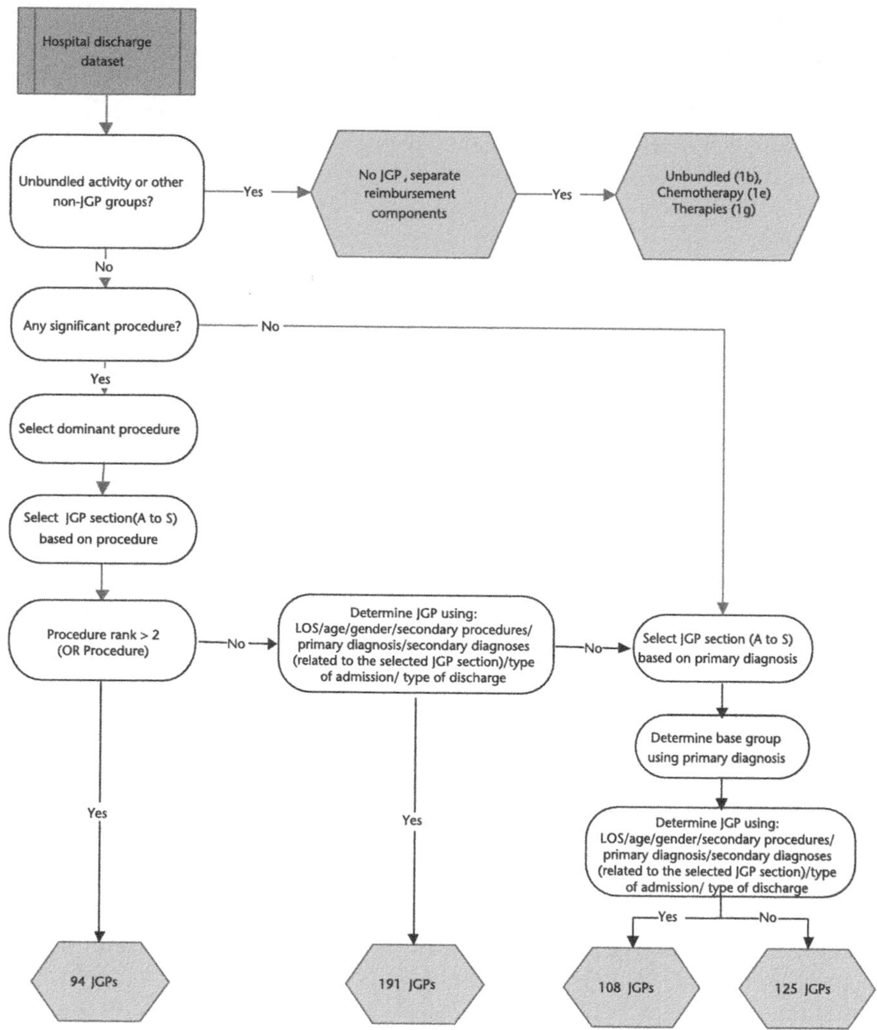

Figure 20.3 JGP grouping algorithm

Source: Compiled by the authors based on grey literature from the NFZ.

Cases without any procedures – or those cases for which a JGP could not be determined by the grouping algorithm described so far – are assigned to the relevant section of the JGP system on the basis of the primary diagnoses of the hospital stay. Subsequently, the primary diagnosis determines a base group. Depending on the primary diagnosis, the JGP can be determined directly (for 108 medical JGPs), or additional conditions may have to be met (for 125 medical JGPs).

Whether a specific secondary diagnosis is considered a to be a complication or co-morbidity (CC) in the grouping process depends on the section of the JGP system concerned. For every section, a list of ICD-10 codes exists that defines

Table 20.4 Differences between British HRGs and Polish JGPs

	British HRGs (Version 3.5)	*Polish JGPs*
Procedure classification system	OPCS	ICD-9-PL
Selection of dominant procedure	Grouper selects highest ranked procedure	Provider selects most relevant procedure of hospital stay
Poly-trauma cases	Included in 'Pre-MDC'-like group	No specific groups. JGP score is inflated depending on the number of affected organs
Paediatric cases	Specific section only for neonates	Separate section for paediatrics
Number of chapters/sections	19	16
Number of groups	610	518

Source: Compiled by the authors based on grey literature from the NFZ.

relevant CCs for the section. In addition, a global list of secondary diagnoses exists, which are considered CCs in all sections.

Each JGP is characterized by a three-digit code. The first digit is a letter indicating the section of the JGP system, for example 'F' is used for diseases of the digestive system (see Table 20.4). The second and third digits are numbers that specify the JGP group, for example 'F83' for appendectomy in uncomplicated cases of appendicitis. In general, lower numbers indicate more complex groups of patients, while higher numbers indicate less-complicated (less-costly) groups of patients. However, there are several important differences between the JGP system and the British HRG system. The most important differences are summarized in Table 20.4.

20.3.3 Data quality and plausibility checks

Hospitals submit all data relevant for reimbursement to the regional branch offices of the NFZ. The NFZ withholds payments in the event that the required information is not complete. Data quality and plausibility are regularly verified: first, health care providers verify their data before sending them to regional branch offices of the NFZ, in order to avoid external auditing. Second, the NFZ verifies that data are complete and checks for plausibility of combinations of diagnoses and procedures. Finally, the NFZ carries out coordinated monitoring by sending out review teams to hospitals, to check patients' medical documentation. If any irregularities are detected, the health care provider must correct its reports and financial penalties are applied.

In October 2009, the Section for Verification and Validation Standards of the NFZ launched a central process of validation and verification of reported data. The aim is to harmonize and automate most processes of validation and verification and to contribute to improved data quality. However, at present, coding problems detected during the process of validation and verification indicate that hospitals still need to improve medical monitoring and controlling in order to improve data quality.

20.3.4 Incentives for up-coding or wrong-coding

Since hospital payment is determined to a large extent by patients' JGPs, hospitals have strong incentives to 'optimize' their coding practices in order to achieve higher payments. However, during data quality checks and controls of patient records at hospitals, the NFZ regularly checks for up- and wrong-coding. If fraudulent coding practices are detected, hospitals may be punished by means of penalties (high fines), or even termination of the contract.

20.4 Cost accounting within hospitals

20.4.1 Regulation

Health care facilities are obliged to produce cost-accounting statements according to the rules set out in an Ordinance of the Minister of Health and Social Policy.[1] However, this document does not specify in detail how health care providers should carry out their cost accounting. Consequently, significant discrepancies exist in the methods of calculating costs between particular service providers.

Given the lack of consistent cost-accounting data, the JGP system is currently not directly related to the costs of hospital services. The only available information on costs of hospital services in Poland is selective. Some hospitals collect cost information on particular medical care episodes and voluntarily submit it to the NFZ. The NFZ may use this information in the process of setting payment rate(s), but does not use it in a systematic way.

20.4.2 Main characteristics of the cost-accounting system

Recently, the NFZ has launched an initiative to establish a cost database. The idea is that about 15 hospitals will collect data on the costs of selected treatment episodes included in the JGP system. The initiative will allow hospitals to know more about their cost structures in comparison to other hospitals. Hospitals that want to participate in the project must fulfil certain requirements. They must:

- comply with the aforementioned Ordinance of the Minister of Health and Social Policy (Dz.U.98.164.1194);
- allocate overhead costs to direct cost centres through a step-down cost-accounting approach;
- estimate costs of sub-ward cost centres (ORs, doctors' rooms for the provision of services for numerous wards, diagnostic laboratories, and so on);
- estimate total costs at direct cost centres; that is, costs at medical departments engaged in the provision of services to patients;
- collect patient-level data on certain consumed resources (drugs, high-cost materials, diagnostic tests, and so on);
- disaggregate costs according to defined cost groups: labour, drugs, diagnostic tests, medical materials, and overheads.

As a result, hospitals should be able to provide information about (1) per diem costs (both 'hotel' costs and care costs), (2) average costs per patient, (3) costs of medical procedures, and (4) costs of services provided by hospital wards for other wards or outside the hospital. In order to standardize the methods of gathering the data from selected service providers, the NFZ has prepared a web-based application which will facilitate the sharing of information.

20.5 JGPs for hospital financing

20.5.1 Role of JGP-based hospital payment in the overall financing of hospitals

All hospitals in Poland that have contracts with the NFZ are financed through the JGP system. The same conditions apply to all hospitals, irrespective of ownership status, hospital type, or regional differences. The system applies to all patients, including day cases, except for psychiatric and most rehabilitative care patients. Payments under the JGP system are supposed to cover the full costs (capital, personnel, overheads, and so on, except costs of major investments) of all services provided by hospitals between admission and discharge of the patient. However, hospitals may receive additional funds for investments from regional governments, for teaching from the Ministry of Science and Higher Education, and from patients for add-on services, such as for a sole-occupancy treatment room.

No information is available on the budget structure of hospitals. However, it is assumed that public funds contracted from the NFZ constitute more than 60 per cent of hospitals' total budgets.

20.5.2 Calculation of JGP scores and trimming

As described in subsection 20.2.2, calculation of JGP scores was based mainly on information about prices of services from the old catalogue of hospital products and the assumed relative frequency of these services within one JGP (in the years 2006–2007). In addition, the ratio of JGP scores was compared with the price ratio of comparable HRGs, while taking into account particularities of the Polish health care system. In particular, the costs of intensive care treatment were included in the most complex groups of patients and costs of medical equipment were considered.

Scores per JGP differ according to the type of admission of the patient. For example, in general, JGP scores are lower for planned hospital admissions or day-care treatment episodes than for unplanned hospital admissions. Table 20.5 shows an example of different scores, according to the type of admission, for a selected group of JGPs.

In order to adequately remunerate hospitals for treating cases with very high costs (outliers), the JGP system provides supplementary payments for cases with a 'very long' lengths of stay (LOS outliers). These cases are identified using an upper LOS threshold, beyond which cases are to be considered to be outliers.

Table 20.5 Example of JGP scores and supplementary points for selected JGP groups

JGP	*Name*	*JGP score*			*Upper LOS threshold*	*< 2-day stay score*	*Per diem surcharge*
		General admission	*Planned admission*	*Day care*			
G24	Cholecystectomy with CCs	71	70	69	–	–	–
G25	Cholecystecomy	63	60	57	–	–	–
N34	Minor surgical intervention on infants and babies	57	–	–	10	11	5

Source: President of the National Health Fund, Order No. 69/2009/DSOZ on defining conditions of concluding and executing such contracts as hospital treatment, 3 November 2009.

The threshold is defined through a non-parametric trimming method based on the interquartile range, and is applied only to certain JGPs:

upper LOS threshold = Q3+1,5*(Q3–Q1),
where:
Q1 is the LOS of the first quartile of patients within a particular JGP and
Q3 is the LOS of the third quartile of patients within a particular JGP

Beyond this threshold, the JGP score is increased by a per diem-based supplementary point value that amounts to 80 per cent of the average per diem value per day below the upper LOS threshold. This is because it is assumed that beyond the upper LOS threshold, the intensity of care is lower. However, upper LOS thresholds are not calculated for planned hospitalizations and day-care treatment episodes.

For certain JGPs the system identifies short-stay outliers; namely, cases in which the patient should usually stay in hospital for more than one day (in accordance with standard medical practice). If these cases are discharged after only one day, hospitals do not receive the full JGP-based payment. Instead, the JGP score is reduced for these lower length-of-stay outliers to 20 per cent of the full JGP score (except in the case of death of a patient during the first day of hospital stay). Table 20.5 shows an example of a JGP score for lower length-of-stay outliers within a particular JGP.

20.5.3 JGP-based hospital payment

Before hospital payment takes place, the regional branch offices of the NFZ check whether JGPs reported by the provider are consistent with the scope of their contracts. For example, if a hospital has grouped a patient into a surgical JGP but does not have the right to provide the procedure, the patient is reclassified by the NFZ into a JGP that was specified in the contract.

Figure 20.4 illustrates the calculation of hospital payment under the JGP-based hospital payment system in Poland. Hospital payment is determined, on the one hand, by basic score points for the JGP (1a) or basic scores for unbundled services (1b), chemotherapy (1e) or therapeutic programmes (for

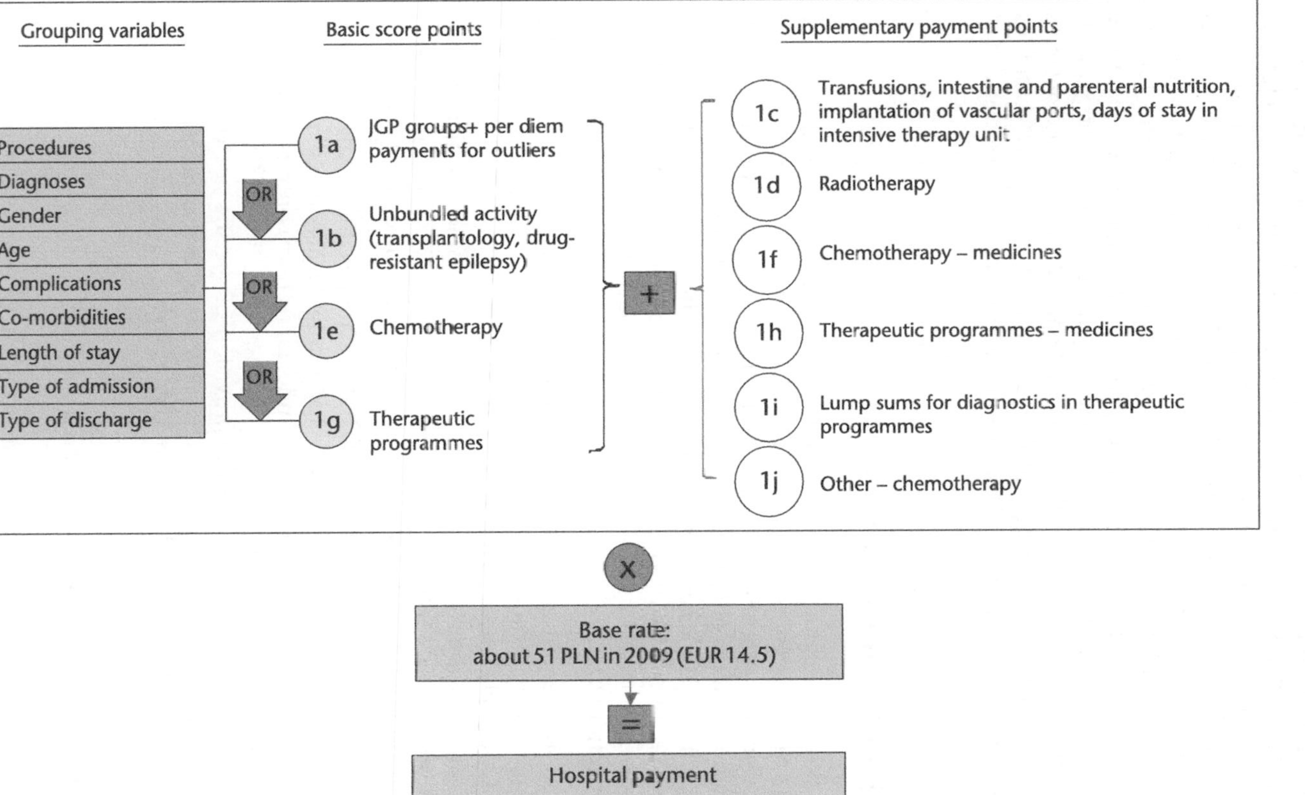

Figure 20.4 Calculation of hospital payment in the era of JGPs

Source: NFZ, 2010.

example, treatment of chronic hepatitis) (1g). On the other hand, additional points are added to the score as supplementary payments for specific services (1c, 1d, 1f, 1h–j). For chemotherapy (1e) or therapeutic programmes (1g), the basic score points are supposed to cover the costs of the stay in hospital, whereas the supplementary payment points 1f or 1h pay for specific medicines or diagnostic evaluations. There are 429 such supplementary payments for a range of specific high-cost drugs or procedures. The sum of points for the JGP score, plus supplementary payment points, is multiplied by a base rate (point value) in order to calculate hospital payment for a specific patient. The base rate was PLN 51 (about €14.5) in 2009 and 2010. The rate depends on the total available NFZ budget and is determined through negotiations between the NFZ, the Ministry of Health and representatives of associations of medical professionals.

20.5.4 Quality-related adjustments

The JGP system does not adjust the hospital payment for specific quality indicators. All hospitals receive the same amount of money (fixed) for each JGP, which means that hospitals face strong incentives to lower their costs. This could potentially compromise the quality of care. However, the quality of hospitals is taken into account by the NFZ prior to the conclusion of contracts with hospitals. In particular, the NFZ considers two types of quality standards – these are implemented by health care providers of their own accord and are not legally binding:[2]

1. International Organization for Standardization (ISO) certificates (ISO 14001, 9001) that certify organizational quality standards of management processes, but not medical standards;
2. accreditation by the National Center for Quality Assessment, which assesses quality on the basis of measurable (structure, process and outcome) indicators. The indicators are dynamic and subject to periodical modifications.

In addition, further structural quality standards are specified in the 'Acts and regulations of the Minister of Health'.[3] For example, personnel must have certain qualifications, equipment must undergo regular controls, and floor space must comply with certain criteria. Furthermore, the NFZ verifies that Ministry of Health requirements for the provision of specific services are met before determining the scope of contracts with hospitals, that is, before deciding which services the hospital will be allowed to provide.

20.6 New/innovative technologies

As a result of the 'Act on health care benefits financed from public funds'[4] the AOTM was established. Hospitals, pharmaceutical companies and manufactures of medical equipment can apply to the AOTM with a proposal for a new technology. The agency assesses applications and makes recommendations regarding whether or not a specific technological innovation should be included in the list of public health care benefits that is published by the Minister of Health. As part of the assessment, the AOTM establishes the level of superiority of the new technology compared to existing treatment options, and assesses possible ways of financing it, along with conditions for implementation. In the process, the AOTM holds meetings with a Consultative Council composed of 12 members who are experts in the assessment of health care technologies. The Council meets once a month and can approve a new technology through majority vote. Subsequently, the president of the AOTM must consult with legal experts and with the NFZ President in order to ensure that the financial impact of introducing a specific technology does not compromise the financial stability of the NFZ. The final decision regarding whether or not to incorporate a new technology into the list of health care benefits is made by the Ministry of Health.

Unlike in other countries (see Chapter 9), there is no system to specifically encourage the adoption of innovations, for example through additional payments for the use of certain technologies. If a specific technology is included in the list of public health care benefits, it is either financed through an existing JGP, or a new JGP is created to account for the higher costs of the new technology. Alternatively, high-cost drugs or procedures can be added to one of the lists for supplementary payments, for example 1c, 1d, 1f, 1h–j (see Figure 20.4).

20.7 Evaluation of the JGP system

20.7.1 *Official evaluations*

The pilot testing of JGPs in early 2008 has been the only official evaluation of the JGP system thus far. However, the main objectives at the time were to test coding practices, the practical functioning of the JGP grouper algorithm and the possibility of paying providers using JGPs (Paszkiewicz, 2008). In addition, the pilot study generated information that facilitated the improvement of the classification of medical procedures and JGP characteristics. The effects of the introduction of JGPs on quality or efficiency of health care service provision were not assessed during the pilot study and still remain unknown.

20.7.2 *Authors' assessment*

The main advantage of the Polish JGP system is that it contributes to transparency in the hospital sector. Grouping algorithms are publicly available and the payment system is based on transparent procedures. In addition, the JGP system contributes to increased availability of data relating to hospital activity, by enforcing coding of diagnoses and procedures and grouping this information into JGPs.

However, important shortcomings persist: cost accounting and collection of cost data are not standardized in Poland, and cost information is not systematically used to determine payment rates. This means that payment rates do not necessarily reflect the costs of service provision. Hospital payments for certain services may be too generous, while other services are not financed sufficiently. Consequently, hospital payments may be considered unfair; they may provide the wrong incentives and could lead to unintended behaviour patterns on the part of providers (see Chapter 6 of this volume). Furthermore, the system does not take into account structural differences between providers, even though these differences may have a significant impact on providers' costs of service provision (Busse et al., 2008).

20.8 Outlook: Future developments and reform

In 2011 the NFZ plans to implement a new change-management system. This will be the most significant alteration of the JGP system since its introduction in 2008. The change-management system is intended to provide a regulatory framework for the process of updating the JGP system. Three main characteristics of the change-management system are as follows: (1) updates to the system will occur no more than twice a year; (2) the JGP patient classification system will be updated on the basis of statistical analyses of length of stay and cost data; and (3) cost data will be used to determine payment rates.

An interesting feature of the proposed change-management process is that it is intended to create two lists: one detailing the most frequently performed JGPs, and another itemizing the JGPs with the highest expenditures. Updates to the JGP patient classification system (for example, splitting of groups, creating new groups, and so on) will focus on the most important JGPs from the two lists. In terms of the payment rate-setting procedure, various projects are currently in the process of improving cost-accounting practices in health facilities, supported by the Ministry of Health and the European Commission. If cost-accounting standards can be sufficiently improved, payment rates will be more closely related to the costs of service provision in Polish hospitals. Furthermore, plans exist to depart from the uniform applicability of a national base rate and to introduce structural and quality adjustments for certain hospitals.

Another major development is that the NFZ plans to gradually extend the JGP system to other areas of care, such as rehabilitation and psychiatry. As mentioned in subsection 20.2.2, the introduction of JGPs for cardiological and neurological rehabilitation in October 2010 forms part of this broader process.

In conclusion, the JGP system is still at a relatively early stage in Poland. The planned change-management system aims to continuously improve the JGP system to better reflect Polish health care patterns and costs of service provision. It seems very likely that JGP-based hospital payment will provide adequate reimbursement to hospitals in the long term, and will thus contribute to improved quality and efficiency of hospital care in Poland.

20.9 Notes

1 Ordinance of the Minister of Health and Social Policy on special principles of cost accounting in public health care facilities, 22 December 1998 (Dz. U. of 1998: No. 164, item 1194 as amended); and Ordinance of the Minister of Health and Social Policy on

guaranteed hospital treatment benefits, 29 August 2009 (Dz. U. of 2009: No. 140, item 1143 as amended).

2 President of the National Health Fund, Order No. 73/2009/DSOZ on defining assessment criteria for offers, 13 November 2009.

3 • Ordinance of the Minister of Health of 3 March 2004 sets forth the requirements which need to be met by the premises and equipment of a medical diagnostic laboratory with special focus on the sanitary condition of the premises and equipment, as well as technical and substantive requirements for the staff and the manager of the laboratory. (Dz.U. No. 43, item 408 of 2004 as amended)
  • Ordinance of the Minister of Health of 23 March 2006 sets forth the quality standards for medical diagnostic and microbiological laboratories as regards the operations of medical laboratory diagnostics, assessment of their quality and diagnostic value and laboratory interpretation and authorization of test results. (Dz.U. No. 61, item 435 of 2006 as amended)
  • Ordinance of the Minister of Health of 27 March 2008 concerning minimum requirements for health care units which provide medical services consisting of X-ray diagnostics, interventional radiology and radioisotope diagnostics and treatment of non-cancerous diseases (Dz. U. 2008, No. 59, item 365)
  • Ordinance of the Minister of Health of 29 March 1999 concerning the qualifications of personnel at various positions in public health care institutions. (Dz. U. 1999, No. 30, item 300).

4 Act on health care benefits financed from public funds, 27 August 2004 (Dz. U. of 2008, No 164, item 1027, as amended).

5 President of the National Health Fund, Order No 69/2009/DSOZ on defining conditions of concluding and executing such contracts as hospital treatment, 3 November 2009.

20.10 References

Busse, R., Schreyögg, J., Smith, P.C. (2008). Variability in health care treatment costs among nine EU countries – results from the HealthBASKET project. *Health Economics*, 17(Suppl. 1):1–8.

Central Statistical Office (2007). *Basic Data on Health Care, Day Places and Outpatients in Hospital Wards*. Warsaw: Central Statistical Office.

Central Statistical Office (2008). *Basic Data on Health Care, Day Places and Outpatients in Hospital Wards*. Warsaw: Central Statistical Office.

Central Statistical Office (2009a). *Basic Data on Health Care, Day Places and Outpatients in Hospital Wards*. Warsaw: Central Statistical Office.

Central Statistical Office (2009b). *Statistical Yearbook of the Republic of Poland 2009*. Warsaw: Central Statistical Office (http://www.stat.gov.pl/cps/rde/xbcr/gus/PUBL_rs_rocznik_statystyczny_rp_2009.pdf, accessed 7 January 2010).

European Commission (2009). *Eurostat: Health Care Expenditure (Data in focus 26/2008)*. Luxembourg: Statistical Office of the European Commission (http://epp.eurostat.ec.europa.eu/statistics_explained/index.php/Healthcare_expenditure#Further_Eurostat_information, accessed 15 November 2010).

Gilewski, D. (2010). *Jednorodne Grupy Pacjentów. Podstawy systemu [Diagnosis-Related Groups: Basics]*. Warsaw: National Health Fund (NFZ).

Kozierkiewicz, A. (2008). *Koło ratunkowe dla szpitali. Od doświadczeń do modelu [A Lifeline for Hospitals. From Experience to a Recipe for Restructuring]*. Poznan: Termedia Publishing House.

Kozierkiewicz, A. (2009). *Jednorodne Grupy Pacjentów. Przewodnik po systemie [Diagnosis-Related Groups: Guide Through the System]*. Warsaw: National Health Fund (NFZ).

Kozierkiewicz, A., Stamirski, M., Stylo, W., Trabka, W. (2006). The definition of prices for inpatient care in Poland in the absence of cost data. *Health Care Management Science*, 9(3):281–6.

Kuszewski, K., Gericke, C. (2005). *Health Systems in Transition: Poland*. Copenhagen: WHO Regional Office for Europe on behalf of the European Observatory on Health Systems and Policies.

Ministry of Health (2008). *Health Care Financing in Poland* [in Polish]. Green Paper II, version 3. Warsaw: Ministry of Health of the Republic of Poland (http://www.mz.gov.pl/wwwfiles/ma_struktura/docs/zielona_ksiega_06012009.pdf, accessed 12 January 2010).

NFZ (2010). *Annual Business Reports 2009*. Warsaw: National Health Fund (NFZ) (http://www.nfz.gov.pl/new/index.php?katnr=3&dzialnr=10&artnr=4126, accessed 25 October 2010).

Paszkiewicz, J. (2008). Efekt JGP [DRG effect]. *Menedżer zdrowia*, 10:42–9.

Schreyögg, J., Stargardt, T., Tiemann, O., Busse, R. (2006). Methods to determine reimbursement rates for diagnosis related groups (DRG): a comparison of nine European countries. *Health Care Management Science*, 9(3):215–23.

Świderek, M. (2009). Comparative analysis of DRG systems in the EU countries. *Acta Universitatis Lodziensis, Folia Oeconomica*: 303–15.

chapter twenty one

Portugal: Results of 25 years of experience with DRGs

Céu Mateus

21.1 Hospital services and the role of DRGs in Portugal

21.1.1 The Portuguese health system

Since 1979 the Portuguese health care system has been based on a National Health Service (NHS) structure financed by general taxation, characterized by universal coverage and access to care that is mostly free at the point of use. The state is committed to achieving equity, and to promoting efficiency, quality and accountability in the Portuguese health care system (Assembleia da República, 1990). However, the Portuguese NHS has never conformed to the general characteristics of the Beveridge model of health care, mainly due to the incomplete transition from a previously fragmented social insurance system. Occupation-based insurance schemes that existed in 1979 are yet to be integrated into the NHS (Barros & de Almeida Simões, 2007). These schemes benefit from additional public funding and provide additional coverage to around 25 per cent of the population, who enjoy double coverage.

The Portuguese health care system is mainly financed through the state budget (around 75 per cent; Barros & de Almeida Simões, 2007), that is, through taxes. Since the early 1980s, total health expenditure has increased steadily and Portugal is at present among the highest spenders in the European Union (EU) in terms of health care expenditure as a percentage of gross domestic product (GDP) (above 10 per cent), in comparison with other countries that have NHS-based systems (OECD, 2008). Private financing accounted for around 25 per cent of total expenditure in 2006 (OECD, 2008), corresponding mainly to out-of-pocket payments for specialty visits, pharmaceuticals, dental care and physiotherapy.

All patients are assigned to an NHS general practitioner (GP) within their area of residence. Primary care GPs are expected to act as gatekeepers and refer patients to secondary care provided by medical specialists. However, access to emergency services is not restricted, contributing to an imperfect gatekeeping system. A large private sector co-exists with the NHS and its role was explicitly recognized in the 1990 NHS law that instituted a mixed health care system (Assembleia da República, 1990). Consequently, the public and private sectors are both involved in the delivery of health care, with the private sector mainly responsible for carrying out specialist visits, elective surgery, ancillary tests and kidney dialysis.

The central government level still exerts most powers according to the tradition of centralized management. Regional Health Administrations manage the provision of primary care and are responsible for state reimbursement of prescribed drugs to the Pharmacies Association. The Central Administration of the Health System (ACSS) is an agency of the Ministry of Health, principally responsible for managing NHS financial resources for primary and hospital care. It also produces statistical information and regulates information technology (IT) both in hospitals and health care centres.

A detailed description of the Portuguese health system – including an overview of key institutions, relationships between the public and private sectors, modes of payment used for different providers and services – is beyond the scope of this chapter but can be found in Barros & de Almeida Simões (2007).

21.1.2 Hospital services in Portugal

Hospital services are provided by both the public and private sectors. Statistics on the number of beds in the private sector are not available for the whole country. The number of public and private hospitals (according to the last five years of data available) is presented in Table 21.1.

In 2007 the number of patients discharged per bed was 37 and (in NHS hospitals only, including mental health care facilities) the average length of stay (ALOS) corresponded to 7.7 days (DGS, 2008). The occupancy rate was close to 79 per cent, but higher in medical specialties than in surgical ones, despite existing waiting lists for surgeries.

NHS hospitals are owned by the state but are managed as independent institutions that are allowed to make profits and run deficits. However, deficits are generally compensated by the Ministry of Health if they threaten the financial viability of hospitals. Hospitals provide elective and non-elective care, ambulatory surgery, maternity services, diagnostic procedures, ancillary tests,

Table 21.1 Number of NHS (public) and private hospitals, 2003–2007

Year	*NHS*	*Private*	*Total*
2003	114	90	204
2004	116	93	209
2005	111	93	204
2006	107	93	200
2007	99	99	198

Source: INE, 2009.

and accident and emergency services. Non-acute psychiatric inpatient and outpatient services are mostly provided by psychiatric hospitals.

Private hospitals provide care to private patients, whether or not they are covered by occupational schemes or private insurance. Private hospitals charge patients a fee for each service according to costs incurred but can also negotiate fees with occupational schemes or insurance plans.

Inpatient services and ambulatory surgery provided at NHS hospitals, except psychiatric hospitals, are paid on the basis of diagnosis-related groups (DRGs). On the one hand, DRGs have been used since the late 1980s to determine DRG-based case payments from occupation-based and other insurance schemes to hospitals. On the other hand, the NHS has used DRGs since 1997 for DRG-based hospital budget allocation. Other hospital services (day care, specialist consultations, emergency services, high-cost drugs and so on) are paid on the basis of fee-for-service with a volume cap that is negotiated between the hospital and the ACSS.

21.1.3 Purpose of the DRG system

When DRGs were first introduced in Portuguese hospitals through a pilot study in 1984, the Ministry of Health had two main objectives. Urbano and colleagues (1993) who were leading the introduction process at the Ministry of Health have recalled that:

> [T]he first objective of the project was to create an integrated information system for hospital management based on a set of necessary and uniform data, which would allow all levels of management to measure and control their productivity, support their decision-making, make plans and budgets, and establish equitable financing criteria. The second objective was to develop an information system that could efficiently collect, treat, analyse, and transmit information within hospitals, between hospitals and central departments, and among central departments.

In summary, the two objectives were to (1) improve resource allocation, and (2) increase transparency. However, the main goal of introducing DRGs was to rationalize the allocation of resources to NHS hospitals by more closely linking resources for inpatient care to hospital output (as measured through DRGs). According to Dismuke & Sena (2001), the Portuguese Ministry of Health sought to encourage a more efficient utilization of resources in public hospitals in order to increase productivity and to curb the uncontrolled growth of public expenditure in the health care sector.

21.2 Development and updates of the DRG system

21.2.1 The current DRG system at a glance

A non-modified version of All Patient (AP-)DRGs (Version 21.0) was imported in 2006. There is only one DRG system in Portugal that applies to all NHS hospitals and all patients (inpatients and ambulatory surgery), except outpatients and patients treated in psychiatric and rehabilitation care settings. Private hospitals are not included in the system.

The current AP-DRG system defines 669 DRGs within 25 Major Diagnostic Categories (MDCs), each corresponding to one organ or physiological system, and one Pre-MDC (including high-cost cases such as transplantations). The DRG system is supervised and maintained by the ACSS within the Ministry of Health.

DRGs are used for DRG-based hospital budget allocation from the NHS to hospitals and for DRG-based case payment from third-party payers. DRG-based hospital budget allocations amount to about 75–85 per cent of total hospital inpatient budgets. The rest corresponds to DRG-based hospital payments from third-party payers. In order to control overall spending, the national base rate can be adjusted to ensure that total hospital payment does not exceed the available budget.

21.2.2 Development of the DRG system

In 1984 the Portuguese Ministry of Health started a pilot project to study the feasibility of implementing United States Health Care Financing Administration (HCFA-)DRGs as a measure of hospital output. The results of the pilot study were seen to be encouraging, and a decision was made to extend the system to all public acute care hospitals. The implementation process followed a centralized top-down approach (from the Ministry of Health to the hospitals). Given the centralization of the Portuguese political system, and the fact that the Ministry of Health owns the majority of hospitals, hospitals had to comply with the decision to introduce DRGs.

Implementation originally started in the Ministry of Health and was spread to NHS hospitals through the involvement of physicians and hospital managers in selected hospitals. A small team led by hospital managers working at the Ministry of Health (initially João Urbano and, after his departure, Margarida Bentes) worked in close cooperation with the Secretary of State for Health. Margarida Bentes was the most influential person regarding the implementation of DRGs in Portugal.

After the pilot study it was decided to adopt HCFA-DRGs to the Portuguese setting, without any adaptation. Several versions of HCFA-DRGs have been used (see Table 21.2). In 2006, the Ministry of Health decided to switch to Version 21.0 of the AP-DRG system, which was developed for use in hospitals in the United States for the calendar year 2004.

The first release of the AP-DRGs was Version 5.0, developed by 3M™ Health Information Systems in the 1980s. In the United States it was effective for the 1988 calendar year. As described in the *All Patient DRG Definitions Manual* (3M, 2003, p. 12) 'the process of forming the DRGs was highly iterative, involving a combination of statistical results from test data with clinical judgement'. AP-DRG Version 21.0 was imported to Portugal without modifications.

The most significant Portuguese development concerning the use of DRGs was that in 1996 a process was initiated to adapt DRGs for the classification of

Table 21.2 Versions of DRG groupers used in Portugal

DRG system	HCFA-DRG Version 4.0	HCFA-DRG Version 6.0	HCFA-DRG Version 10.0	HCFA-DRG Version 15.0	HCFA-DRG Version 16.0	AP-DRG Version 21.0
Date	1984–1989	1990–1993	1994–1998	1998–2000	2001–2006	2006–2011
Purpose	Pilot study	Information system, DRG-based case payments from third parties				
		–		DRG-based budget allocation		
Data used for deveopment	None: the grouper is not developed in Portugal. Cost weights have been adapted based on Maryland cost weights and the Portuguese hospital cost database					
Number of DRGs	470	477	491	503	511	669
Included services	All inpatient care			All inpatient care and ambulatory surgery		
	Excluding: outpatient care, and psychiatric and rehabilitation care					
Included costs	None	Full costs: including recurrent and capital costs, and costs of research and teaching in relevant hospital; excluding certain high-cost drugs				
Applied to	Participating hospitals	All NHS hospitals				

ambulatory surgery procedures (Bentes et al., 1996; Mateus & Valente, 2000). The rationale for this lay in the growing trend to shift care from inpatient to ambulatory settings and an ever-growing number of ambulatory surgery procedures being financed through DRGs as short-stay outlier or inlier admissions, depending on the low trim-point of the relevant DRG. From the viewpoint of the payer (the Ministry of Health itself), this was a clear distortion of the inpatient DRG system, considering that it was neither designed nor intended to classify ambulatory surgery procedures.

Based on a list developed by the Irish Department of Health and a survey of 56 selected hospitals, a set of 33 DRGs was selected from existing HCFA-DRGs as being eligible to classify ambulatory surgery procedures based on four criteria: physician's responses; homogeneity of the DRG's content; reported volume of zero day stays for the most common selected procedure code above 30 per cent; and, in addition, the low trim-point for the DRG in question had to be less than or equal to two days, to preserve face validity. To ensure validity and acceptability of results, panels of physicians were assembled and through consensus techniques a final list of 38 HCFA-DRGs were selected as 'ambulatory surgery DRGs' (five other DRGs were included with the original set of 33).

Subsequently, a price was computed for each ambulatory surgery DRG according to the Portuguese DRG cost/weight model (see subsection 21.5.2). Hospital costs were separated into those that could be assumed to vary with length of stay (e.g. physician, hotel) and those which were likely to be similar for each inpatient admission in the same DRG (e.g. laboratory, pharmacy). The price of each ambulatory surgery DRG was established according to the following price components of the corresponding inpatient DRG: 100 per cent of operating room (OR) cost; 100 per cent of physician cost for one day; 100 per cent of hotel and nursing costs for one day; 100 per cent of administration cost for one day; 80 per cent of the cost of supplies; 25 per cent of imaging and laboratory costs; 25 per cent of the cost of the relevant drugs for the procedure; zero per cent of intensive care unit (ICU) and other ancillary costs.

The first prices were published in 1998 and used for funding in the same year. More recently, a similar methodology has been used to select a list of specific therapeutic medical procedures that are eligible to be carried out in day-care settings.

DRGs were introduced for hospital payment from third-party payers in 1988. Starting in 1997, DRGs were also progressively introduced for the calculation of hospital budget allocations from the NHS (see subsection 21.5.3). Since 2002, the total NHS inpatient budget has been allocated through DRG-based hospital budget allocations.

21.2.3 Data used for development and updates of the DRG system

All DRG systems that have been in use in Portugal were purchased from abroad, and no Portuguese data were used to develop these systems. For the selection of

Table 21.3 Sources of data for the calculation of Portuguese prices by DRG

Variable	*Country*	*Source*
Costs	Portugal	Hospitals cost database (ACSS)
Relative weights	United States	Maryland cost weights
Inpatient discharges	Portugal	DRG database (ACSS)
National base rate	Portugal	Ministry of Health

ambulatory surgery DRGs only, information about Portuguese ambulatory care patterns was considered.

Table 21.3 presents sources of information that are considered for the calculation of Portuguese cost weights and for setting the national base rate. Portuguese DRG cost weights are calculated using Maryland cost weights (see subsection 21.5.2) and data from the national hospital costs database at ACSS, which contains information about treatment costs in all NHS hospitals (see section 21.4). Cost information is forwarded electronically to the national database, which is maintained and updated by the data unit at ACSS. Cost data from the database are also used to calculate Portuguese cost weights for ambulatory surgery DRGs.

Another important database used for the calculation of Portuguese cost weights is the DRG database at ACCS. The database contains all information from the uniform minimum basic datasets (UMBDS) of all NHS hospitals in the country. The national base rate is set by the Ministry of Health but the decision is based on information relating to the average costs of the average patient for a given year.

21.2.4 Regularity and method of system updates

The 3M™ Health Information System regularly updates the AP-DRG system in order to account for changes of the ICD-9-CM (WHO International Classification of Diseases 9th revision, Clinical Modification), or to adjust the system to new developments in medical technology or to changing practice patterns. A variety of statistical techniques are used to ensure optimal redesign and to maintain and improve quality and statistical coherence of the grouper.

Imported DRG systems have always been implemented in Portugal without any changes to the grouping algorithms developed in the United States. No system of regular updates of the DRG system exists in Portugal. DRG cost weights are recalculated at irregular intervals. The base rate is usually revised every 18 months. However, there is always a time lag of at least two years between the year of the data and the year of application of new DRG cost weights in hospitals. For example, hospital cost data from the year 2009 were analysed during the year 2010 in order to define the national base rate used for hospital payment in 2011.

21.3 The current patient classification system

21.3.1 Information used to classify patients

After a patient is discharged from hospital, the information on her/his medical record is abstracted to the UMBDS according to the coding rules. All patients are classified into AP-DRGs on the basis of the principal diagnosis, secondary diagnoses, procedures, age, sex and discharge status (3M, 2003).

Since the beginning of the first pilot project, diagnoses and procedures have always been coded through ICD-9-CM and coding activities have been carried out by trained physicians within hospitals.

21.3.2 Classification algorithm

Hospitals group every discharged patient into exactly one DRG using a computerized grouping software. The AP-DRG system defines 669 DRGs within 25 MDCs and one Pre-MDC. Figure 21.1 illustrates the grouping algorithm. In a first step, the grouping algorithm checks an exception hierarchy that specifies certain cases, which are separated during the Pre-MDC process (see Table 21.4). The Pre-MDC process defines specific high-cost procedures (such as transplants) that lead to direct classification of patients into certain DRGs within the Pre-MDC, or it assigns cases to MDCs on the basis of certain criteria other than their principal diagnosis. All cases that do not have conditions specified in the exception hierarchy are classified into MDCs on the basis of their principal diagnosis.

Within MDCs, the algorithm groups cases into a 'surgical' partition or a 'medical' partition according to whether an OR procedure was performed during the hospital stay. At the partition level, cases with secondary diagnoses

Table 21.4 AP-DRG hierarchy in the pre-MDC process

Exception Hierarchy	*MDC / AP-DRG Assignment*
Liver transplant	Assign to AP-DRG 480
Lung transplant	Assign to AP-DRG 795
Simultaneous kidney/pancreas transplant	Assign to AP-DRG 805
Pancreas transplant	Assign to AP-DRG 829
Heart transplant	Assign to AP-DRG 103
Kidney transplant	Assign to AP-DRG 302
Allogenic bone marrow transplant	Assign to AP-DRG 803
Autologous bone marrow transplant	Assign to AP-DRG 804
Age less than 29 days	Assign to MDC 15
Principal diagnosis of HIV or secondary diagnoses of HIV and principal diagnosis of HIV-related condition	Assign to MDC 24
ECMO or tracheostomy	Assign to AP-DRG 482 or 483
Principal diagnosis of trauma and at least two significant traumas from different body sites	Assign to MDC 25
Principal diagnosis	Assign to MDCs 1–14, 16–23

Source: 3M, 2003.

Note: ECMO: extracorporeal membrane oxygen.

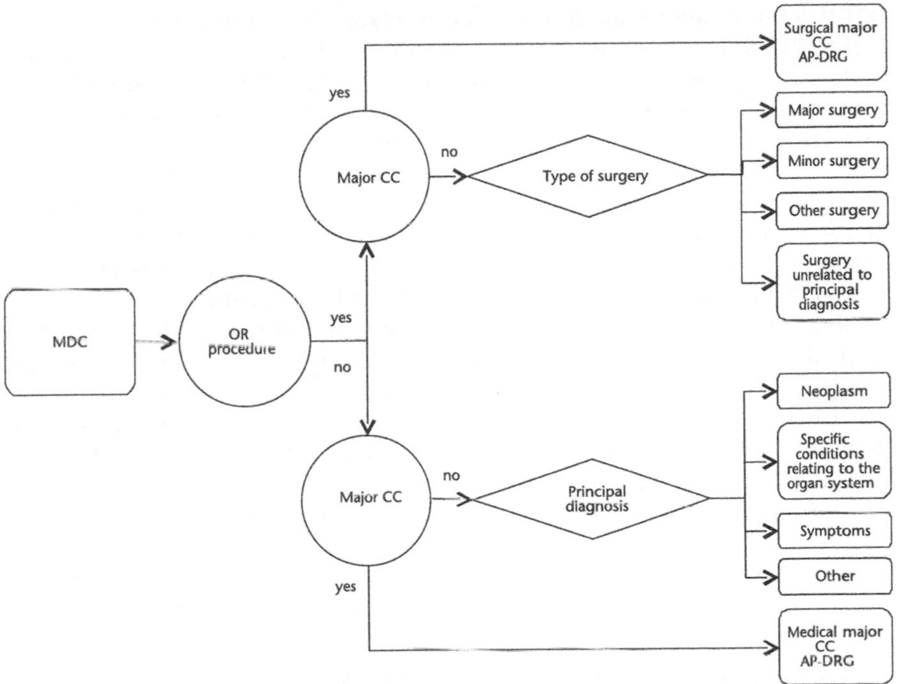

Figure 21.1 AP-DRG (Version 21.0) classification algorithm

Source: 3M, 2003.

that are considered a 'major CC' (major complication and/or co-morbidity) are separated and combined into a small number of medical or surgical 'major CC' groups. All other surgical cases are grouped into a surgical 'class' based on the highest ranked OR procedure or into the 'unrelated surgery' class in the event that the procedure is unrelated to the principal diagnosis. 'Classes' are similar to base-DRGs in other DRG systems in that they comprise patients with similar characteristics (see Chapter 4). Medical cases are grouped into medical classes (e.g. neoplasm, or symptoms and special conditions relating to the organ system). Both partitions also include a residual class for infrequent cases or those that are not well defined. In the last step of the grouping algorithm, classes can be split in order to increase economic homogeneity of the final DRGs based on age, discharge type, body weight (neonates) and secondary diagnoses that are considered to be 'CCs'. Both the 'CC list' and the 'major CC list' are globally defined with exclusions and adjustments at the principal diagnosis level (3M, 2003). There are 303 DRGs in the surgical partition and 364 DRGs in the medical partition.

21.3.3 Data quality and plausibility checks

High-quality data are essential for any DRG system. In Portugal, coding is carried out by physicians who are voluntarily trained as coders. A hospital-wide framework for data evaluation was put in place early in the process of introducing DRGs (Bentes et al., 1997). Since 1995, internal and external hospital clinical coding audits have been carried out on a regular basis. Each hospital has assigned an internal auditor who coordinates the data-collection process and supervises the clinical coding of physician coders within hospitals. An external clinical coding auditing team – composed of eight physicians and a senior manager from ACSS – has been appointed to promote, support and monitor clinical coding audit activity at the hospitals. In addition, the external auditing team conducts site visits and verifies patient records in order to assess whether the classification of patients into DRGs has been carried out correctly.

Clinical coding audits are supported by computer software, which identifies the main data errors and inconsistencies in samples of hospital records. The software returns information about the average number of codes per record, the percentage of invalid codes for diagnoses, procedures and administrative data, and coding errors (e.g. opposite codes), as well as alerting the users to coding problems or deficient information within the medical records (e.g. diagnosis and procedure duplication, unspecified principal diagnosis) and atypical lengths of stay.

By the end of 2009 a web portal completely devoted to coding issues was made available.[1]

21.3.4 Incentives for up- or wrong-coding

As more complex DRGs have a higher cost weight, hospitals are incentivized to code all existing secondary diagnoses of their patients. However, there is also an incentive to engage in up-coding (see Chapter 6), although the periodic coding audits that are carried out strongly disincentivize this behaviour. During the external clinical coding audits that took place between 2006 and 2008, one third of the records presented critical non-conformities. Nevertheless, only 11 per cent had errors leading to a change of the original DRG, and the change was not always for a less complex group.

It is worth noting that as part of the financing criteria for 1998, the final quality coding score of each individual hospital has been considered for adjustments to the preliminary budget (in terms of premiums/penalties), thus creating incentives for data-quality improvement. The impact of the premiums/penalties was below 1 per cent of the inpatient budget of the hospital, and this was a one-off adjustment.

21.4 Cost accounting within hospitals

21.4.1 Regulation

It is mandatory for all NHS hospitals to report their activity and costs annually to ACSS. Since 1995 an NHS Costing Manual has been in place and sets out the mandatory practice of costing to be applied in NHS hospitals (IGIF, 2007). With the implementation of the Costing Manual, the collection and production of costing information presents a greater degree of consistency.

Clinical costing standards cover acute inpatient care, consultations, day-case treatments, emergency visits and ancillary tests. In January 2010 more detail was introduced for mental care services and psychiatric hospitals also had to collect costing information according to the Costing Manual regulations.

21.4.2 Main characteristics of the cost-accounting system

The range of costs included in accounting terms corresponds to the full cost of the provision of all services borne by the hospital. Therefore, all operating expenses, staff costs and capital costs are included. As usual, total costs should be reconciled to the financial costs of the provider for the previous financial year.

Costs are calculated using a top-down approach because information on itemized resource use by individual patients is not collected at NHS hospitals. The Costing Manual (IGIF, 2007) specifies that hospitals should group their costs into five homogenous sections (see Table 21.5), which are cost centres within hospitals, created to absorb direct costs and to allocate indirect costs (IGIF, 2007).

Costs are allocated to cost centres in the principal section, following a step-down approach that includes four steps (see Figure 21.2), as detailed here.

1. First step: imputation of direct costs into principal, auxiliary and administrative sections.
2. Second step: allocation of total costs of the administrative sections to the auxiliary and principal sections.
3. Third step: allocation of total costs of general support auxiliary sections to the sections that benefit from their activities.
4. Fourth step: allocation of total costs of clinical support auxiliary sections to the sections that benefit from their activities.

Table 21.5 Homogenous sections and cost centres

Homogenous sections	*Relevant cost centres*
1. Principal sections	Clinical inpatient services, e.g. medical specialties, surgical specialties, obstetrics, radiotherapy, ICU, transplant unit Clinical ambulatory services, e.g. day-case treatments, ambulatory surgery, outpatients, emergency care
2. Auxiliary sections of clinical support	Diagnostic and therapeutic tests Anaesthesiology OR Other clinical support services
3. Auxiliary sections of general support	Buildings and equipment services Hotel services
4. Administrative sections	Administration and board, e.g. accountancy, management Technical and administrative services
5. Non-imputable	Costs not associated with activities of other sections, e.g. tests ordered by other hospitals

Source: IGIF, 2007.

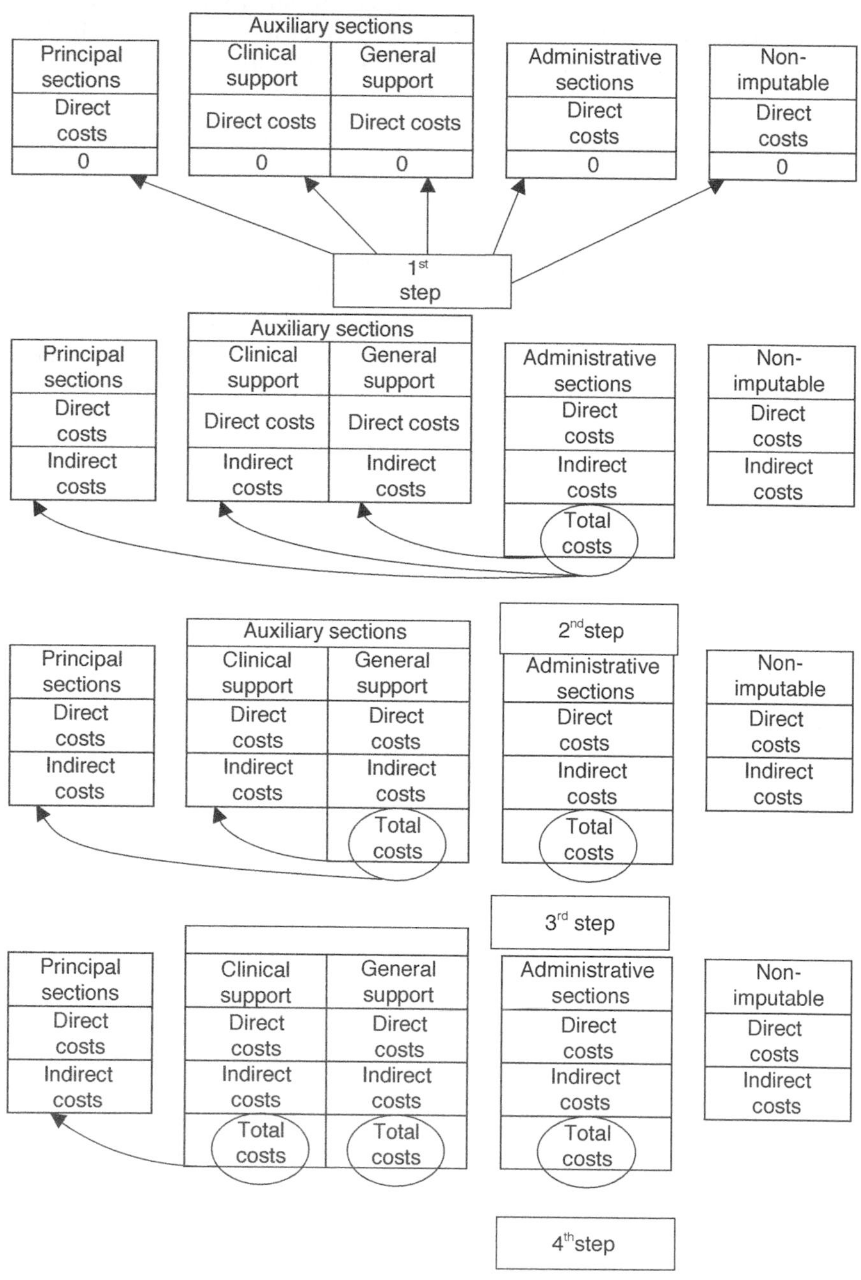

Figure 21.2 Structure/rules for cost allocation

Source: IGIF, 2007.

First-level costs – direct costs – are directly associated to a homogenous section because they are a direct result of its activity. Second-, third-, and fourth-level costs – indirect costs – have to be apportioned to the principal sections that use the services they provide according to the reciprocal distribution method (IGIF, 2007).

Hospitals report their costs for all sections (principal, auxiliary and administrative) to the national hospital cost database that is used for the DRG cost/weight calculation model. A working group was established in 1997 in order to improve the linkage between the hospitals' cost accounting and the DRG cost/weight calculation model. For all hospitals, items to be included in each cost centre were reviewed in order to ensure greater comparability within costs included in the model. However, the hospitals' cost-accounting systems still use different reporting criteria, which impacts negatively on the DRG cost/weight calculation model.

21.5 DRG-based hospital payment in Portugal

21.5.1 Range of services and costs included in DRG-based hospital payment

For payment of hospital activities, DRG use in Portugal is threefold: (1) calculation of a prospective global budget for inpatient care (accounting for about 75–85 per cent of total NHS hospital inpatient revenues); (2) DRG-based case payment for care provided to beneficiaries of occupation-based schemes and insurance companies (mainly for traffic accidents and occupational injuries); (3) DRG-based case payment for surgical procedures included in the waiting list recovery programme. Outpatient care, rehabilitation and psychiatric care are not included in the system. Furthermore, hospital payment of private hospitals is not based on DRGs.

DRG-based budgets or DRG-based case payments cover the full costs of treatment of a patient in a particular DRG, including recurrent costs such as salaries of medical doctors, and capital costs. There are no specific adjustments for research and teaching activities, which are supposed to be financed through additional budgets from other ministries. Nevertheless, a proportion of the higher costs of teaching and research are supposed to be taken into account through the adjustments that are in place for different groups of hospitals (see subsection 21.5.3).

21.5.2 Calculation of DRG cost weights

Calculation of national Portuguese cost weights suffers from the inexistence of data relating to per-patient costs in NHS hospitals. However, a Portuguese DRG cost/weight calculation model is in place that adjusts original AP-DRG cost weights to the Portuguese context using Maryland cost weights and information contained in the national hospital cost database and the national DRG database (see section 21.2.3). Maryland cost weights are developed by the

Maryland Cost Review Program and provide a set of internal cost weights that reflect the costs of one service relative to other services within each DRG. By assuming that Portuguese hospitals have the same pattern of service use as hospitals in Maryland, but at different levels, it is possible to determine the relative costs of each service that comprise total hospital costs by DRG (see also Chapter 22 of this volume).

The shortcoming of this methodology lies in assuming an identical profile of treatment in Portugal and in Maryland in the United States. Since 1994, panels of physicians (by MDC) have convened at the ACSS when necessary to validate Portuguese cost weights estimated through the DRG cost/weight calculation model.

In order to account for cases with extremely long or short length of stay, calculated cost weights apply only to cases falling within specified length-of-stay thresholds. These thresholds are calculated on the basis of an inter-quartile method using length-of-stay data from the national DRG database.

The national base rate is determined by the Ministry of Health on the basis of the 'calculated base rate' for the previous year (e.g. 2009), and the available budget for the next year (e.g. 2011). The calculated base rate is the quotient between the total costs of a given year and the total number of discharges for the same year, and it expresses the average costs for the average patient for that year. When setting the value of the national base rate, the Ministry of Health bears in mind its impact on third-party payers' budgets and on the expenditure of the NHS. The base rate is used to calculate the hospitals' budgets and the DRG tariff for third-party payers (see subsection 21.5.3). After changes in cost weights or base rates, the model is recalibrated in order to ensure a national casemix index (CMI) of one.

21.5.3 DRGs for hospital payment

DRG-based budget allocation from the NHS

Key components of the DRG-based budget allocation model are the hospital casemix indices, hospital adjustment rates and the total number of discharges. However, it should also be kept in mind that the amount spent under the DRG funding system cannot exceed the national budget for inpatient care and, frequently, it is necessary to adjust the national base rate to conform to that constraint. The hospital inpatient budget (H_i) is calculated by multiplying the number of standardized NHS inpatients the hospital is expected to treat during the budget year (*t*) (predicted equivalent discharges)[2] multiplied by its CMI in the year before last (*t-2*) and multiplied by the group base rate. Hospital groups are defined normatively based on the number and diversity of specialties they can provide, among other criteria. The group base rate is determined to a certain percentage based on the hospitals' base rates within the group (that is, the average costs of the average patient treated in each hospital), with the remaining proportion based on the national base rate.

$$H_i = CMI_{(t-2)} \times \sum \textit{predicted equivalent discharges} \times \textit{group base rate}$$

Table 21.6 Percentage of funding based on DRGs

Year	*DRG (%)*	*Previous year's budget (%)*	*Limit of losses*
1997	10	90	Zero
1998	20	80	No limit
1999	30	70	No limit
2000	30	70	Zero
2001	40	60	Zero
2002	50	50	n/a

Note: n/a: not available.

Hospital budgets for the year 2011 were defined on the basis of the hospitals' CMIs in the year 2009.

Since 2003, DRGs have been used to set the total amount of each NHS hospital's inpatient budget. However, between 1997 and 2002 they were introduced gradually with a progressively increasing share of the budget being determined through DRGs (Table 21.6). For some years, the Ministry of Health decided to limit losses to zero; that is, it was decided not to reduce the budgets from one year to another.

DRG-based case payments from third-party payers

In order to receive DRG-based hospital payments for a given month, hospitals must provide information to third-party payers about the number and type of DRGs that were provided to their patients. The payment for every DRG is based on the official tariff, which is determined by multiplying the applicable DRG cost weight with the current national base rate. Payments are adjusted to account for both long-stay and short-stay outliers. Long-stay outliers are paid, after the high trim-point (according to the relevant DRG), at a daily rate that is identical for all DRGs. For short-stay outliers, the payment corresponds to the number of days multiplied by the day price for the DRG. The payment is the same to all NHS hospitals, regardless of the type of hospital (specialty hospitals or general hospitals).

21.5.4 Quality-related adjustments

According to the goals set in the contracts between the ACSS and hospitals, the hospitals can receive a bonus if the percentage of readmissions in the first five days after discharge remains under a defined threshold. The share of ambulatory surgery procedures as a percentage of the total programmed surgical procedures and the ALOS are also considered for the calculation of bonuses.

21.5.5 Main incentives for hospitals

One of the main goals related to the introduction of DRGs for hospital payment was to improve efficiency through increased activity and shorter ALOS and, therefore, to reduce waiting times. The other goal was to control the growth of public expenditure in the health care sector. As hospitals are paid according to the number and type of DRGs that they provide, DRGs encourage hospitals to cut costs, to reduce length of stay and to treat more patients. Analysis of the evolution of the number of patients treated and of the ALOS seems to confirm these expectations (see section 21.7).

21.6 New/innovative technologies

Innovative drugs and devices not included in any DRG are treated on an ad-hoc basis. Physicians remain responsible for decisions related to need. However, physicians must justify their decisions to the hospital's board or to the Drugs and Therapeutics Committee. Usually, clinical criteria prevail. There are no disincentives for hospitals to use new or innovative technologies, as hospital budgets are not fixed and there are no penalties if hospitals incur a deficit.

21.7 Evaluation of the DRG system in Portugal

21.7.1 Existing evaluations

Since the introduction of DRGs, the ALOS has been decreasing in Portuguese NHS hospitals, while the number of patients discharged shows the opposite trend (Table 21.7). This could indicate increasing efficiency in the treatment process, especially as occupancy rates have been constant at around 75 per cent (Bentes et al., 2004).

It should be noted that data for the last two years originate from a different source, which might explain the increase observed in the inpatients' ALOS. Furthermore, the number of patients being treated in ambulatory settings has been rising, which certainly indicates that the complexity/severity of cases being treated in inpatient settings has also been increasing.

In Table 21.7, the cost weights from 1998 were used for the computation of the CMI in each year presented. This explains why the CMI is 1 for the year 1998 and higher for all subsequent years. With that information in mind it can be ascertained that the complexity of cases being treated in Portuguese NHS hospitals has been increasing.

As was the case in the United States, after the first ten years with a DRG-based hospital payment system, in Portugal some of the interest in evaluations of the system has also vanished. Mateus (2008) provides a review of previous evaluations. In summary, the results found in Portugal were similar to those in the United States or Australia; namely, a decrement in the ALOS, and an increase in the CMI and in the number of discharged patients. More patients are being treated, which could indicate efficiency gains.

21.7.2 Author's assessment

After 25 years we can now say that the implementation of DRGs in Portugal has been a success. Not only have NHS hospitals since the late 1980s been billing

Table 21.7 Cases treated, ALOS and CMI in the period 1997–2006

	1997	*1998*	*1999*	*2000*	*2001*	*2002*	*2003*	*2004*	*2005**	*2006**
Inpatient discharges	810 979	818 513	839 393	899 935	895 836	892 607	900 415	876 385	970 146	958 606
Ambulatory surgeries	20 237	20 334	24 850	26 857	37 356	47 735	63 366	77 821	80 417	90 487
Total	831 216	838 847	864 243	926 792	933 592	940 342	963 781	954 206	1 050 563	1 049 093
ALOS (inpatient only)	7.5	7.5	7.3	7.1	7.1	7.0	6.8	6.8	7.2	7.2
CMI	0.99	1.00	1.02	1.04	1.07	1.08	1.08	1.10	1.12	1.13

Sources: IGIF, 2005; * ACSS, 2007.

third-party payers based on DRGs, but also, since the late 1990s, DRG-based hospital budget allocation has been used for the funding of NHS inpatient activity. More patients are being treated in a shorter time, and DRGs have proved to be a helpful cost-control mechanism (Mateus, 2008; Barros & de Almeida Simões, 2007).

Moreover, the creation of the DRG database with morbidity information and treatment profiles of the Portuguese population has great potential in terms of informing decision-makers. Yet, it has remained unused, apart from in three major fields: hospital funding, hospital comparisons, and the setting of national tariffs for inpatient and ambulatory surgery care. In the author's opinion, information from the DRG database could be useful in the design of national health plans and health care policy: to profile morbidity characteristics of the Portuguese population at national and regional levels; to organize provision of care according to need; to target areas for utilization review and quality assurance; and to control the achievement of goals set in existing national health plans for different pathologies. Furthermore, data collected in patient registries could be used – as pointed out by Noe and colleagues (2005) – to support health economics research in certain areas, such as identifying of practice patterns and evaluating variations based on setting, examining regional differences, conducting population sub-group analyses, determining the characteristics of high- or low-cost patients, and so on.

It would be a major achievement to develop national cost weights, and a sample of representative hospitals should be sought. Encouraging private hospitals to code their inpatient activity with the DRGs would be another worthwhile step. The private sector is becoming increasingly more important in the provision of care and there is no justification for the non-reporting of their activity.

21.8 Outlook: Future developments and reform

21.8.1 Trends in hospital service (or general health care) delivery

According to the latest available data, hospital inpatient care is still very important in Portugal and ambulatory surgery represents no more than 10 per cent of inpatient activity. Services provided in non-inpatient settings are funded on a fee-for-service basis. The number of hospitals being built (both public and private) sends a signal that, at the least at the planning level, inpatient care is and will continue to be important in the provision of health care in Portugal.

21.8.2 Trends in DRG application and coverage

The use of DRGs for hospital payment and budget allocation has been evolving since its implementation. In the mid-1990s two pilot studies were carried out concerning the adaptation of Ambulatory Patient Groups (APGs) to the Portuguese context. The results obtained from both studies were very promising;

however, APGs were never implemented due to a lack of political will. Currently, ambulatory activity (consultations and ancillary services) is financed on a fee-for-service basis, which is the preferred method of payment of hospital managers and physicians. Therefore, there is strong opposition from hospitals to the implementation of APGs.

Studies have been carried out regarding the feasibility of using a patient classification system suited for mental health care settings. No decision has been made regarding the grouper to be used, but both the system implemented in the United States and those being developed in Canada (System for Classification of In-Patient Psychiatry)[3] and Australia (Mental Health Classification And Service Costs)[4] are being closely analysed.

Due to the development of a National Network of Nursing Homes in Portugal, interest is also being raised in the implementation of a patient classification system for rehabilitation care. At present, care is financed by a per diem payment that reflects neither the characteristics of the patients nor of the facilities.

It can be expected that increasingly more fields of care will be covered by DRG-like systems for funding and for information purposes. Portugal was one of the earliest countries in Europe to adopt DRGs for inpatient care and it is likely that it will also be one of the pioneers in the use of patient classification systems for other types of care.

21.9 Notes

1 Available only in Portuguese (http://portalcodgdh.min-saude.pt, accessed 10 July 2011).
2 Equivalent discharges correspond to the total number of inpatient episodes obtained after standardizing outlier lengths of stay (below or above the low and high trim-points) in each DRG with equivalent lengths of stay in terms of the 'normal' episodes (those with lengths of stay within the trim-points). Patients with short-stay admissions are accounted for as less than one; patients with long-stay admissions are accounted for as more than one; and those with episodes involving lengths of stay within the trim-points are accounted for as one.
3 See the Canadian Institute for Health Information web site (http://secure.cihi.ca, accessed 10 July 2011).
4 See the Australian Government Department of Health and Ageing web site (http://www.health.gov.au, accessed 10 July 2011).

21.10 References

3M (2003). *All Patient DRG Definitions Manual (Version 21.0)*. St. Paul, MN: 3M Health Information Systems.

ACSS (2007). *Sistema Classificação de Doentes em Grupos de Diagnósticos Homogéneos (GDH). Informação de Retorno: Ano 2006 [Patient Classification System into Diagnosis-Related Groups (DRGs). Feedback Reports: Year 2006]*. Lisbon: Administração Central do Sistema de Saúde.

Assembleia da República (1990). Lei 48/90: Lei de Bases da Saúde [Law 48/90: Basic Law on Health]. *Diário República*, 195:3452–9.

Barros, P., de Almeida Simões, J. (2007). Portugal: Health system review. *Health Systems in Transition*, 9(5):1–140.

Bentes, M., Dias, C.M., Sakellarides, C., Bankauskaite, V. (2004). *Health Care Systems in Transition: Portugal*. Copenhagen, WHO Regional Office for Europe on behalf of the European Observatory on Health Systems and Policies.

Bentes, M., Valente, M.C., Mateus, C., Estevens, S. (1997). Feedback and audit: ingredients for quality improvement. *Proceedings of the 13th PCS/E International Working Conference, Florence, 1–3 October*.

Bentes, M., Mateus, C., Estevens, S., Valente, M.C., Veertres, J. (1996). Towards a more comprehensive financing system for the Portuguese NHS hospitals. *Proceedings of the 12th International PCS/E Working Conference, Sidney, 19–21 September*.

DGS (2008). *Centros de Saúde e Hospitais: Recursos e Produção do SNS: Ano de 2007 [Health Care Centres and Hospitals: NHS Resources and Results: Year 2007]*. Lisbon: Direcção-Geral da Saúde.

Dismuke, C.E., Sena, V. (2001). Is there a trade-off between quality and productivity? The case of diagnostic technologies in Portugal. *Annals of Operations Research*, 107(1–4): 101–16.

IGIF (2005). *National DRG Database*. Lisbon: Instituto de Gestão Informática e Financeira & Departamento de Desenvolvimento de Sistemas de Financiamento e de Gestão (DDSFG)

IGIF (2007). *Plano de Contabilidade Analítica dos Hospitais (3rd edition) [Hospitals' Accounts Plan]*. Lisbon: Instituto de Gestão Informática e Financeira.

INE (2009). *Indicadores Sociais 2008 [Social Indicators 2008]*. Lisbon: Instituto Nacional de Estatística.

Mateus, C. (2008). Casemix implementation in Portugal, in J.R. Kimberly, G. de Pouvourville, T. D'Aunno, eds. *The Globalization of Managerial Innovation in Health Care*. Cambridge: Cambridge University Press.

Mateus, C., Valente, M.C. (2000). The impact of ambulatory surgery DRGs. *Proceedings of the 16th PCS/E International Working Conference, Groningen, 27–30 September*.

Noe, L., Larson, L., Trotter, J. (2005). Utilizing patient registries to support health economics research: integrating observational data with economic analyses, models, and other applications. *ISPOR CONNECTIONS*, 11(5):6–8.

OECD (2008). *OECD Health Data 2008*. Paris: Organisation for Economic Co-operation and Development.

Urbano, J., Bentes, M., Vertrees, J.C. (1993). Portugal: national commitment and the implementation of DRGs, in J.R. Kimberly, G. de Pouvourville et al., eds. *The Migration of Managerial Innovation*. San Francisco, CA: Jossey-Bass Inc.

chapter twenty two

Spain: A case study on diversity of DRG use – The Catalan experience

Francesc Cots, Xavier Salvador, Pietro Chiarello, Montse Bustins and Xavier Castells

22.1 Hospital services and the role of DRGs in Spain

22.1.1 The Spanish health system

The Spanish 1978 Constitution granted all citizens the right to health protection and care, and this was confirmed by the 1986 General Health Care Act (GHCA). The GHCA specified the basic features of the Spanish health care system, such as public financing and universal access to public health care services free of charge at the point of use. Furthermore, it recognized the devolution of health care responsibilities to the Autonomous Communities (ACs), that is, to the Spanish regions, which is an important characteristic of the Spanish health care system today.

In 2007, total health expenditures amounted to €1980 per capita per year, which corresponds to 8.4 per cent of gross domestic product (GDP) (European Commission, 2011). Public expenditures (mostly financed through general taxation) are the most significant source of finance in the Spanish health system as they account for roughly 72 per cent of total health expenditures. Household out-of-pocket expenditures account for about 22 per cent of total health expenditures and are mostly spent on services not covered by the public system (for example, dental care and services provided by private specialists). In addition, an increasing share of the population (25 per cent in 2007) holds private health insurance coverage (López Casasnovas, 2008), which pays for care provided in the private sector.

On the one hand, the main responsibilities of the central Government still include setting the general framework for coordination and financing of the National Health Service (NHS), defining the basic NHS benefits package, regulating pharmaceuticals, and coordinating medical education (Durán et al., 2006). On the other hand, each of the 17 ACs has a Regional Health Service that is responsible for purchasing and provision of health care. In addition, ACs develop public health policies, and are entitled to extend the basic NHS benefits package (Health Information Institute, 2010).

Most importantly, the central Government collects income taxes and value-added tax (VAT) and allocates health budgets to the Health Service of each AC on a simple per capita allocation basis which includes criteria for adjusting the allocation, such as the proportion of the elderly population and insularity. In addition, each AC is free to collect additional resources through marginal add-on taxes on income.

Besides the general per capita allocations, the central Government also finances the Health Cohesion Fund, which was created in 2002 and accounts for less than 1 per cent of public health expenditures. The Cohesion Fund is managed by the NHS and aims to assure equal access to health care for the entire Spanish population. In order to do so, the Fund allocates resources to ACs that provide care to patients from ACs in which certain services defined by the Ministry of Health are not available (mostly high-technology services).

Each AC has developed its own structures and financing mechanisms. This chapter focuses on Catalonia in particular, as it was the first AC to adopt diagnosis-related groups (DRGs) for casemix analyses, management and hospital financing (HOPE, 2006). In Catalonia, in 2007, total health expenditures were at 7.4 per cent of GDP (CatSalut, 2010), of which 67.2 per cent were paid from public sources.

22.1.2 Hospital services in Spain and Catalonia

Spain

About 40 per cent of total health expenditures in Spain are spent on hospital care, almost exclusively (93 per cent) from public sources (European Commission, 2011). There are about 770 hospitals in Spain, of which 591 are acute care hospitals. Some 42 per cent of acute care hospitals are public (247). They represent 72 per cent of all acute care beds, with their average being greater than that of private hospitals (380 beds and 105 beds, respectively).

In general, the private sector offers services which are excluded from the public benefits package. It has specialized in areas such as plastic surgery and certain elective procedures for which waiting lists exist in the public sector.

As the responsibility for purchasing and provision of health care lies with the ACs, the central Government is not directly involved in the financing of hospital care. Instead, all resources (per capita allocations and Cohesion Fund resources) are channelled through the ACs' Regional Health Services, which have set up different organizational structures and management tools for the purchasing and provision of hospital care.

Catalonia

ACs differed greatly in terms of the availability of public health care infrastructures at the time of devolution. In some ACs the existing number of public hospitals (and their capacity) was adequate for the task; in others less so. In Catalonia, public health centres and hospitals were mostly concentrated in major cities. Therefore, in order to ensure universal availability of services a Public Hospital Network (*Xarxa Hospitàlaria d'Utilització Pública*, XHUP) was created by incorporating hospitals from a wide range of owners, including several town councils, the Red Cross, the Catholic Church and private charity societies.

In the XHUP there are 68 hospitals with an average of 237 beds (Table 22.1). Just 10 of the hospitals are directly owned by the Health Care Department and they constitute the Catalan Health Care Institute (ICS). The remaining hospitals have different owners (some of them private non-profit-making entities) and they are represented by two hospital associations: the Consorci de Salut i Social de Catalunya and the Unió Catalana d'Hospitals.

The private sector is relatively important as it represents about 20 per cent of discharges and 15 per cent of beds. Private care tends to be primarily used for obstetric services (perceived to offer higher comfort and room quality), for elective surgery (in order to avoid waiting lists), and for specialties with no public coverage, such as cosmetic surgery and dental care.

Hospitals do not only provide inpatient care: In 2007, over 10 million ambulatory care specialist visits took place at public hospitals. Primary care is provided through a public network organized on a territorial basis. Within the primary care network, each person is assigned to a general practitioner (GP), who has a coordinating role with the XHUP and who refers patients to hospital specialist

Table 22.1 Acute hospitals in Catalonia

Acute hospital activity XHUP 2007	*XHUP*	*%*	*Private network*	*%*	*Total*
Hospitals	68	63.0	40	37.0	108
Beds	16 119	85.5	2 813	14.5	18 932
Occupancy rate (%)	83.8	–	63.8	–	80.7
Staff	42 624	90.4	4.512	9.6	47 136
Staff/Number of beds	2.6	–	1.5	–	2.5
Discharges	725 108	79.7	184 864	20.3	909 972
Total bed days	4 932 360	87.4	709 004	12.6	5 641 364
Ambulatory visits	10 061 109	89.1	1 232 137	10.9	11 293 246
Emergencies	3 923 380	85.2	679 619	14.8	4 602 999
Publicly financed discharges	665 755	99.9	475	0.1	666 230
Publicly financed discharges/ Total discharges (%)	92.7	–	0.3	–	83.9
Expenditures	4 960 000	90.9	495 000*	9.1	5 455 000
Revenues	4 917 000	91.6	450 000*	8.4	5 367 000

Sources: Authors' own compilation based on EESRI, 2007 and CatSalut, 2007.

* Includes mixed acute, social and mental health care centres.

ambulatory care. In addition, major ambulatory surgery (MAS) has increased significantly since the mid-1990s and accounted for 15 per cent of all hospital discharges and 40 per cent of total surgical activity in 2007 (CatSalut, 2007).

The current hospital payment system in Catalonia has been in place since 1997 and is the same for the entire XHUP, independent of hospital ownership. Global inpatient budgets are set on the basis of DRGs and structural indicators. Additional budgets are distributed to hospitals for specific health programmes, capital investments, research and education. Inpatient hospital treatment accounts for the largest share of total hospital revenues. Outpatient consultations are paid through a flat fee per visit that differs according to the structural characteristics of the hospital. Emergency care is paid for by means of a fee-for-service system, whereby the fee is adjusted according to the structural characteristics of the hospital. 'Specific techniques' are financed through additional payments (see subsection 22.5.1 for further details).

22.1.3 Purpose of the DRG systems in Spain and Catalonia

Spain

National use of All-Patient (AP)-DRGs in Spain has two main purposes: (1) performance assessments and benchmarking, and (2) enabling DRG-based case payments from the Cohesion Fund to the ACs.

The casemix index (CMI) and the length of stay per DRG are the basic indicators of hospital scorecards used for performance assessments and benchmarking. Most ACs and the national Government give hospitals feedback in terms of national and regional DRG norms. The use of DRGs to evaluate efficiency is quite popular, and in some cases it is related to the evaluation of contract programmes. However, the most extensive and important uses of benchmarking come from private companies (IASIST, 2008).

The Cohesion Fund uses AP-DRGs to compensate ACs for care provided within their hospitals to patients from other ACs. As already mentioned, the Cohesion Fund was introduced in 2002 to assure equal access to public sector hospital services for the entire Spanish population. However, prior to receiving treatment in another AC, patients must seek authorization from their home AC. The Cohesion Fund does not compensate ACs for emergency care provided in their hospitals to patients from other ACs.

Catalonia

In Catalonia, DRGs have been used since 1997 to adjust hospital payments. Since the year 2000, 35 per cent of hospital inpatient budgets have been related to DRGs. Before the introduction of DRGs as a tool for hospital payment, the Catalan Health Service used the UBA (Basic Care Unit) model, which paid hospitals an equal amount of money per equivalent hospital stay (Brosa & Agusti, 2009). The purpose of the introduction of DRGs for hospital payment was to ensure an enhanced measure of hospital activity that would contribute to making hospital payment more closely related to performance (Cots &

Castells, 2001). Using DRGs was thought to encourage efficiency, improve data quality, and facilitate hospital management.

22.2 Development and updates of the DRG systems

22.2.1 The current DRG systems at a glance

All ACs provide to the Ministry of Health their minimum basic datasets (MBDS) detailing hospital activity, grouped using 3M AP-DRGs (current version 25), as is the standard defined at national level. National data from hospital patients grouped with AP-DRGs are used to analyse the casemix and for benchmarking. There are no national modifications of the imported AP-DRG system to the number of DRGs, nor to the algorithms used.

In Catalonia, all XHUP hospitals are required to group their discharges (inpatient and MAS) using Centers for Medicare and Medicaid Services (CMS)-DRGs. The CHS uses CMS-DRGs in order to adjust hospital budgets (see section 22.5). However, all Catalan hospitals also have to report on AP-DRGs, which are used to analyse efficiency, and to compare Catalan hospitals with the rest of Spain.

22.2.2 Development of the DRG systems

Spain has not developed a national DRG system but has relied on different DRG systems imported from abroad. In the 1990s, Spanish authorities decided to use imported DRG systems as there was no reliable cost-accounting information available in Spain that would have allowed a Spanish national DRG system to be developed. Only very few Spanish hospitals have a complete bottom-up cost-accounting system (as explained in section 22.4).

Spain

Table 22.2 provides an overview of the main facts relating to the national-level use of DRGs in Spain. AP-DRGs were introduced in 1999 for the benchmarking of hospitals. Since then, copies of the MBDS of all Spanish hospitals are transmitted to the national Ministry of Health, which uses the information to group discharges into DRGs. Every year, hospital activity data for all Spanish hospitals are reported by the Ministry of Health using AP-DRGs.

Since 2002, imported AP-DRG cost weights have been adjusted to the Spanish context by using cost-accounting information from an increasingly large sample of Spanish hospitals to calculate national tariffs. The original sample for the calculation of national AP-DRG tariffs included 19 hospitals, increasing to 30 in 2008. Hospitals were deliberately selected in order to be representative of all national public hospitals. However, the sample only includes one Catalan hospital, which means that wage and price differences between ACs are not adequately reflected in the estimated national AP-DRG tariffs. Hospitals

Table 22.2 Main facts about the use of DRGs in Spain

	National/ Intercommunities				
DRG system	AP-DRG v. 14.1	AP-DRG v. 18.0	AP-DRG v. 21.0	AP-DRG v. 23.0	AP-DRG v. 25.0
Date of introduction	1999	2002	2006	2008	2010
(Main) Purpose	Analysis/benchmarking of hospital data at national level				
	–	DRG-based case payments for compensation of intercommunity activity through the Cohesion Fund			
Data used for development	Grouping algorithm: Completely imported. National DRG tariffs: Data at cost centre level form a sample of 18 hospitals		Grouping algorithm: Completely imported. National DRG tariffs: Data at cost centre level form a sample of 30 hospitals		
Number of DRGs	644	656	670	676	684
Applied to	MBDS of all hospitals of the NHS (inpatient and MAS care)				
	–	ACs (to compensate patient mobility)			
Included services	All inpatient care, excluding psychiatric and long-term care	Benchmarking: all inpatient care (excluding psychiatric and long-term care) DRG-based case payments: elective high-complexity patients treated in non-resident ACs			
Included costs	–	Capital and recurrent costs			

participating in the data sample must follow a standardized cost-accounting methodology (see section 22.4 for more details).

Catalonia

Since 1985 some initiatives introduced United States Health Care Financing Administration (HCFA)-DRGs in the CHS (Ibern, 1991). However, it was not until 1997 that the Catalan Health Authority decided to officially introduce CMS-DRGs to the CHS (see Table 22.3).

The CMS-DRG system is not modified for use in Catalan hospitals, and unadjusted CMS-DRG cost weights are used for hospital payment. However, CMS-DRGs and AP-DRGs are used in Catalonia not only for inpatient care but also to group high-profile emergencies and MAS.

Since 1999, when data from all Spanish hospitals started being transmitted to the national Ministry of Health, data from Catalan hospitals were included in the national dataset. However, only in 2006 did the CHS start using AP-DRGs for casemix analysis at the regional level. Since then, the CHS has grouped patients discharged from XHUP hospitals using AP-DRGs. The CHS produces annual AP-DRG reports for every hospital to facilitate performance comparisons and to benchmark hospitals.

Table 22.3 Main facts about the use of DRGs in Catalonia

	Catalonia								
	1st set						*2nd set*		
DRG system	HCFA-DRGs (now CMS-DRG) v. 13.0	CMS v. 16.0	CMS v. 18.0	CMS v. 20.0	CMS v. 22.0	CMS v. 24.0	AP-DRG v. 21.0	AP-DRG v. 23.0	AP-DRG v. 25.0
Date of introduction	1997	2000	2002	2004	2006	2008–2010	2006	2008	2010
(Main) Purpose	Adjust the allocation of global budgets						Hospital benchmarking		
Data used for development	None (completely imported)								
Number of DRGs	492	499	499	510	520	538	670	676	684
Applied to	XHUPs						XHUPs		
Included services	Inpatients, MAS and high-profile emergencies, excluding psychiatric and long-term care						As in the rest of Spain		
Included costs	DRGs determine 35% of hospital inpatient budgets						n/a		

Note: n/a: not applicable.

22.2.3 Data used for development and updates of the DRG systems

All DRG versions in use in Spain and Catalonia have been imported from the United States. Their algorithms were not developed in Spain.

National use of AP-DRGs for benchmarking and performance comparison relies on imported cost weights. However, in order to adapt AP-DRGs for intercommunity hospital payment, national tariffs have been calculated based on United States cost weights and cost data from an increasingly large sample of Spanish hospitals.

Over the last few years, cost data used for updates were always two years old: tariffs in use in 2008 and 2009 were based on cost data from the year 2006; tariffs in use since 2010 are based on cost data from the year 2008.

22.2.4 Regularity and method of system updates

In Spain as a whole (all ACs), DRG systems are updated every other year; that is, every two years a new version of AP-DRGs (CMS-DRGs in Catalonia) is imported from the United States. A new AP-DRG version is purchased every other year by the Ministry of Health from 3M Health Information Systems. In addition, ACs and individual hospitals purchase AP-DRGs according to their needs. In Catalonia, CMS-DRGs are also purchased from 3M Health Information Systems.

For the last update of national AP-DRG tariffs, a new version of AP-DRGs (version 25) was imported at the end of 2008. Then cost data from the hospital sample were grouped using AP-DRGs during the year 2009 in order to calculate tariffs for the year 2010. Consequently, in 2010 a version of AP-DRGs was used that had been introduced in the United States two years earlier. In Catalonia, CMS-DRGs are always two years old as they are introduced in the United States two years prior to their import to Catalonia.

Both AP- and CMS- (in Catalonia) DRG systems require that information about diagnoses and procedures is coded using the WHO International Classification of Diseases (ICD) 9th revision – clinical modification (ICD-9-CM), which is a United States-modified version of the ICD. As each version of the DRG systems is based on a specific ICD-9-CM version, a new ICD-9-CM version is always imported, together with the new DRG systems.

22.3 The current patient classification systems

22.3.1 Information used to classify patients

Every hospital in Spain produces a standardized minimum basic dataset (CMBD), which provides information on demographic characteristics of each patient, length of stay, type of admission, discharge destination, discharging department, and diagnoses and procedures coded using the ICD-9-CM. This information is transmitted to the Regional Health Authority (for example, the Conselleria de Salut in Catalonia), which forwards the data to the national

Ministry of Health. The national Ministry of Health extracts the necessary information from the national dataset in order to group patients into AP-DRGs.

In Catalonia, the Conselleria de Salut uses the same data from the CMBD to group patients into AP- and CMS-DRGs.

22.3.2 Classification algorithm

Since the general grouping algorithm of AP-DRGs is presented in the Portuguese chapter of this volume (see Chapter 21), this section will focus on CMS-DRGs.

Figure 22.1 illustrates the grouping process of the CMS-DRG system: in the first step, the grouper checks for invalid or implausible data and classifies patients into Error DRGs. Subsequently, cases are assigned into one of 25 major diagnostic categories (MDCs) on the basis of their principal diagnosis, with each MDC corresponding to a single organ system or etiology. However, there are a certain number of high-cost treatments (such as transplantations), which are reclassified into a Pre-MDC DRG on the basis of the performed procedure, without considering the principal diagnosis. Within each MDC, the presence of a surgical intervention assigns patients into the surgical 'partition', and its corresponding class (for example, Major Surgery), according to the procedure.

If no procedure was performed, cases are assigned to the medical 'partition' and to one of four classes (such as Neoplasms), according to the principal diagnosis. In the last step, the presence of certain secondary diagnoses that are considered to be complications and co-morbidities (CCs) is checked, and the final DRG is determined based on CCs, age of the patient, weight of the newborn (where relevant), and discharge status. This is similar to the process in the AP-DRG system, but the CMS-DRG system does not differentiate between major CCs and other CCs (see Chapter 4 of this volume).

There are a total of 281 DRGs in the medical partition and 255 in the surgical partition. Each DRG is characterized by a three-digit number, for example DRG 167 (appendectomy without complicated diagnosis, without CCs). The numbers are counted from DRG 001 to DRG 578 and do not indicate the MDC or the partition.

22.3.3 Data quality and plausibility checks

Spain

The Spanish Ministry of Health audits the cost-accounting information provided by the hospitals for the calculation of national AP-DRG tariffs (Spanish Ministry of Health and Consumption, 2008). For these hospitals a systematic auditing process is undertaken when the CMBD is submitted to the national Ministry of Health. The Ministry of Health verifies the plausibility of clinical data and the cost information provided. In addition, the Ministry performs site visits and checks patient records within hospitals, to ensure that the information provided is correct.

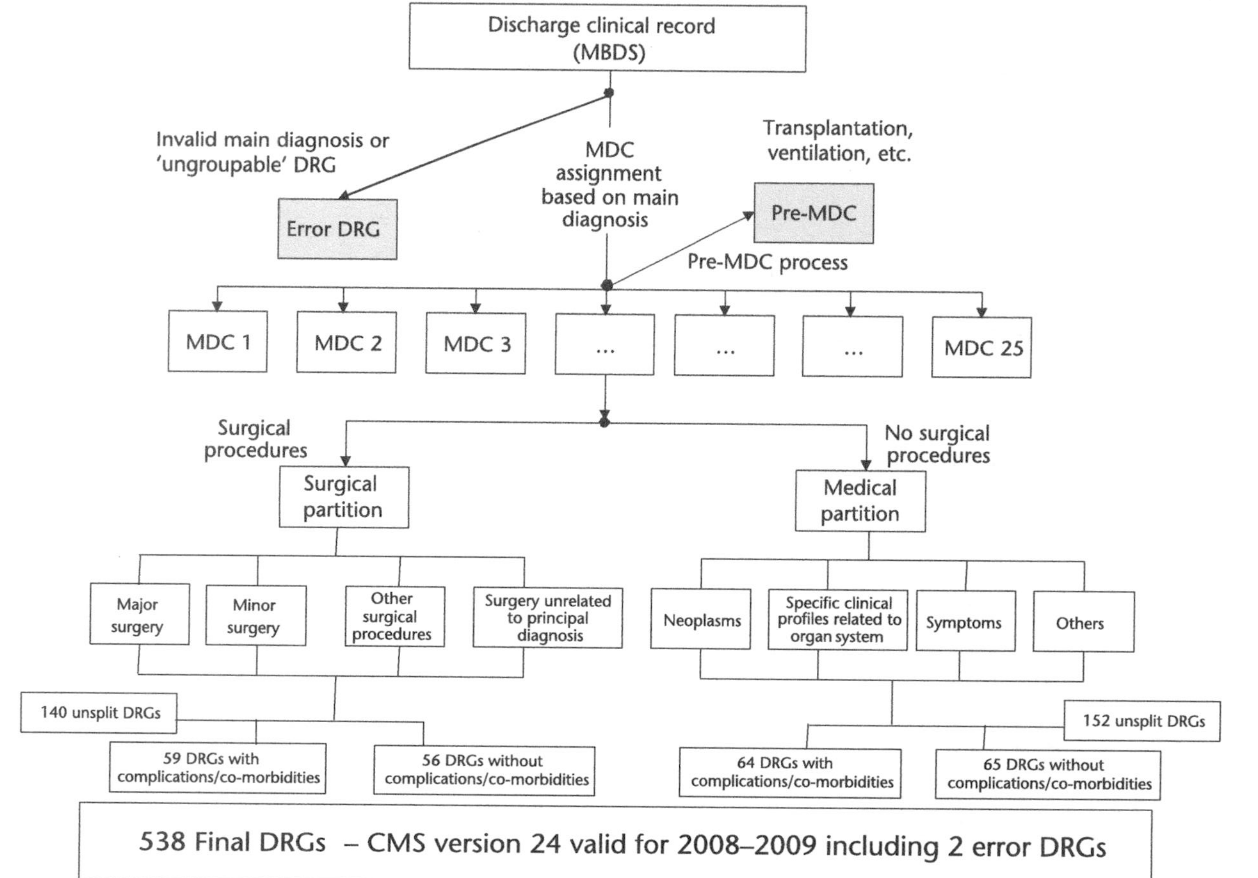

Figure 22.1 CMS-DRG version 24 grouping algorithm

22.3.4 Incentives for up- or wrong-coding

Catalonia

Since hospital payment depends partly on classification of patients into DRGs, hospitals have moderately strong incentives to 'up-code' their patients. In order to ensure that fraudulent practices are avoided, the CHS regularly carries out random auditing of hospital records to verify consistency between internal patient records and those reported. However, even when unusual coding practices are detected, auditing is oriented towards improving the quality of coding, rather than towards imposing sanctions.

22.4 Cost accounting within hospitals

22.4.1 Regulation

There are no national regulations mandating hospitals to use a specific cost-accounting system. However, given that the responsibility for the public health care system lies with the ACs, some ACs have defined minimum cost-accounting standards for their hospitals, requiring them to generate patient-level cost data (for example Catalonia and Cantabria).

In Catalonia, the Central de Balanços, which is a department of the CHS, provides hospitals with regulations relating to the production of financial statements (CatSalut, 1992). Furthermore, some (mostly private) hospitals collect patient-level cost information in order to improve hospital management.

As already mentioned, in 2008 a sample of 30 hospitals collected cost data for the calculation of Spanish AP-DRG tariffs. Hospitals participating in the sample were required to have at least a top-down cost-accounting system.

22.4.2 Main characteristics of cost-accounting systems in Spain

There are only few hospitals which have complete patient-level cost information. Different cost-accounting models are in use in Spain.

Before 2002 there was the GECLIF model (Financial and Clinical Management) of INSALUD (the former national centre of the Ministry of Health). The model was developed at national level within some projects that aimed to calculate costs per department (SIGNO I and SIGNO II – still used in a few hospitals) (González Pérez, 2008) in order to determine costs per DRG (INSALUD, 2001a, b).

At present, GESCOT™ – developed by a private consulting firm (SAVAC S.L.) and based on the GECLIF model – is one of the most common and most consistently used accounting systems in Spanish hospitals. It can determine costs per patient if hospitals have a fully functioning and high-quality information system, allocating costs to each patient according to each care service received. It means that the Health Information System must register each service, patient and cost centre at which the service is provided. The advantage of GESCOT™ is that it has a strong and valid imputation system, based on matricial distribution between cost centres, namely the Structural, Intermediate and Final cost centres.

In addition to these systems, some ACs have started introducing and developing their own cost-accounting systems, the most important of which are listed here.

- COANh, by the Andalusian Health Service, extended to the XHUP since 1995, uses a full costing system that employs reciprocal imputation in attributing costs between different types of cost centres.
- ALDABIDE, by the Basque Health Service, implemented in 1994 and updated in 1996 and 1998, aims to calculate costs at the department level.
- SIE has been implemented by the AC of Valencia since 1992.

Table 22.4 summarizes the four main cost-accounting systems in Spain, the methodology of cost imputation to final cost centres (that is, whether reciprocal imputation or mixed imputation with iterations (loop or matricial imputation) is used); and whether the model is able to provide patient costs through direct allocation to patients (that is, whether the system includes a bottom-up cost-accounting module).

Table 22.4 shows that relevant differences exist in imputation methodologies between different cost-accounting systems. GESCOT™ has the same structure within all hospitals for the first step of the cost-accounting process – that is, the primary cost-distribution method (top-down approach) – and each of these hospitals has developed a different final attribution structure, according to the level of detail of the activity information system.

Monge (2003b) surveyed hospitals employing the presented accounting systems and found that almost 40 per cent of polled hospitals declared using their own accounting systems, and that they were characterized by imprecise

Table 22.4 Main Spanish cost-accounting systems

Accounting system	*Cost categories*	*Methodology*	*Level of aggregation*
GESCOT™	Staff costs Goods and services Structural services Secondary services	Reciprocal imputations	Bottom up
COANh	Staff costs Goods and services Structural services Secondary services	Reciprocal imputations	Top down
ALDABIDE	Staff costs Goods and services Structural services Secondary services	Mixed, with iterations between cost centres of the same level	Top down
SIE	Staff costs Goods and services	Mixed, with iterations between cost centres of the same level	Top down

imputing methods and parameters, as well as slow information processing with manual dataset capture and management.

SAVAC Consultants S.L., provider of GESCOT™, estimate that – out of the almost 130 Spanish (public and private) hospitals using the GECLIF-derived cost-accounting system (GESCOT™) – only a few of them (around 15) can calculate costs per patient in accordance with a secondary cost distribution (bottom-up) process from final cost centres to patients.

22.5 DRGs for hospital payment

22.5.1 Range of services and costs included in DRG-based hospital payment

Spain

In general, AP-DRGs are only used for determining payments from the Cohesion Fund to compensate ACs for treating inpatients from other ACs. Payments from the Cohesion Fund are made mostly on behalf of small ACs that do not have the capacity to treat highly complex cases. In these cases, patients are treated electively in hospitals of other ACs, after authorization has been obtained from the Regional Health Authority where the patient lives. Payments from the Cohesion Fund are supposed to include all costs categories, that is, capital costs (for example, buildings and equipment) and running costs (for example, personnel and supplies).

Catalonia

In Catalonia, CMS-DRGs are used to determine DRG-based budgets for all hospitals within the public network, which includes many non-profit-making organizations. DRGs are used not only for inpatient activity (hospitalization), but also for MAS and high-profile emergencies (stays of longer than 12 hours, deaths or transfers to other hospitals). In general terms, DRGs include only acute care and do not cover psychiatric and long-term care. The inclusion of MAS was a political decision designed to provide a powerful incentive to set surgery in an outpatient setting, as one of the measures to reduce waiting lists, as well as to reduce costs.

About 15–20 per cent of total revenues in Catalan hospitals are related to the DRG-based CMI (relative resource intensity, RRI), which means that incentives to use DRGs are only moderate or weak. A much larger share of hospital revenues is determined by the hospitals' structural characteristics – namely its equipment, size, and so on – which influence payments not only for inpatient care but also for outpatient care and emergency care.

Non-surgical day cases are financed through fee-for-service prices, adjusted at the hospital level. Outpatient consultations are paid by means of a flat fee per visit, which is supposed to cover all possible following visits, and differs according to the structural characteristics of the hospital. Emergency care is financed by a fixed price that is adjusted according to the structural characteristics of the hospital.

Hospitals receive additional funding for teaching and research. Furthermore, certain specific techniques are paid for on a fee-for-service basis (such as radiotherapy sessions), while others are financed through specific budget allocations (such as breast cancer screening programmes). Furthermore, a specific fund exists that finances surgical activity related to waiting list reduction and a programme to cope with emergency pressure in the winter. There are also additional payments for high-complexity treatments and diagnostic tests, such as radiotherapy, neuroradiology, catheterization and dialysis.

22.5.2 Calculation of DRG prices/cost weights

Spain

As already mentioned, Spanish national tariffs are calculated by adapting American AP-DRG cost weights on the basis of cost information from 30 Spanish hospitals. To elaborate these datasets and relative hospital-level costs, first a top-down cost allocation is realized in order to estimate costs of 11 'partial cost centres' (Operating Room, Radiology, Laboratory, Pharmacy, Medical Services, Intensive Care, Other Hospitalization Costs, Other Intermediate Hospitalization Costs, Medical Staff, Functional Costs, and Overheads).

Hospital cost-accounting systems perform a top-down process using a limited amount of clinical data. Once the top-down distribution to the 11 partial cost centres is completed, American DRG weights are used to value the cost of each patient and calculate an average cost per DRG (Falguera Martínez-Alarcón, 2001). The main weakness of this system is that it calculates an estimated, rather than real, cost per patient (Table 22.5).

Table 22.5 Evaluation of unit cost using internal DRG weights

	CC_1	$\ldots CC_i$	$\ldots CC_{11}$
DRG_1	$N_1 * W_{1\text{-}1}$	$N_1 * W_{i\text{-}1}$	$N_1 * W_{11\text{-}1}$
...			
DRG_j	$N_j * W_{1\text{-}j}$	$N_j * W_{i\text{-}j}$	$N_j * W_{11\text{-}j}$
...			
DRG_{886}	$N_{886} * W_{1\text{-}886}$	$N_{886} * W_{i\text{-}886}$	$N_{886} * W_{11\text{-}886}$
Total weighted activity	$\mathbf{TW_1=\Sigma(N_j * W_{i=j})}$	$\mathbf{TW_i=\Sigma(N_j * W_{1\text{-}j})}$	$\mathbf{TW_{11}=\Sigma(N_j * W_{11\text{-}j})}$ $\mathbf{UC_{11}= TCOST_{11}/}$
Unit cost 1 to 11	$\mathbf{UC_1 = TCOST_1 / TW_1}$	$\mathbf{UC_i = TCOST_i / TW_i}$	$\mathbf{TW_{11}}$
Cost per DRG$_j$	$\mathbf{CDRG_j= \Sigma(UC_i * W_{i\text{-}j})}$		

$\mathbf{CC_i}$ is a partial cost centre

$\mathbf{W_{i\text{-}j}}$ is the internal (partial) DRG weight for DRG_j and the partial cost centre CC_i

$\mathbf{N_j}$ is the total number of patients classified into DRG_j

$\mathbf{TCOST_i}$ is the total cost for the partial cost centre CC_i

$\mathbf{UC_i}$ is the unit cost for the internal (partial) cost weight W_i

$\mathbf{CDRG_j}$ is the cost in Euros for DRG_j

The imputation is realized for each discharge (by its length of stay) and for each 'partial cost centre'. The weights are based on information about costs for these partial cost centres from a large number of American datasets, which are supposed to be statistically representative (Spanish Ministry of Health and Consumption, 2008).

By multiplying the number of cases (N_j) in each DRG (DRG_j) with an internal AP-DRG cost weight ($W_{i\text{-}j}$), the total weighted activity is calculated for each partial cost centre. Subsequently, the total costs of each partial cost centre (W_i) (derived from the top-down cost allocation) are divided by its total weighted activity to calculate a partial unit cost and then assigned to each discharge, for which a total cost can be calculated. Consequently, average costs for each AP-DRG can be calculated, which are used for setting national AP-DRG tariffs.

Catalonia

In Catalonia, the original CMS-DRG cost weights are used. However, in the process of determining hospital budgets, CMS-DRG cost weights are used only as an indicator of the RRI of cases within one hospital compared to the RRI of cases in the entire XHUP.

22.5.3 DRGs in actual hospital payment

Spain

The process before payment from the Cohesion Fund takes place can be described as consisting of several steps: (1) authorization must be obtained from the AC in which the patient is living; (2) the patient is transferred to another AC for treatment; (3) after treatment has been completed, the hospital is paid on the basis of the normal system of payment applicable in the hospital's own AC; (4) the Cohesion Fund compensates the AC in which the patient was treated for the provided services.

In order to determine payment to a specific AC, the MBDS of all non-resident patients treated in the AC are submitted to the Cohesion Fund at the end of the year. The Cohesion Fund groups the patient information from the CMBD into AP-DRGs, and pays hospitals on the basis of the national tariff, which is the same for all ACs.

Catalonia

The current Catalan hospital payment system relies on two types of information in order to determine global hospital budgets: (1) the RRI of cases treated by the hospital (measured through CMS-DRGs), and (2) each hospital's structural characteristics. Based on these two types of information, hospitals are paid for the number of discharges contracted by the CHS.

Figure 22.2 shows how the RRI of cases treated by a hospital is accounted for in the payment system: first, the CMI is calculated for each hospital by dividing the sum of all CMS-DRG cost weights of all patients treated by the hospital in

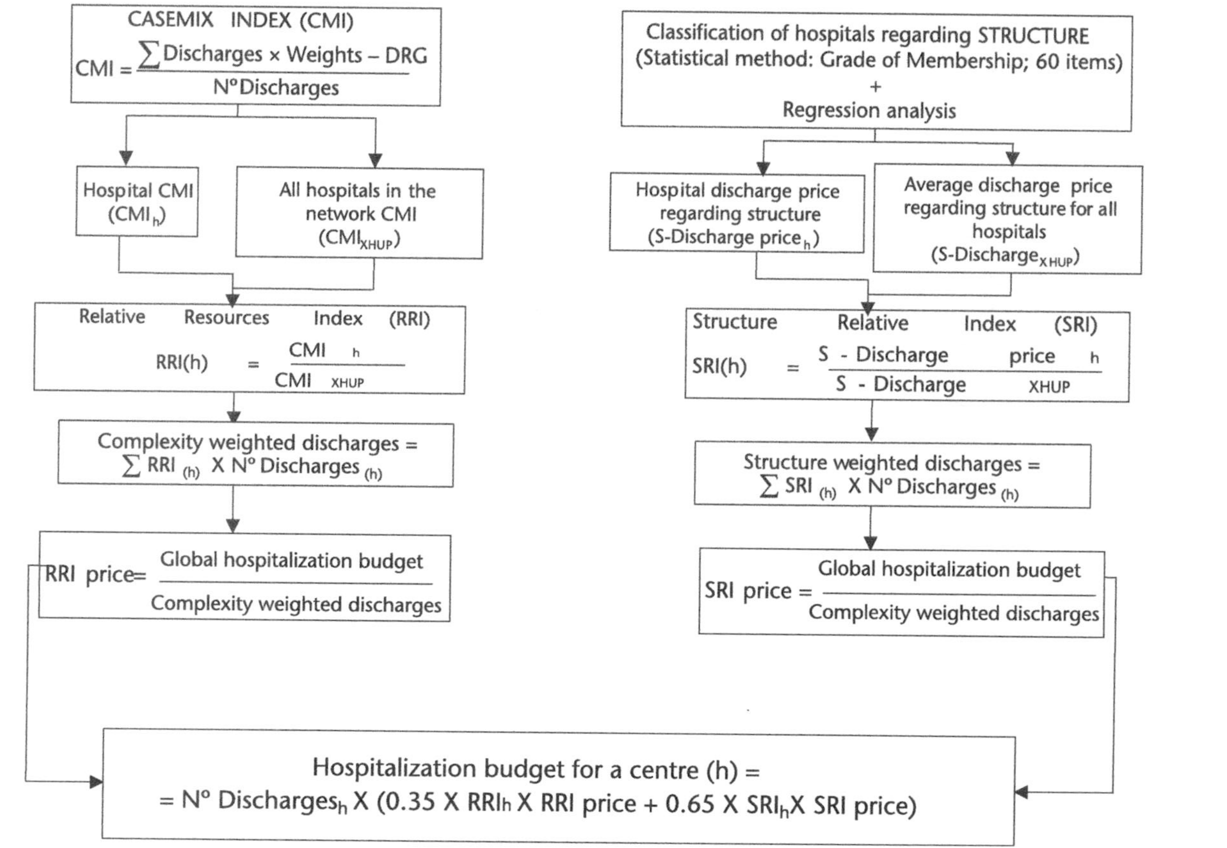

Figure 22.2 The hospital payment system in Catalonia

Source: Adapted from Sánchez-Martínez et al., 2006.

the previous year by the number of total patients treated. Accordingly, the CMI of the entire XHUP is calculated (Sánchez-Martínez et al., 2006). Second, each hospital's CMI is divided by the casemix of the XHUP in order to determine the RRI of patients treated in each hospital. Third, the complexity of all discharges within the XHUP is determined by summing the product of the RRI of each hospital (RRI_h), multiplied by the number of discharges in the hospital. Finally, the price per RRI (RRI price) is calculated by dividing the predetermined global hospitalization budget by the sum of complexity-weighted discharges of the XHUP.

In order to account for the structural characteristics of each hospital, a structural relative index (SRI) is calculated by the CHS for each hospital every four years. First, different structural groups are defined (for example, university hospitals, specialized hospitals), and structural weights are assigned to each group. Then, each hospital is classified into one or more of these structural groups, and its Grade of Membership to the group is determined through regression analysis. Finally, the SRI is computed for each hospital by applying the Grade of Membership proportions to the mean structural weight of each group.

In order to calculate DRG-based hospital budgets, the RRI and the SRI are multiplied by the RRI price and the SRI price, which are established by the CHS and updated every year. Hospital budgets for the year 2010 were determined on the basis of hospital activity data for the period from July 2008 to June 2009.

When CMS DRGs were introduced in 1997, the CHS planned to gradually reduce the weight of the SRI and to increase the weight of the RRI. However, the weight of the RRI has been increased only once (in the year 2000), from 30 per cent to 35 per cent. Consequently, the hospital structure (the SRI) still determines 65 per cent of hospital payment. Apparently, the current weight attached to the RRI is not significant enough to motivate hospitals to attract more complex patients, as the complexity of patients (measured through CMS-DRGs) is responsible for only 35 per cent of hospital payment. Figure 22.3 shows the distribution of RRI values for each hospital within the network of public hospitals in Catalonia.

22.5.4 Quality-related adjustments

There are no quality-related adjustments to hospital payments on the basis of DRGs. In general, it is assumed that certain structural characteristics of hospitals – such as teaching status – imply higher quality and higher costs. However, these costs are not reflected in the DRG weight but are accounted for in the structural payment components of the Catalan hospital financing system.

22.5.5 Main incentives for hospitals

Since hospital payment is only partly based on DRGs, hospitals have only moderate incentives to up-code their patients (especially to increase the number and severity of secondary diagnoses).

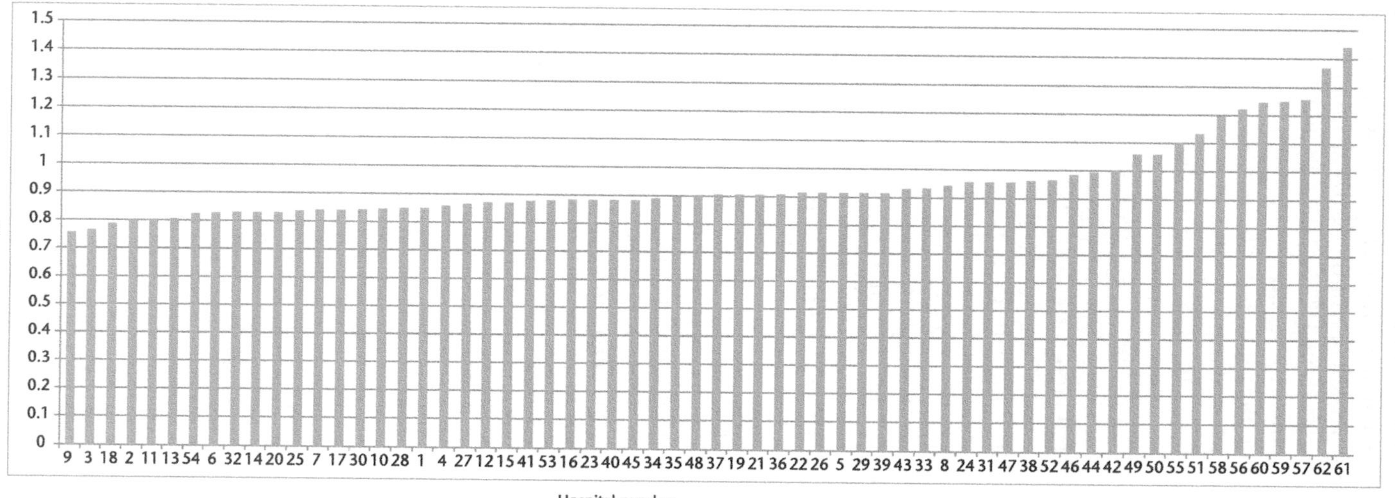

Figure 22.3 Relative resource intensity values for Catalan hospitals, 2009

Source: Secretaria Tècnica UCH, 2009.

'Present on admission' flags are not used in the Spanish coding system, and the DRG system is unable to discriminate between secondary diagnoses representing genuine co-morbidities and secondary diagnoses, reflecting complications as a result of medical errors or negligence. However, it remains unclear whether this inability to discriminate between different types of secondary diagnoses has a negative effect on treatment quality. The fact that hospitals have received the same payment for surgical procedures performed in an ambulatory setting (MAS) as for those surgical patients treated as inpatients has been a strong incentive to substitute inpatient surgery with MAS.

22.6 New/innovative technologies

Providers (for example, teaching hospitals) are entitled to make use of any health technology on the market. However, in order to receive additional payments for a specific new technology that is more costly than an existing one, hospitals need to apply to the CHS for funding. Unfortunately, there is not a clearly specified process of steps required in order for hospitals to receive additional payment. Applications by hospitals proposing the introduction of a specific technology can be either accepted by the CHS or rejected, depending on the available evidence on effectiveness and costs of the new technology.

The costs of initial applications of new technologies are usually borne by providers (such as teaching hospitals) and 'the industry' in general (namely, pharmaceutical companies or medical device manufacturers). Eventually, the technology is either included in the general benefits basket and paid for as with any other activity, or it is added to a list of certain approved innovative services to be financed from a specific fund for certain techniques and specific procedures (Brosa & Agusti, 2009).

Treatments and procedures that are financed through additional (fee-for-service) payments are generally delivered in day-care settings, and include high-complexity treatments and diagnostic tests, such as radiotherapy, stereotactic radiosurgery and neuroradiology, cardiac or hepatic catheterism, as well as highly technical care procedures such as those in urology departments and care of patients with renal failure.

In general, as hospital payment is only partially based on DRGs, the DRG-based incentives and disincentives relating to introducing new technologies (see Chapter 9) are thought to be of only moderate strength in Catalonia.

22.7 Evaluation of DRG systems in Spain

22.7.1 Official evaluations

Spain

The Spanish Ministry of Health oversees the development of AP-DRGs and, recently, has also been pilot testing International Refined (IR)-DRGs. The Ministry publishes data and information about casemix and costs based on AP-DRGs (Spanish Ministry of Health and Consumption, 2008).

Recently, the potential to change to the IR-DRG system has been discussed, as this would provide the opportunity to include in one DRG-based system also non-surgical outpatient activity and emergency care.

Catalonia

The CHS has used HCFA- and later CMS-DRGs since the first introduction of DRGs in Catalonia in 1997. It did not make the change to the AP-DRG system used in the rest of the country because the change would have brought about significant changes in the distribution of resources among hospitals.

22.7.2 Authors' assessment of successes and problems

Spain

Spain has adopted a foreign DRG system based on the notion that it was too small to develop its own system. Several articles have been published by the authors of this chapter criticizing the adoption of a foreign DRG system. However, given the difficulty of developing and updating a national DRG system, and given the increasing interest in cross-border comparisons of hospital performance, the adoption of a foreign system does not seem to be such a bad choice.

If Spanish authorities seek to adopt a DRG system that explicitly considers outpatient care, Spain can migrate to the IR-DRG system without any significant cost. Currently, a project is under way, which aims to estimate national Spanish cost weights for IR-DRGs, using detailed patient-level cost data from a sample of hospitals following a common bottom-up cost-accounting methodology. Therefore, once these national cost weights are available, a change to IR-DRGs would also have the advantage that IR-DRGs would better reflect Spanish practice patterns.

Yet, any DRG system has the limitation that it only partially reflects the entire patient health care process. DRGs are always related to only one hospital stay and ignore care provided prior to admission or after discharge.

Catalonia

Almost 85 per cent of hospital financing remains related to structural indicators (SRI or prices for medical day cases, outpatient visits and emergencies based on structural levels) (Brosa & Agusti, 2009). Only 15–20 per cent of hospital revenues are related to the DRG-based RRI index. Consequently, the Catalan system of adjusting hospital payment on the basis of DRGs carries only moderate incentives, whether these are intended (to increase efficiency) or unintended (to engage in up-coding). Since hospital revenues are mostly determined by their SRI, hospitals are more likely to focus on introducing new and advanced technologies in order to increase their SRI, rather than focusing on improving performance as measured by DRGs.

The importance of structural financing components can be partly explained by the fact that outliers are not accounted for in the Catalan hospital financing system. Teaching hospitals tend to have a higher rate of outliers (Cots et al., 2003). Increasing the share of DRG-based payment in total hospital revenues would mean that hospitals would not receive adequate payments if they have a high rate of outliers. If the CHS wanted to increase the importance of DRG-based financing, it would need to find a way of paying hospitals for treating outliers. Until then, the SRI ensures that those hospitals that are likely to treat a large share of outlier patients (for example, teaching hospitals) receive sufficient funding to cover their associated costs.

22.8 Outlook: Future developments and reform

The most significant trend in health care delivery in Spain (including Catalonia) is the increasing importance of outpatient care in hospital activity. Consequently, there is a need for the health care system to develop and use management tools that better fit with the new patterns of service delivery. In this context, adoption of the IR-DRG system would be a step forward. IR-DRGs have been specifically developed to better integrate outpatient activity with inpatient activity. Unfortunately, the benefits of the process of moving towards IR-DRGs at the national level are not being sufficiently promoted in Spain.

Furthermore, there is an increasing awareness of the need to coordinate hospital-level care with primary care and long-term care. Consequently, there has been a lot of interest in per capita grouping algorithms, such as Adjusted Clinical Groups (Sicras-Mainar & Navarro-Artieda, 2009) or Clinical Risk Groups (Inoriza et al., 2009). Currently, the CHS is focusing on a project for the development of per capita grouping mechanisms (Brosa & Agusti, 2009).

Until now, sufficiently detailed information about treatment costs in Spanish hospitals – to inform decisions relating to DRG system development – has remained unavailable. Ten Spanish hospitals have now built a cost database[1] for per-patient cost information, which has been used to provide information for the EuroDRG project. The intention is to regularly update the database with new cost information, with consistent input from a greater number of participating hospitals, and to make it accessible for use by other hospitals, researchers and benchmarking projects.

In the Spanish context, which includes the specific case of Catalonia, there is marked stagnation in the development of patient classification systems. The current hospital financing system does not require refined per-patient cost information. The division of regulating, financing, purchasing and supplying functions of the health care system has not been consolidated, even though this separation was clearly specified in national legislation. DRGs are and will probably continue to be used as tools to generate quality indicators (efficiency and effectiveness), but they also continue to have a minor impact on the management of the health care system and its transformation.

The inability to make changes is a significant aspect of this stagnation. Although the 17 Spanish ACs could independently introduce changes in patient classification systems, the overall health system requires homogeneity in its health care model. An active process of improvement is hampered by the duplication of responsibilities among the different levels of government, namely the

ACs and central Government. A joint national and regional effort would be required in order to progress to a better DRG system and to use it more consistently for hospital payment.

22.9 Note

1 See the *Red Española de Costes Hospitalarios* (Spanish Network of Hospital Costs) web site (www.rechosp.org, accessed 10 July 2011).

22.10 References

Brosa, F., Agusti, E. (2009). *Public Health Care Payment Systems in Catalonia, 1981–2009 (Historical Evolution and Future Perspectives).* Barcelona: Servei Català de la Salut, Generalitat de Catalunya Departament de Salut (http://www10.gencat.net/catsalut/archivos/publicacions/planif_sanit/sistemes_pagament_angles.pdf, accessed 10 July 2011).

CatSalut (1992). *La Central de Balanços del Servei Català de la Salut [Central Institute of Financial Statements of the Catalan Health Service].* Barcelona: Servei Català de la Salut, Departament de Sanitat i Seguretat Social (http://www10.gencat.cat/catsalut/archivos/central_balancos/informe_3_cat.pdf, accessed 10 July 2011).

CatSalut (2007). *Activitat asistencial de la xarxa sanitària de Catalunya. Any 2007 [Health Care Activity of the Catalan Health Network].* Barcelona: Servei Català de la Salut, Generalitat de Catalunya Departament de Salut (http://www10.gencat.cat/catsalut/archivos/cmbd/cmbd_07.pdf, accessed 27 July 2011).

CatSalut (2010). *La Salut com a sector econòmic de Catalunya [Health Care as an Economic Sector of Catalonia. Catalan Health Service].* Barcelona: Servei Català de la Salut, Generalitat de Catalunya Departament de Salut (http://www10.gencat.cat/catsalut/archivos/publicacions/econo_sanitaria/informes/informe_10_cat.pdf, accessed 10 July 2011).

Cots, F., Castells, X. (2001). Cómo pagamos a nuestros hospitales. La referencia de Cataluña y el contrapunto desde Andalucía [How we pay our hospitals. The point of reference of Catalonia and the counterpoint from Anadalusia]. *Gaceta Sanitaria*, 15(2):172–81.

Cots, F., Elvira, D., Castells, X., Dalmau, E. (2000). Medicare's DRG-weights in a European environment: the Spanish experience. *Health Policy*, 51:31–47.

Cots, F., Elvira, D., Castells, X., Saez, M. (2003). Relevance of outlier cases in casemix systems and evaluation of trimming methods. *Health Care Management Science*, 6(1):27–35.

Durán, A., Lara, J.L., van Waveren, M. (2006). Spain: health system review. *Health Systems in Transition*, 8(4):1–208 (http://www.euro.who.int/__data/assets/pdf_file/0005/96386/E89491.pdf, accessed 10 July 2011).

EESRI (Servei d'Informació i Estudis) (2007). *Informació estadística de l'assistència Hospitalària. Catalunya 2007* [*Statistical Information on Hospital Care. Catalonia 2007*]. Barcelona: Generalitat de Catalunya Departament de Salut (http://www.gencat.cat/salut/depsalut/html/ca/xifres/eesri07.pdf, accessed 10 July 2011).

European Commission (2011). *Eurostat: Database on Health Care Expenditure* (February update). Luxembourg: European Commission (http://epp.eurostat.ec.europa.eu/portal/page/portal/statistics/search_database, accessed 27 July 2011).

Falguera Martínez-Alarcón, J. (2001). *La contabilidad de gestión en los centros sanitarios* [*Management Accounting in Health Care Centres*] (Thesis). Barcelona: Universitat Pompeu Fabra.

González Pérez, J.G. (2008). *Informe SEIS: La gestión de los medicamentos en los Servicios de Salud. Sistemas de gestión de costes, beneficios y oportunidades de desarrollo con las TIC [Informe SEIS: Drug Management in Health Care Services: Cost-Accounting Systems. Advantages and Development Opportunities with ICT Tools]*. Madrid: Sociedad Española de Informática de la Salud.

Health Information Institute (2010). *National Health System Spain 2010*. Madrid: Ministry of Health and Social Policy, Health Information Institute (http://www.msps.es/organizacion/sns/docs/sns2010/Main.pdf, accessed 10 July 2011).

HOPE (2006). *DRGs as a Financing Tool*. Brussels: European Hospital and Healthcare Federation (http://www.hope.be/05eventsandpublications/docpublications/77_drg_report/77_drg_report_2006.pdf, accessed 10 July 2011).

IASIST (2008). *Top 20. What is it?* Barcelona: IASIST S.A, UBM Medica (http://www.iasist.com/en/top--20, accessed 10 July 2011).

Ibern, P. (1991). The development of cost information by DRG – experience in a Barcelona hospital. *Health Policy*, 17:179–94.

Inoriza, J.M., Coderch, J., Carreras, M. et al. (2009). Measuring the severity and resource utilization of hospitalized and ambulatory patients. *Gaceta Sanitaria*, 23(1):29–37.

INSALUD (2001a). *Gestión clínico-financiera y coste por proceso [Clinical-Financial Management and Cost Per Process]*. Madrid: Instituto Nacional de la Salud.

INSALUD (2001b). *Resultados de la Gestión Analítica en los hospitales del INSALUD [Results of Analytical Accounting Management in INSALUD Hospitals]*. Madrid: Instituto Nacional de la Salud.

López Casasnovas, G. (2008). *El paper de l'assegurament sanitari i de la medicina privada en els sistemes públics de salut. Reflexions per a l'elaboració d'una política sanitària nacional [The Role of Health Insurance and Private Medicine in Public Health Systems. Considerations for National Health Policy-Making]*. Barcelona: Universitat Pompeu Fabra Centre de Recerca en Economia i Salut.

Monge, P. (2003a). Estudio comparativo de los diferentes sistemas o modelos de costes implantados en los hospitales públicos españoles [Comparative study of different cost-accounting systems implemented in Spanish public hospitals]. *Revista Iberoamericana de Contabilidad de Gestión*, 2:13–42.

Monge, P. (2003b). Ventajas e inconvenientes de los diversos sistemas de costes implantados en los hospitales españoles [Advantages and disadvantages of the different cost-accounting systems implemented in Spanish public hospitals]. *Boletín Económico de Información Comercial Española*, 2764:17–25.

Sánchez-Martínez, F., Abellán-Perpiñán, J.M., Martínez-Pérez, J.E., Puig-Junoy, J. (2006). Cost accounting and public reimbursement schemes in Spanish hospitals. *Health Care Management Science*, 9:225–32.

Secretaria Tècnica UCH (2009). *Anàlisi de l'evolució del preu alta i dels valors IRR i IRE període 1999–2009 en el conjunt de centres de la XHUP [Analysis of the Evolution of SRI and RRI Prices and SRI and RRI Values for the Hospitals of the Public Hospitals Network of Catalonia]*. Barcelona: Unió Catalana d'Hospitals.

Sicras-Mainar, A., Navarro-Artieda, R. (2009). Validating the adjusted clinical groups [ACG] casemix system in a Spanish population setting: a multicenter study. *Gaceta Sanitaria*, 23(3):228–31.

Spanish Ministry of Health and Consumption (2008). *Análisis y desarrollo de los GDR en el Sistema Nacional de Salud [Analysis and Development of DRGs in the National Health System]*. Madrid: Spanish Ministry of Health and Consumption (http://www.msc.es/en/estadEstudios/estadisticas/inforRecopilaciones/anaDesarrolloGDR.htm, accessed 10 July 2011).

chapter twenty three

The Netherlands: The Diagnose Behandeling Combinaties

Siok Swan Tan, Martin van Ineveld, Ken Redekop and Leona Hakkaart-van Roijen

23.1 Hospital services and the role of Diagnose Behandeling Combinaties in the Netherlands

23.1.1 The Dutch health care system

The Dutch health care system is mostly health insurance based and is divided into three compartments (Stolk & Rutten, 2005; Schäfer et al., 2010; Enthoven & van de Ven, 2007). The first compartment consists of a compulsory social health insurance scheme, which provides continuous long-term care for those with chronic conditions and short-term home nursing care for acute conditions. This social health insurance scheme is regulated in the Exceptional Medical Expenses Act (*Algemene Wet Bijzondere Ziektekosten*, AWBZ). The AWBZ is mainly financed through income-dependent contributions. Care is provided after needs assessment has taken place, and is subject to a complicated system of cost-sharing.

The second compartment consists of a social health insurance scheme covering the whole population for 'basic health insurance'. Since January 2006, previously existing public sickness funds and private health insurance schemes have been integrated into one compulsory scheme, which is regulated by the Health Insurance Act (*Zorgverzekeringswet*, ZVW) (Schut & Hassink, 2002). Health insurers must offer a standard benefits package including most curative medical care (general practitioners (GPs), medical specialists, short-term hospital care). All Dutch citizens contribute to this scheme in two ways. First, they pay a flat-rate premium directly to the health insurer of their choice. Second, an income-dependent employer contribution is deducted through their payroll and transferred to the Health Insurance Fund. The resources from this Fund are then allocated among the health insurers according to a risk-adjustment system. A 'health care allowance' should partly compensate lower-income individuals for their health insurance costs.

The third compartment consists of complementary voluntary health insurance (VHI), which may cover health services that are not covered under the AWBZ and the ZVW. Prevention and social support are not part of the compulsory social health insurance or VHI, but are mainly financed through general taxation.

Three independent institutions under the Ministry of Health, Welfare and Sport (*Volksgezondheid, Welzijn en Sport*, VWS) are central actors in terms of supervision and regulation of the Dutch health care system. The first is the Healthcare Inspectorate (*Inspectie voor de Gezondheidszorg*; IGZ), which monitors and controls the quality of health care services, prevention measures and medical products. The second is the Dutch Healthcare Authority (*Nederlandse Zorg autoriteit*; NZa), which determines the financial framework, budgets and tariffs, as well as advising the VWS on setting the conditions for regulated competition. The third institution is the Healthcare Insurance Board (*College Voor Zorgverzekeringen*; CVZ), which advises the VWS on benefits package issues and monitors compliance with the AWBZ and the ZVW.

In 2005, total health care expenditure amounted to about €68 billion, which is equal to about 12 per cent of the country's gross domestic product (GDP). The Dutch health care system is predominantly financed by the AWBZ (about 27 per cent) and the ZVW (41 per cent). Only 4 per cent is financed by VHI. Other sources of financing include out-of-pocket expenses (10 per cent), the VWS (13 per cent) and health care-related profit-making and non-profit-making organizations (5 per cent).

In general, the Dutch health care delivery system is divided into 11 sectors. The hospital sector is the most significant sector in terms of expenditure (26 per cent in 2005). Other important sectors include elderly care institutions (19 per cent), social service institutions (12 per cent) and suppliers of pharmaceuticals and medical aids (12 per cent). The 'other health care providers' sector (3.4 per cent) comprises, amongst others, Independent Treatment Centres (*Zelfstandige Behandel Centra*; ZBCs) and private clinics (Poos et al., 2008).

23.1.2 Hospital services in the Netherlands

Inpatient care and day care are only provided by hospitals. In 2009, there were 8 university hospitals, 85 general hospitals, 32 specialized hospitals and 23 rehabilitation centres in the Netherlands. The specialized hospitals comprised 1 abortion clinic, 4 audiology centres, 3 dialysis centres, 2 epilepsy centres, 10 integral cancer centres, 4 radiotherapy centres, 3 asthma centres and 5 other specialized hospitals. All hospitals work on a non-profit basis but may provide services excluded from the standard benefits package, which are reimbursed by VHI.

Table 23.1 presents some key figures for university and general hospitals in 2009 (Kiwa Prismant, 2010). The number of inpatient days in 2009 amounted

Table 23.1 Key figures for university and general hospitals in 2009

	University hospitals	*General hospitals*
Number of hospitals	8	85
< 200 beds	0	9
200–300 beds	0	15
300–400 beds	0	22
400–600 beds	0	18
> 600 beds	8	21
Inpatient admissions * 1000	235	1 653
Inpatient days * 1000	1 709	9 125
Inpatient stay duration	7.3	5.5
Day-care admissions * 1000	226	1 627
Outpatient visits * 1000	3 142	24 257

Source: Kiwa Prismant, 2010.

to 1 709 000 at university hospitals and 9 125 000 at general hospitals, with average length of stay (ALOS) durations of 7.3 and 5.5 days, respectively. The number of hospital admissions increased while the ALOS has decreased in recent years. This is largely due to an increase in the number of day-care admissions (38 per cent between 2005 and 2009). The number of first outpatient visits increased by 10 per cent between 2005 and 2009.

Although day care and outpatient visits were traditionally only provided by hospitals, competition between health care providers is now encouraged by allowing ZBCs free access to the hospital care market. Figure 23.1 depicts the role of hospitals and ZBCs in the delivery of hospital services. Whereas hospitals

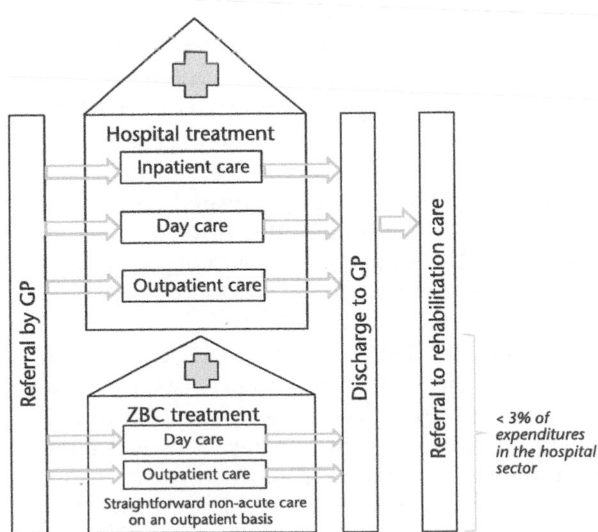

Figure 23.1 Role of hospitals and ZBCs in the delivery of hospital services

provide the whole spectrum of day care and outpatient care, ZBCs usually only provide straightforward non-acute day care and outpatient care, which requires cooperation between at least two medical specialists working on a non-profit-making basis. ZBCs deliver care included in the basic health insurance (ZVW), but also engage in services covered by VHI. In order to remain competitive over the years, many hospitals have established ZBCs. These treatment centres only account for less than 3 per cent of expenditure in the hospital sector, but the number of ZBCs has rapidly increased from 79 in 2005 to 195 in 2009 (Kiwa Prismant, 2010). Private clinics provide private medical specialist care, which is not covered by the social health insurance scheme. They are not included in the scope of this chapter.

Structural reforms of the health care sector in recent years have entailed substantial changes in the financing and budgeting of health care providers. Hospitals in the Netherlands are independent and are contracted by health insurers through either collective or selective contracts. Before 2005, budgeting and financing systems were mainly targeted towards controlling health care expenditure. Incentives to increase production or to produce health services more efficiently were mainly absent (Oostenbrink & Rutten, 2006). In order to provide stronger incentives for efficiency and quality, a new system for the payment of hospitals and ZBCs was introduced in February 2005. The new system relies on a self-developed system of diagnosis–treatment combinations (*Diagnose Behandeling Combinaties*; DBCs) as the basis of payment for care provided by medical specialists and hospitals.

23.1.3 Purpose of the DBC system

The main purpose of the introduction of the DBC system was to reform hospital payment to facilitate negotiations (in particular on quality) between purchasers and providers by defining the products of hospitals (that is, DBCs) (van Ineveld et al., 2006; van de Ven & Schut, 2009). DBCs were believed to provide a concise definition of hospital products as the basis for selective contracts. However, only a small selection of DBCs (list B DBCs) were freely negotiable when the new system was introduced. For the majority of DBCs (list A DBCs), hospitals received a fixed amount per treated case within the framework of a collective contract. In the future, the Government aims to gradually increase the share of list B DBCs to about 70 per cent, as it wishes to increase the share of hospital services for which hospitals and providers can negotiate regarding quality.

Since the introduction of DBCs in the Netherlands, benchmarking has become increasingly important. Average resource-use profiles are calculated for list A DBCs on the basis of resource-use and cost-accounting data collected in Dutch hospitals. These resource-use profiles have become an important external benchmark for individual hospitals. In addition, other benchmarking tools have been developed; for example, the Association of Dutch Health Insurers annually publishes a guide containing hospital performance indicators relating to list B DBCs, to support its members.

23.2 Developing and updating the DBC system

23.2.1 The DBC system at a glance

There is only one national DBC system in the Netherlands, which is centrally regulated and monitored by 'DBC onderhoud' (DBC-O), a governmental institution specifically set up for that task. The system is used to enable DRG-type payment of all hospitals and ZBCs in the country, including payment of psychiatric care services since 2008 and rehabilitation care at hospitals and rehabilitation centres since 2009.

In contrast to DRGs in other countries, most DBCs stretch from the first contact with a medical specialist to treatment completion (Steinbusch et al., 2007). These DBCs, referred to as *'regular care'* DBCs, could include one or more inpatient admissions in addition to several outpatient visits and post-discharge follow-up care during the same year.

Next to *'regular care'* DBCs, two other important types of DBC exist (Figure 23.2). The first type, referred to as *'continuation of regular care'* DBCs, is opened to replace a *'regular care'* DBC when treatment exceeds 365 days. The second type, referred to as *'inpatient without days'* DBCs, is opened in addition to a *'regular care'* DBC when a patient requires treatment which is medically not related to the *'regular care'* DBC for which they are initially admitted. For example, a patient admitted for chronic non-specific lung disease could require an appendectomy. In this case, a *'regular care'* DBC is opened for lung disease and an *'inpatient without days'* DBC for appendectomy. *'Inpatient without days'* DBCs narrowly define specific hospital stays similar to those defined by other DRG systems.

DBCs belong to one of two lists: currently, about 67 per cent of DBCs belong to list A and 33 per cent to list B. List B DBCs are supposed to comprise high-incidence cases with sufficiently homogeneous resource-consumption patterns, such as hip and knee replacement, diabetes mellitus, cataract and inguinal hernia repair. Hospital payment is different for list A DBCs and list B DBCs (see subsection 23.5.2).

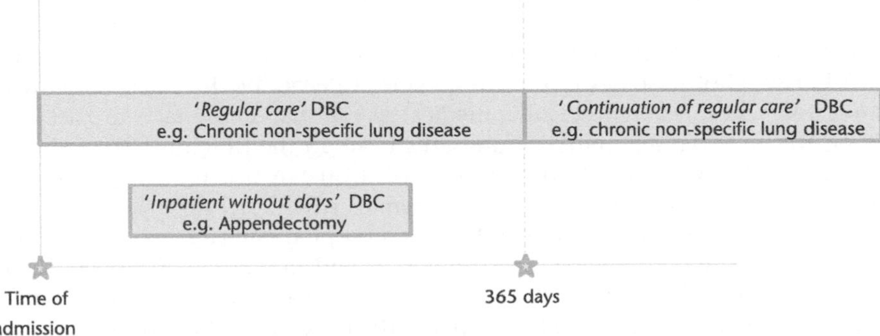

Figure 23.2 Fictional overview of types of DBCs

Table 23.2 Traditional DRGs versus DBCs

Difference	*Typical DRG systems*	*DBC system until 2010*
Defined hospital product	One hospital admission or outpatient contact	One diagnosis–treatment combination (may include several hospital admissions or outpatient contacts)
Number of DRGs/DBCs per patient	One per patient (but exceptions exist)	Several per patient
Level of detail/precision of the system	Aggregated system < 3000 DRGs	Detailed system > 30 000 DBCs
Selection of DRG/DBC	Assigned by computerized grouping algorithm after hospital discharge	Medical specialist opens DBC upon first diagnosis

Table 23.2 presents some of the main differences between typical DRG systems and the DBC system. While DRG systems generally define different types of hospital admissions or outpatient contacts, the DBC system defines different types of diagnosis–treatment combinations. Consequently, all hospital services related to this diagnosis–treatment combination during one year are included in only one DBC. While DRG systems typically assign one DRG per patient according to the most important diagnosis or procedure, the DBC system uses several DBCs per patient if several diagnoses require treatment. As opposed to DRG-based systems, which often consist of between 600 and 2000 DRGs, the DBC system currently comprises about 30 000 DBCs.

In addition, the current DBC system does not entail a computerized grouping algorithm. The medical specialist decides which DBC is applicable and manually opens this DBC upon first diagnosis. It is possible to change the DBC registration during the treatment process. However, a new generation of DBCs is forthcoming in which some aspects of traditional DRG systems are covered (see subsection 23.8).

23.2.2 Development of the DBC system

In the late 1990s, a simplified version of the All Patient (AP)-DRG system was tested at six pilot hospitals in the Netherlands to examine the extent to which the system was able to reflect Dutch medical specialist and hospital care patterns. Given the growing importance of outpatient care in the Dutch health care system, the inability of the AP-DRG system to adequately account for outpatient cases was seen as a major deficit of the system. Furthermore, since patients were grouped by administrative staff members after hospital discharge, rather than by medical specialists, interpretational differences and mistakes were perceived to be problematic (Custers et al., 2007; Zuurbier & Krabbe-Alkemade, 2007). Therefore, health insurers and hospitals initiated the development of DBCs. Medical specialists' associations defined DBCs for each medical specialty. A representative sample of 23 'frontrunner' hospitals registered detailed resource-use and cost data for all inpatient and outpatient hospital services according to the DBC system.

DBC tariffs comprise two separate components (Beersen et al., 2005; Zuurbier & Krabbe-Alkemade, 2007): (1) the *honorarium component* for the payment of specialists; and (2) the *hospital cost component* for the payment of all relevant hospital services. For the calculation of the honorarium component, the 'norm-time' was determined for each DBC. The 'norm-time' is supposed to reflect the time requirements of medical specialists to perform all relevant tasks related to a DBC. The time was estimated from hospitals' administrative databases and validated by expert opinion. The 'norm-time' was then multiplied with a fixed fee per hour of €135.50 to calculate the honorarium component (Folpmers & de Bruijn, 2004). With respect to list A DBCs, the hospital cost component was determined based on the resource-use and cost data of the hospital services at the 23 'frontrunner' hospitals; average resource-use profiles were multiplied with national unit costs (see subsection 23.4.2). Hospital services were categorized into 15 resource-use categories, as presented in Table 23.3. National unit costs for these hospital services included wages, equipment, overheads and – since 2009 – capital costs (see subsection 23.4.2). With respect to list B DBCs, the hospital cost component results from negotiations between health insurers and hospitals (see subsection 23.5.2).

Since February 2005, the DBC system has been continuously updated through revisions and additions that are implemented without the definition of new versions of the system. Table 23.4 shows some main facts relating to the DBC system upon first introduction (2005) and the current version (2010). At the introduction of the DBC system, each diagnosis and treatment combination was appointed one DBC for the first outpatient visit only, and one DBC for all related hospital services with the exception of the first outpatient visit. The number of DBCs amounted to about 100 000, of which about 90 per cent were list A DBCs. List A DBC tariffs excluded capital costs.

In the current version of the DBC system, the classification of patients has been simplified. The number of DBCs has been substantially reduced from about 100 000 to 30 000, of which about 67 per cent relate to list A DBCs. Each

Table 23.3 Hospital services resource-use categories

Inpatient days
Intensive care days
Day-care hours
Outpatient and emergency room visits
Laboratory services
Medical imaging services
Medical devices
Surgical procedures
Diagnostic activities
Microbiological and parasitological services
Pathological services
Blood products
Paramedical and supportive services
Rehabilitation services
Other services

Source: DBC-O, 2011.

Table 23.4 The main facts relating to the DBC versions, at its introduction (2005) and the current version

	1st DBC version	*Present DBC version*
Date of introduction	2005	2010
(Main) Purpose	Hospital payment	Hospital payment, benchmarking
Source	Self-developed	Self-developed
Data used for development	Resource use and unit costs of 23 'frontrunner' hospitals	Resource use of *all* hospitals; unit costs of 15–25 'frontrunner' hospitals
Services included	Whole spectrum of inpatient and outpatient care, *excluding* psychiatric and rehabilitation care	Whole spectrum of inpatient and outpatient care, *including* psychiatric and rehabilitation care
Cost categories included	Recurrent costs, *excluding* costs of education, teaching, research and commercial exploitation	Recurrent costs and capital costs, *excluding* costs of education, teaching, research and commercial exploitation
Number of DBCs	± 100 000; list A: 90%; list B: 10%	± 30 000; list A: 67%; list B: 33%
Applied to	All hospitals and ZBCs	All hospitals and ZBCs

diagnosis and treatment combination is now appointed one single DBC covering all related hospital services, including the first outpatient visit. In addition, DBCs were rearranged, for example, by reducing the number of categories to describe the 'type of care' and 'treatment' dimensions (see subsection 23.3.2). The hospital cost component for list A DBC tariffs is currently determined from detailed resource-use profiles of *all* hospitals and cost data derived from 15–25 'frontrunner' hospitals. In addition, the hospital cost component now includes capital costs.

An increasing share of DBCs is progressively being moved from list A to list B, which is in line with the original purpose of the DBC system (see subsection 23.1.3). There are six main criteria which must be met by a list A DBC in order for it to be transferred (DBC-O, 2009). The DBC must: (1) be is characterized by sufficiently homogeneous levels of resource consumption; (2) have a sufficiently high volume of cases; (3) be sufficiently spread amongst health care providers; (4) involve predictable non-acute care. In addition, (5) the transfer must be supported by medical specialists and hospitals; and (6) all list A DBCs defined on the basis of the same diagnosis must meet these criteria.

23.2.3 Data used for development and updates of the DBC system

Regarding the aforementioned honorarium component, the 'norm time' is updated based on time studies and validated by expert opinion (Oostenbrink & Rutten, 2006). The fixed fee per hour is set by the NZa.

The hospital cost component of list A DBCs is determined and updated by

DBC-O on the basis of a database that is maintained by a subdivision of DBC-O, called the 'DBC information system' (DBC-DIS). The database contains two datasets: (1) resource-use information from the minimum basic datasets (MBDS) collected by all hospitals; and (2) unit cost information from a varying number of 15–25 'frontrunner' hospitals (see subsection 23.4.2). Figure 23.3 depicts the data-collection process from medical specialists to the national database at the DBC-DIS. From the opening of a DBC by a medical specialist, resource use per DBC and per treated case is collected and integrated into one hospital database. The registration system also records the DBC for which a hospital service is performed. After integration of the data at DBC-DIS, technical feedback is provided to medical specialists to assure high-quality data.

23.2.4 Regularity and method of system updates

Regularity and method of updating the DBC classification system

Medical specialists' associations notify DBC-O when problems arise in classifying DBCs, as DBC-O is responsible for the irregular but continuous updating of the DBC classification system. DBC-O is also the gatekeeper for innovation in the DBC system (see section 23.6). DBCs may be merged, split or created. Examples include the recent reduction in the number of DBCs (see subsection 23.2.2) and the introduction of a new generation of DBCs (see section 23.8). Updating is based on feedback from medical specialists' associations and information from the national DBC-DIS database.

Regularity and method of updating tariffs

As already mentioned, the norm-time relating to the honorarium component is updated at irregular intervals. The fixed fee per hour is re-examined annually and updated when necessary. The hospital cost component of list A DBCs is recalculated annually, or as necessary, by multiplying the average resource-use profile and national unit costs. An example of a fictional resource-use profile for a specific DBC ('surgery/ regular care// arthrosis knee/ surgery with clinical episode') is provided in Table 23.5. The calculation of unit costs per service is described in section 23.4.

There is always a time-lag of at least two years between the year of the data and the year of application of tariffs in hospitals. For example, hospital resource-use and cost data from the year 2009 will be analysed during the years 2010 and 2011 in order to define the DBC hospital cost component that will be used for hospital payment in 2012.

23.3 The current patient classification system

23.3.1 Information used to classify patients

A medical specialist is consulted to decide which DBC is applicable and (s)he manually opens the DBC upon first diagnosis by specifying five types of

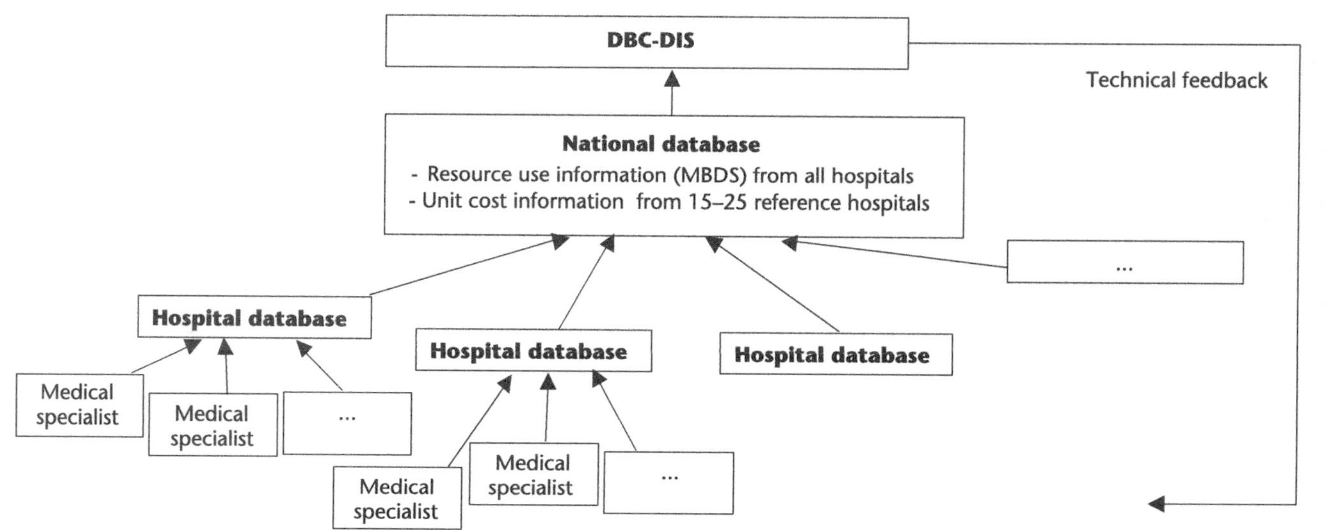

Figure 23.3 Data-collection process for the national database

Table 23.5 Fictional average resource-use profile for the DBC 'surgery regular care/ arthrosis knee surgery with clinical episode'

Hospital services	*% of patients receiving this hospital service*	*Average resource-use for patients receiving this hospital service*	*Average resource-use for all patients*
Inpatient days	100	6.0	6.0
Outpatient visits	100	8.0	8.0
Laboratory services	100	1.0	1.0
Medical imaging services			
X-ray thorax	50	1.0	0.5
X-ray knee/lower leg	100	2.0	2.0
X-ray hip joint	50	1.0	0.5
MRI hip/lower leg	10	1.0	0.1
Surgical procedures			
Surgery dislocation	100	1.0	1.0
Paramedical and supportive services			
Physiotherapy	100	2.0	2.0

Source: Zorgverzekeraars Nederland, 2004.

Notes: For instance, 50 per cent of the patients received X-ray thorax examinations; the average number of X-ray thorax examinations for these patients was 1.0; the average number of X-ray thorax examinations for all patients was 0.5.

information called 'dimensions' of a DBC (van Beek et al., 2005): (1) medical specialty; (2) type of care; (3) demand for care; (4) diagnosis; (5) treatment axis (setting and nature).

Thus, the information used to classify patients includes clinical and resource-use data. The DBC system does not distinguish between principal and secondary diagnoses. If a patient has a second diagnosis that requires treatment, this second diagnosis will be classified into a separate DBC (see subsection 23.2.1).

23.3.2 Classification algorithm

Classification of patients follows the order of the five dimensions: (1) the medical specialty is specified through a four-digit code; (2) a two-digit code for the type of care is added to the first four digits; (3) the demand for care is indicated for certain medical specialties; (4) the diagnosis is specified by adding another three-digit code; and (5) the treatment axis is defined by the last three digits of the DBC. An illustrative example of the patient classification for patients with appendicitis treated in a surgery department is provided in Table 23.6.

Medical specialty

Patients can be classified into one of 27 medical specialties (codes 0301 to 1900). For patients with appendicitis treated in a surgery department, the 'medical specialty' code would be 0303//// (surgery////).

Table 23.6 The patient classification system logic: Surgery example

Medical specialty	*Type of care*	*Demand for care*	*Diagnosis*	*Treatment axis*
0303 Surgery	11 Regular care 21 Continuation of regular care	*Not applicable*	113 Appendicitis	201 Open-surgery outpatient 202 Open-surgery in day care 203 Open-surgery with clinical episode(s) 204 Single outpatient with procedure 206 *Inpatient without days* Open-surgery with clinical episode(s) 301 Endo-surgery outpatient 302 Endo-surgery in day care 303 Endo-surgery with clinical episode(s) 306 *Inpatient without days* Endo-surgery with clinical episode(s)

Type of care

Currently, two categories are used to describe the 'type of care' dimension: 'regular care' (code 11) and 'continuation of regular care' (code 21). For patients with appendicitis, the code would be 0303/11/// (surgery/ regular care///).

Demand for care

The 'demand for care' dimension is only used for a limited number of medical specialties (namely, plastic surgery, urology, gastroenterology and radiotherapy). The dimension specifies demand for care which is expected to result in higher than average resource consumption. For the medical specialty 'plastic surgery', the 'demand for care' dimension distinguishes '≥ two procedures in the same surgical area', 'extensive crush injury within the surgical area', 'congenital impediments within the surgical area', 'requirement of a second surgeon' and 'children ≤ 10 years of age'.

Diagnosis

The 'diagnosis' dimension describes the diagnosis of the patient in medical terms. The classification of diagnoses is based on the International Classification of Diseases 10th revision (ICD-10) coding, even though the ICD-10 codes are not used in the codification of DBCs. For patients with appendicitis, the 'diagnosis' code would be 0303/11//113/ (surgery/ regular care// appendicitis/).

Treatment axis

The 'treatment axis' dimension expresses the 'treatment setting' and 'treatment nature'. The 'treatment setting' is either 'outpatient', 'in day care' or 'with clinical episode(s)'. The subdivision of 'treatment nature' varies by medical specialty and may, for instance, specify whether treatment concerns an 'open-surgery' or a laparoscopic procedure. The number of treatment axes varies from 6 for the medical specialties 'gastroenterology' and 'paediatrics' to over 60 for the medical specialty 'internal medicine'. For patients presenting with appendicitis, the 'treatment axis' code could, for example, be:

0303/11//113/201 (surgery/ regular care// appendicitis/ open-surgery outpatient); 0303/11//113/202 (surgery/ regular care// appendicitis/ open-surgery in day care); or 0303/11//113/203 (surgery/ regular care// appendicitis/ open-surgery with clinical episode(s)).

23.3.3 Data quality and plausibility checks

The DBC-DIS performs data quality and plausibility checks relating to developing and updating the DBC system. These annual checks take place at the national level and comprise the technical validation of the information from the MBDS in the national database (technical correctness, comprehensiveness and functional correctness). There is no system of external data audits.

23.3.4 Incentives for up- or wrong-coding

Although up-coding has been described as a potential threat to the DBC system, the Dutch system seems to be less sensitive to up-coding compared to DRG systems in the United States and Australia (Steinbusch, 2007). The relative strength of the Dutch system is related to the use of classification criteria that are aligned with clinical practice, the fact that DBCs are opened upon diagnosis, and the fact that hospitals generally operate as non-profit-making institutions.

23.4 Cost accounting within hospitals

23.4.1 Regulations

Cost accounting is not mandatory for the majority of Dutch hospitals, which only provide their MBDS to the DBC-DIS. However, the 15–25 'frontrunner' hospitals must follow a uniform product costing model, which was developed during the DBC system's introductory period (Zuurbier & Krabbe-Alkemade, 2007).

23.4.2 Main characteristics of the cost-accounting system

All frontrunner hospitals have to allocate all relevant hospital costs to individual hospital services. Relevant hospital costs include wages, equipment, overheads and capital costs (see subsection 23.2.2). Hospital costs relating to education, teaching, research and commercial exploitation are not considered relevant because they are not financed by the DBC system.

Allocating relevant hospital costs from support cost centres to final cost centres

Hospital departments producing hospital services are called 'final cost centres'. These include, among others: inpatient and outpatient clinics, laboratories, operating rooms (ORs) and radiology departments. Departments not providing patient care are called 'support cost centres'. These include, among others: departments for administration, personnel, billing, communications, finance, security and availability in case of emergencies. Costs of support cost centres may also be referred to as overheads.

In the first step, relevant hospital costs are allocated from support cost centres to final cost centres. Hospitals are free to choose the allocation method for the assignment of hospital costs from support cost centres to final cost centres. As the allocation method was found to have only a minor impact on individual patient's costs (Zuurbier & Krabbe-Alkemade, 2007), hospitals commonly use simple direct allocation, in which the costs of support cost centres are assigned to the final cost centres without interaction between support cost centres (Finkler et al., 2007; Horngren et al., 2005). The product costing model contains specifications regarding the allocation base to be used for each cost centre; for example, the area (m^2) to allocate costs of accommodation, or the number of full-time equivalents to allocate the costs of administration.

Allocating relevant hospital costs from final cost centres to hospital services

Once the costs of support cost centres are assigned to final cost centres, the total costs of each final cost centre can be assigned to individual hospital services, such as inpatient days, intensive care days, laboratory services, medical imaging services and surgical procedures (see Table 23.3). Weighting statistics are used to assign relevant hospital costs from final cost centres to hospital services. They differ between final cost centres according to the type of service they produce. An example of such a weighting statistic is the average time of surgical interventions to distribute the cost of the final 'OR' cost centre to these interventions. The NZa determines the national unit costs of about 4500 hospital services from the weighted average across the 15–25 'frontrunner' hospitals. National unit costs are determined with a lag-time of at least two years. The tariffs for 2012 will be based on the national unit costs of 2009.

23.5 DBCs for hospital payment

23.5.1 Range of services and costs included in DBC-type hospital payment

Inpatient and outpatient hospital care of all hospitals and ZBCs (including psychiatric and rehabilitation care) is fully financed according to the DBC system logic. One exception concerns some very expensive and orphan drugs for which the NZa provides hospitals with additional funding (80 per cent of the purchase price for expensive drugs and 100 per cent of the purchase price for orphan drugs) (Rodenburg-van Dieten, 2005). Other relevant sources of financing for hospitals exist but do not relate to hospital care, such as education, teaching, research and commercial exploitation. These sources accounted for 15.9 per cent of total hospital revenues in 2009 (Kiwa Prismant, 2010).

23.5.2 Calculation of DBC tariffs

DBC tariffs consist of two parts: (1) the *honorarium component* and (2) the *hospital cost component*. The honorarium component is calculated on the basis of a 'norm-time' and a fixed fee per hour both for list A and for list B DBCs (see subsections 23.2.2 to 23.2.4). For list A DBCs, the hospital cost component is calculated on the basis of average resource-use profiles from all hospitals and unit costs calculated through the product costing model described in subsection 23.4.2. A fictional example to illustrate the cost calculation of the hospital cost component for the DBC 'surgery/ regular care// appendicitis/ surgery with clinical episode' is provided in Table 23.7.

The tariff for the hospital cost component of list B DBCs is negotiated between hospitals and insurers. Insurers are not obliged to contract all hospitals for list B DBCs, and may employ different DBC prices for different hospitals. Likewise, hospitals may negotiate different prices for the same DBC with different insurers. Health insurers and hospitals determine the frequency and terms of agreements. Current practice suggests that negotiations take place annually, but that either party can reopen negotiations if required by the circumstances (van Ineveld et al., 2006). Examples of such circumstances include long waiting lists, increased public attention to a specific health problem or the introduction of very expensive/orphan drugs or medical devices.

23.5.3 DBCs in actual hospital payment

All hospitals in the Netherlands receive a nationally uniform payment per list A DBC and a negotiated hospital-specific payment for list B DBCs. In order to receive payments under the DBC system, hospitals classify all patients into the appropriate DBCs. After treatment is completed, a bill is sent to the patients' health insurer indicating all relevant DBCs. Subsequently, the insurer pays hospitals on the basis of the fixed list A DBC tariffs or the negotiated list B DBC tariffs.

For list A DBCs, prospective budgets determine the total financial volume which hospitals can earn through the provision of DBCs. Budgets are established annually by the NZa based on fixed and variable costs and a variety of parameters, including the hospital's adherent population, the type of facilities, the number of beds and production parameters (such as the number of inpatient days and outpatient visits) (Nederlandse Zorgautoriteit, 2009). Hospitals are fully compensated for the difference between the prospective budget and DBC payments (yield). Consequently, higher production may result in higher costs without additional yield, while lower production results in lower costs but not in lower yield.

Table 23.7 Fictional cost calculation of the hospital cost component

Hospital services	*Total resource use for all patients*	*National unit costs (€)*	*Total costs (€)*	*Average costs per patient (€)*[a]
Inpatient days	1 250	296	370 083	1 341
Outpatient visits	864	43	37 147	135
Day-care hours	1 029	34	35 002	127
Laboratory services				
Urine screening	560	2	1 121	4
Ureum	836	1	836	3
Creatinine	974	2	1 949	7
Leucocytes	781	1	781	3
Medical imaging services				
X-ray thorax	615	52	32 005	116
X-ray abdomen	781	52	40 616	147
CT abdomen	144	228	32 723	119
Echo abdomen	281	83	23 320	84
Surgical procedures				
Appendectomy	276	548	151 248	548
Colon resection	8	1 595	13 207	48
Small intestinal resection	11	1 056	11 658	42
Resection appendicular abscess	6	761	4 201	15
Diagnostic activities				
Diagnostic laparoscopy	41	484	20 038	73
Diagnostic duodenoscopy	14	408	5 630	20
Cysto-/urethrography	6	479	2 644	10
Microbiological and parasitological services	856	33	28 235	102
Paramedical and supportive services				
Physiotherapy	500	31	15 486	56
TOTAL			827 929	3 000

Source: Zuurbier & Krabbe-Alkemade, 2007.

Notes: For the list A DBC: 'surgery/ regular care// appendicitis/ open-surgery with clinical episode'; [a]The average costs per patient add up to the DBC tariff '~ *number of closed DBCs: 276*'.

For list B DBCs, insurers may limit the maximum volume of list B DBCs that a hospital is allowed to produce. That aside, insurers and hospitals may agree upon a lower or higher DBC price if production exceeds a predetermined figure. The hospital's and medical specialists' yield only depends on DBC payments. Consequently, higher production may result in higher costs and additional yield, while a lower level of production directly results in lower costs and lower yield.

The DBC system also applies to 'non-contracted care'; that is, care provided to foreign patients, uninsured patients or patients whose health insurer does not have a contract with the hospital. In these situations, the foreign insurer or the patient must pay the DBC tariff. The tariffs for the honorarium component of list A and B DBCs and for the hospital cost component of list A DBCs are the same both for non-contracted and contracted care. The tariffs for the hospital cost component of list B are determined by the hospital and may differ between contracted and non-contracted care. Hospitals do not have to publish tariffs for contracted care, whereas they are obliged to publish tariffs for non-contracted care.

23.5.4 Quality-related adjustments

For list A DBCs, no quality related adjustments exist. The tariff is the same for all hospitals, regardless of quality. Although the negotiations on list B DBCs were intended to be based on the quality of delivered care, insurers and hospitals currently predominantly negotiate on price and/or production volume (see subsection 23.7).

23.5.5 Main incentives for hospitals

Hospitals are incentivized to keep their costs below the national unit costs for any specific list A DBC. For list B DBCs, hospitals are incentivized to keep costs below negotiated prices. The DBC system therefore offers hospitals an incentive to improve those quality aspects that lead to lower resource consumption. For example, it encourages quality improvements that would lead to fewer unnecessary diagnostic services and to a reduction in the ALOS (Custers et al., 2007).

Quality improvement aimed at reducing complication rates – such as post-operative infections and/or readmission rates – are not stimulated by the DBC system, because the occurrence of complications might lead to a new DBC (Custers et al., 2007). Hospitals could even be incentivized to accept a price below the costs of production for a specific list B DBC, in order to gain a contract with an insurer, and could then try to compensate for the losses by providing profitable list A DBCs to these patients.

23.6 New/innovative technologies

23.6.1 Steps required prior to usage in hospitals

DBC-O is the gatekeeper for innovation in the DBC system. Current regulations require a process of seven steps following an application (for example, from a hospital) before a new technology can be included in the DBC system (VWS, 2009), as detailed here.

1. DBC-O assesses the admissibility, completeness, nature, size and complexity of the application.
2. The CVZ performs a systematic literature review to examine the extent and level of evidence supporting the specific technology.
3. DBC-O assesses the costs, effectiveness, ethical aspects, patient preferences and system consequences of the application.
4. Based on the information acquired from steps 2 and 3, DBC-O decides upon the implementation of the technology in the DBC system.

5. The positive decision by DBC-O is approved by the NZa.
6. The CVZ advises the VWS whether the new technology should be made part of the insurance benefits package.
7. Finally, DBC-O incorporates the new technology into the DBC system.

The seven steps should take no longer than six months from registration of the new treatments (VWS, 2009). At first introduction of the new technology in the DBC system, average resource-use profiles are not yet available and DBC tariffs are based on expert opinion. For the DBC system until 2010, 24 new technologies have been assessed by DBC-O, the NZa and the CVZ. Seven led to new DBCs, four have been merged with existing DBCs, and five were not approved. Eight are still under consideration.

23.6.2 Funding

Currently, new or innovative treatments are introduced into the DBC system twice a year. Until the new technology is incorporated in the DBC system, additional payments exist only for innovative drugs. Since 2006, an innovative drug can be provisionally included on the 'list of expensive drugs' or 'list of orphan drugs' for four years, on the conditions that: (1) added therapeutic value is demonstrated; (2) its expenses account for over 0.5 per cent ('expensive drugs') or 5.0 per cent ('orphan drugs') of the annual hospital drugs budget; and (3) a plan for the assessment of cost–effectiveness in daily clinical practice is approved by the pharmaceutical advisory committee.

23.7 Evaluation of the DBC system in the Netherlands

The main purpose of introducing DBCs was to enable price and quality negotiations between insurers and providers. Although these negotiations were intended to be based on the quality of delivered care, insurers and hospitals currently predominantly negotiate on price and/or production volume. Since 2006, prices for list B DBCs have increased at a lower rate than those for list A DBCs and the health insurers increasingly apply pressure to hospitals to charge even lower prices (van de Ven & Schut, 2009). Table 23.8 depicts the negotiated tariffs in 2007 compared to those in 2004 for seven list B DBCs at four health insurers. List B DBC prices had increased by about 8 per cent in 2007, compared to 2004 tariffs. In general, major price deviations only occurred for a minority of DBCs. More complex and chronic DBCs seem to be less sensitive to market competition. Evidence from recent years suggests that hospitals negotiate on the total budget of the total B segment, rather than on the individual DBC level (van Ineveld et al., 2006).

Insurers have been reluctant to selectively contract with hospitals and to offer preferred hospital contracts to their customers. Aside from the problems of having the right mix of criteria to determine quality, obtaining accurate data, and doing so in a timely manner, there are several limitations for Dutch health insurers that limit their interest in negotiating on quality and to selectively

Table 23.8 Negotiated tariffs in 2007 compared to those of 2004

	N	*2004 tariff (€)*	*Average 2007 tariff (€)*	*Relative price increase (%)*	*Minimum 2007 price*	*Maximum 2007 price*
Inguinal hernia repair	407	2 163	2 254	4.2	1 529	3 088
Diabetes	410	409	483	18.1	385	1 027
Tonsillectomy	409	740	800	8.1	433	1 498
Cataract	407	1 317	1 381	4.8	1 044	1 599
Hip replacement	409	8 561	9 097	6.3	7 603	11 370
Knee replacement	404	10 228	10 746	5.1	9 097	13 000
Spinal disc herniation	354	3 046	3 308	8.6	2 413	5 778

Source: Nederlandse Zorgautoriteit, 2005.

Note: Example of seven list B DBCs at four health insurers.

contract with higher quality hospitals (Custers et al., 2007; van de Ven & Schut, 2009).

- Health insurers are afraid of acquiring a bad reputation if they restrict consumer choice to a limited network of preferred hospitals.
- Patients assume that the quality of care in terms of effectiveness and safety is equal among all hospitals. As a result, insurers have no incentive to negotiate for higher quality (and to pay higher prices) if patients do not appreciate higher quality in contracted hospitals.
- Furthermore, a 'free-rider' problem exists: hospitals have contracts with several insurers. If one single insurer motivates a particular hospital to improve quality, all of this hospital's patients will benefit from the quality improvement, including patients who are insured through other insurers.
- Finally, if an insurer acquires recognition for providing high-quality care, it is likely to enrol a disproportionate share of patients with chronic medical problems.

Unfortunately, information necessary to evaluate the DBC system is not easily accessible. A lot of information is available in the national DBC-DIS database but, at present, only a limited number of actors have access to the database.

23.8 Outlook: Future developments and reform

A new generation of DBCs – the so-called 'DBCs towards transparency' ('*DBCs Op weg naar Transparantie*') – is forthcoming. In the new system, patients will be classified according to a computerized grouping algorithm (see Figure 23.4). The number of DBCs will be substantially reduced from about 30 000 to 4000 by discarding the 'medical specialty' dimension. In addition, expensive/orphan drugs, intensive care and *other products* are to be accounted for by means of treatment related 'add-ons', each with their own tariff. Other products may concern transmural/shared care; namely, hospital services provided in cooperation with medical professionals outside of the hospital (for example, the GP).

Another important feature of the future grouping algorithm is the possibility to consider care intensity for the classification of patients. For example, separate DBCs could be defined for an inpatient stay of up to five days and for over five days. The grouping algorithm is currently being tested, but it is not yet clear when it will be implemented nationwide.

Another future development concerns the transition to a situation in which prospective budgets are solely determined based on production parameters, such as first outpatient visits, first admissions, the number of inpatient days and day-care hours. The transition phase started early 2010 and is expected to last at least three years (Nederlandse Zorgautoriteit, 2009).

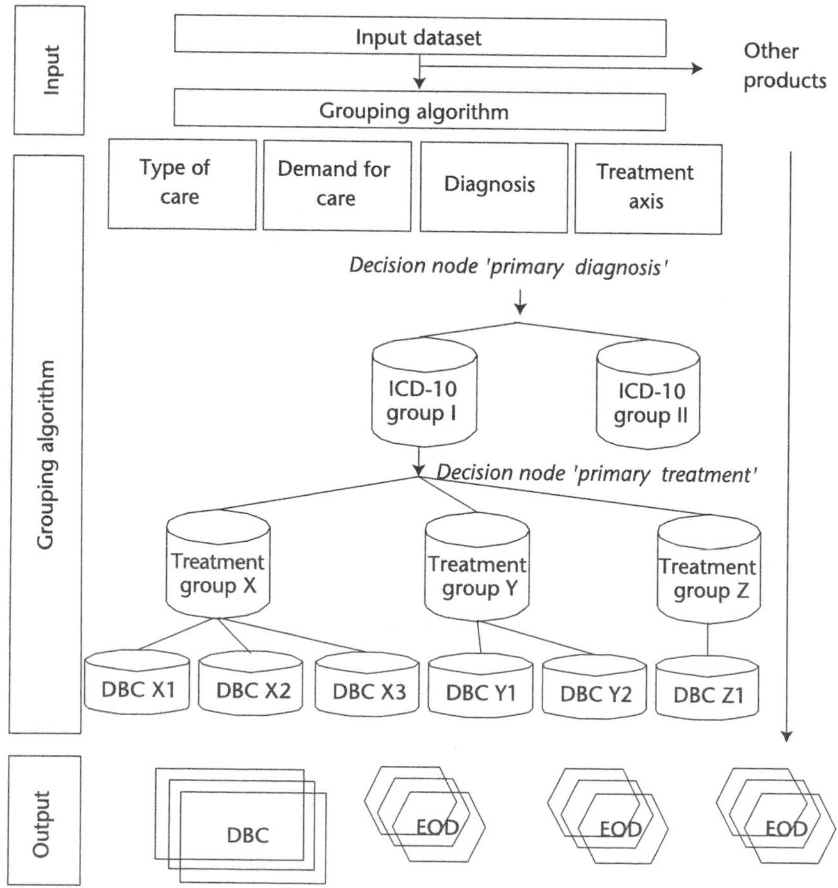

Figure 23.4 The grouping algorithm for the new generation of DBCs

Notes: EOD: 'add-on' expensive/orphan drugs.

It is too early to predict the potential effects of the future developments of the DBC system. Most significantly, the importance of negotiations between hospitals and insurers is bound to increase.

23.9 References

Beersen, N., Redekop, W.K., de Bruijn, J.H.B. et al. (2005). Quality-based social insurance coverage and payment of the application of a high-cost medical therapy: the case of spinal cord stimulation for chronic non-oncologic pain in the Netherlands. *Health Policy*, 71:107–15.

Custers, T., Arah, O.A., Klazinga, N.S. (2007). Is there a business case for quality in the Netherlands? A critical analysis of the recent reforms of the health care system. *Health Policy*, 82:226–39.

DBC-O (2009). *Scenario's invulling B-segment 2011 [B-Segment Composition Scenarios]*. Utrecht: DBC-Onderhoud.

DBC-O (2011). *DBC Onderhoud Diagnose Behandeling Combinatie*. Utrecht: DBC-Onderhoud (www.dbconderhoud.nl, accessed 10 July 2011).

Enthoven, A.C., van de Ven, W.P.M.M. (2007). Going Dutch – managed competition health insurance in the Netherlands. *New England Journal of Medicine*, 357(24):2421–3.

Finkler, S.A., Ward, D.M., Baker, J.J. (2007). *Essentials of Cost Accounting for Health Care Organizations. Third edition*. New York, NY: Aspen Publishers.

Folpmers, M., de Bruijn, J. (2004). Honorering in de Zorg, Overgang naar de nieuwe landelijke DBC-systematiek [Remuneration in Health Care, Transition towards the New National DBC Systematic]. *MCA Tijdschrift voor Organisaties in Control*, 6:18–25.

Horngren, C.T., Datar, S.M., Foster, G. (2005). *Cost Accounting: A Managerial Emphasis. Twelfth edition*. New York, NY: Prentice-Hall, Englewood Cliffs.

Kiwa Prismant (2010). *Kengetallen Nederlandse Ziekenhuizen 2009 [Key Numbers Dutch Hospitals 2009]*. Utrecht: Dutch Hospital Data.

Nederlandse Zorgautoriteit (2005). *Oriënterende monitor ziekenhuis zorg: analyse van de onderhandelingen over het B-segment in 2005 [Exploratory Monitoring of Hospital Care: Analyses of the Negotiation on the B-Segment in 2005]*. Utrecht: Nederlandse Zorgautoriteit.

Nederlandse Zorgautoriteit (2009). *Consultatiedocument Prestatiebekostiging binnen de medisch specialistische zorg [Consultation Document on Remuneration According to Performance within Medical Specialist Care]*. Utrecht: Nederlandse Zorgautoriteit.

Oostenbrink, J.B., Rutten, F.F. (2006). Cost assessment and price setting of inpatient care in the Netherlands. The DBC casemix system. *Health Care Management Science*, 9: 287–94.

Poos, M.J.J.C., Smit, J.M., Groen, J. et al. (2008). *Kosten van ziekten in Nederland [Cost of Illnesses in the Netherlands]*. Bilthoven: National Institute for Public Health and the Environment (RIVM).

Rodenburg-van Dieten, H.E.M. (2005). *Richtlijnen voor farmaco-economisch onderzoek [Guidelines for Pharmaco-Economic Research]*. Diemen: Healthcare Insurance Board (CVZ).

Schäfer, W., Kroneman, M., Boerma, W. et al. (2010). The Netherlands: health system review. *Health Systems in Transition*, 12(1):1–228.

Schut, F.T., Hassink, W.H. (2002). Managed competition and consumer price sensitivity in social health insurance. *Journal of Health Economics*, 21:1009–29.

Steinbusch, P.J.M., Oostenbrink, J.B., Zuurbier, J.J., Schaepkens, F.J.M. (2007). The risk of up-coding in casemix systems: a comparative study. *Health Policy*, 81(2–3):289–99.

Stolk, E.A., Rutten, F.F.H. (2005). The 'health benefit basket' in the Netherlands. *European Journal of Health Economics*, 6:53–7.

Van Beek, L., Goossen, W.T., van der Kloot, W.A. (2005). Linking nursing care to medical diagnoses: heterogeneity of patient groups. *International Journal of Medical Informatics*, 74:926–36.

Van de Ven, W.P.M.M., Schut, F.T. (2009). Managed competition in the Netherlands: still work-in-progress. *Health Economics*, 18:253–5.

Van Ineveld, M., Dohmen, P., Redekop, K. (2006). De startende marktwerking in de gezondheidszorg [The starting market forces in health care]. *Economisch Statistische Berichten*, 91(4494):470–3.

VWS (2009). *Innovaties en DBC's [Innovation and DBCs]. Letter from the Minister of Health, Welfare and Sport to the Second Chamber, 24 March 2009*. The Hague: Minister of Health, Welfare and Sport.

Zorgverzekeraars Nederland (2004). *DBC-inkoopgids 2005, Segment B: Zorgverzekeraars onderhandelen over zorg [DBC Purchase Guide, Segment B: Health Insurers Negotiate on Care]*. Zeist: Zorgverzekeraars Nederland.

Zuurbier, J., Krabbe-Alkemade, Y. (2007). *Onderhandelen over DBC's [Negotiating on DBCs. Second edition]*. Maarssen: Elsevier Gezondheidszorg.

Index